Śiva Sūtras

The Yoga of Supreme Identity

*Text of the Sūtras and the Commentary Vimarśinī of Kṣemarāja
Translated into English with Introduction,
Notes, Running Exposition, Glossary and Index
by*

JAIDEVA SINGH

MOTILAL BANARSIDASS PUBLISHERS
PRIVATE LIMITED • DELHI

First Edition : Delhi, 1979
Reprint : Delhi, 1982, 1983, 1984, 1988,
1990, 1991, 1995, 1998, 2000, 2003

ISBN: 81-208-0406-6 (Cloth)
ISBN: 81-208-0407-4 (Paper)

Also available at:
MOTILAL BANARSIDASS
41 U.A. Bungalow Road, Jawahar Nagar, Delhi 110 007
8 Mahalaxmi Chamber, 22 Bhulabhai Desai Road, Mumbai 400 026
236, 9th Main III Block, Jayanagar, Bangalore 560 011
120 Royapettah High Road, Mylapore, Chennai 600 004
Sanas Plaza, 1302 Baji Rao Road, Pune 411 002
8 Camac Street, Kolkata 700 017
Ashok Rajpath, Patna 800 004
Chowk, Varanasi 221 001

Printed in India
BY JAINENDRA PRAKASH JAIN AT SHRI JAINENDRA PRESS,
A-45 NARAINA, PHASE-I, NEW DELHI 110 028
AND PUBLISHED BY NARENDRA PRAKASH JAIN FOR
MOTILAL BANARSIDASS PUBLISHERS PRIVATE LIMITED,
BUNGALOW ROAD, DELHI 110 007

DEDICATED

with profound respects
to
MM. Dr. Gopinath Kaviraj
who was a source of inspiration in life
And remains a Beacon-light in death.

BLESSING

The ŚIVASŪTRAM is a highly respected treatise of Kashmir Śaivism. It contains the highest truth as expounded by Lord Śiva. One can attain the truth by just understanding the meaning of the sūtras. Śrī Jaideva Singh has done a great service to seekers by translating *Śivasūtra Vimarśinī* into English. Now this great work will be available to people outside India too. May its truth spread in the world.

SWAMI MUKTANANDA

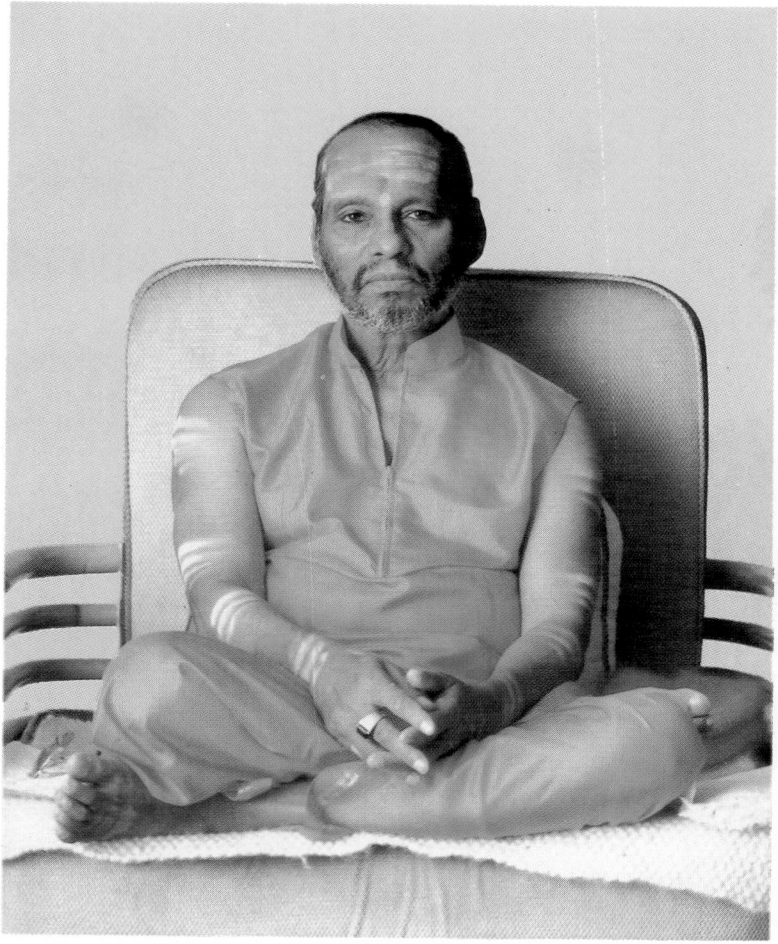

Sadguru Swami Muktananda

PREFACE

A year before his death, my revered Guru MM. Gopinath Kaviraja called me and said, "Recently one translation of Śiva-Sūtras into Hindi and another into English have been brought to my notice. I have been both pained and shocked by the flagrant errors committed by these translators. It is my earnest wish that you prepare another translation of this great book into English."

My Guru's wish was more than a command to me. I looked into the translations referred to. A new interpretation should always be welcome, but when it goes against the very spirit and tradition of the system, it becomes a pernicious procedure. To cite one instance, the 5th sūtra of the first section is worded as 'udyamo Bhairavaḥ'. The word *udyama* has been translated as 'exertion'. The first section deals with Śāmbhava-upāya, Even the veriest tyro of Śaivāgama knows that Śāmbhava upāya has nothing to do with exertion, and so 'udyama' does not and cannot mean exertion in this context. Even the structure and grammar of the Sanskrit language have been twisted and tortured to yield certain pre-conceived meanings. Such preposterous translation is, to say the least, a literary crime.

I had made a promise to carry out the commands of my Guru, but when I tried to understand the text, I found myself at sea. I was afraid of setting pen to paper lest I should do injustice to this great scripture. Kavirāja jī was too ill to teach. So I studied the text word by word with the help of Ācārya Rāmeshvara Jhā who is a great Sanskrit scholaı and fully conversant with Śaivāgama. I am very grateful to him for his help. I felt, however, that I should study it further with the help of one who has been brought up in the Śaivāgama tradition. So I approached my old Guru, Svāmī Lakṣmaṇa Joo of Kashmir who, in spite of his old age and a heavy schedule of engagements with a number of scholars who had gathered round him, kindly agreed to help. He taught me the *sūtras* together with the commentary of Kṣemarāja and gave luminous exposition of some very knotty problems, I am deeply beholden to him for unravelling the meaning of this difficult text.

Kṣemarāja, in the introductory portion of his commentary, says that since many incongruous expositions had been given by the commentaries extant in his time, he undertook to write a new commentary in due conformity with the old tradition. I have, therefore, translated the *sūtras* along with the Vimarśinī commentary of Kṣemarāja. The style of Kṣemarāja is somewhat involved, and so it has been an uphill task to translate his commentary into English. I have tried my best to make the translation as clear and readable as possible.

Four commentaries on *Śiva-sūtras* are available at present, the *Vimarśinī* commentary of Kṣemarāja in prose, the *Śiva-sūtra-vṛtti* by some anonymous author in prose, the *Śiva-sūtra-vārttikam* by Bhāskara in verse, and the *Śiva-sūtra-vārttikam* by Varadarāja in verse.

The *Śiva-sūtra-vṛtti* is so close to *Vimarśinī* that it appears to be either a preliminary draft or a later abstract of the Vimarśinī. There is a strong presumption that the author of the *Vṛtti* was *Kṣemarāja* himself. The *Vārttikam* by Varadarāja is only a rehash of the *Vimarśinī* in Verse. The *Vārttikam* by Bhāskara is an independent commentary. He differs at places from Kṣemarāja. I have indicated this in my notes or exposition wherever necessary. Kṣemarāja's commentary is so detailed and scholarly that it has practically elbowed every other commentary out of existence. I have, therefore, duly followed Kṣemarāja in my exposition.

I have adopted the following plan in the book. Each *sūtra* is given both in Devanāgarī and Roman script. Then the meaning of every word of the *sūtra* is given in English followed by a translation of the whole *sūtra*. This is followed by the Vimarśinī commentary in Sanskrit. The commentary is then translated into English. After this, copious notes are added on important and technical words. Finally, I have given a running exposition of the main ideas of the *sūtra* in my own words.

A long Introduction has been given in the beginning. This is followed by an abstract of each *sūtra*. At the end of the book, a glossary of all the technical terms and Index have been appended.

For me, this work has been a labour of love, without any financial and secretarial assistance whatsoever. My great Guru, MM. Gopinath Kavirāja passed away before the work could be completed. I can now only console myself by dedicating it to his revered memory.

Varanasi.
1-1-1979

JAIDEVA SINGH

TABLE OF CONTENTS

INTRODUCTION

THE MAIN SOURCES OF THE NON-DUALISTIC ŚAIVA SYSTEM OF PHILOSOPHY AND YOGA

The Śaiva system of Philosophy and Yoga is generally known as Āgama. The word Āgama means a traditional doctrine or system which commands faith.

The Śaiva system, in general, is known as Śiva-śāsana or Śivāgama. The non-dualistic Śaiva system of Kashmir is known as Trika-Śāsana or Trika-śāstra or Rahasya-sampradāya. The words *śāsana* and *śāstra* are very significant. Both contain the root *śāsa* which means discipline. Śāsana or Śāstra means teaching containing rules for discipline. A *Śāstra* or *Śāsana* in India never meant merely an intellectual exposition of a particular system. It certainly expounded the fundamental principles of reality but at the same time laid down on the basis of the principles certain rules, certain norms of conduct which had to be observed by those who studied the particular Śāstra. A Śāstra was not simply a way of thought but also a way of life. The Śaiva philosophy of Kashmir is generally called 'Trika Śāstra, because it is philosophy of the triad — (1) Śiva (2) Śakti (3) Nara — the bound soul or (1) *para* — the highest (2) *parāpara* — identity in difference and (3) *apara* — difference.

The literature of the Trika system of Kashmir falls into three categories, viz., (1) the Āgama Śāstra, (2) the Spanda Śāstra and (3) the Pratyabhijñā Śāstra.

Āgama Śāstra :

Āgama Śāstra is considered to be revelation by Śiva. It lays down both the principles and practices of the system. Among the works belonging to the Āgama category may be mentioned the following Tantras.

Mālinīvijaya or Mālinīvijayottara, Svacchanda, Vijñāna Bhairava, Mṛgendra, Netra, Rudra-Yāmala, Śiva-Sūtras, etc.

Most of these taught generally the dualistic doctrine. The most important Āgama of the Trika system was known as the Śiva-Sūtras.

Śiva-Sūtras :

The importance of this work consists in the fact that it was revealed to counter the effects of dualism.[1] It is generally known as Śivopaniṣat-saṅgraha — a compendium containing the secret doctrine revealed by Śiva. This was revealed to Vasugupta.

There are three theories regarding the revelation of the Śiva-Sūtras to Vasugupta.

1. Kallaṭa in the Spanda-vṛtti says that Śiva taught the Śiva-Sūtras in a dream to Vasugupta who was living on Mahādeva mountain in the valley of the Harvan stream behind the Shalimar garden near Śrīnagara.

2. Bhāskara says in his Vārttika on the Śiva-Sūtras that they were revealed to Vasugupta in a dream by a Siddha — a perfected semi-divine being.

3. Kṣemarāja, in his commentary Vimarśinī, maintains that Śiva appeared to Vasugupta in a dream and said, "On the Mahādeva mountain, the secret doctrines are inscribed on a piece of stone. Collecting the doctrines from there, teach them to those who deserve grace." On waking up, Vasugupta went to the place and by a mere touch the particular stone turned up and he found the Śiva-Sūtras inscribed on it.

The particular rock is still called Śaṁkaropala, and it is said that the Sūtras were inscribed on it. (See the plate No. 1). The rock is there, but there is no trace of the sūtras.

The following are the common points in all the theories regarding the discovery of the Śiva-Sūtras.

1. There was no human author of the Sūtras. They originated from Śiva.

2. They were revealed to Vasugupta.

Whether they were revealed to him by Śiva in a dream or by a Siddha or they were found on a rock at the instance of Śiva are matters which are irrelevant to the main issue of the revelation.

1. "कदाचिच्च असौ द्वैतदर्शनाधिवासितप्राये जीवलोके रहस्यसम्प्रदायो मा विच्छेदि इत्याशयतः अनुजिघृक्षापरेण परमशिवेन स्वप्ने उन्मिषित-प्रतिभः कृतः।
S.S.V.P.5.

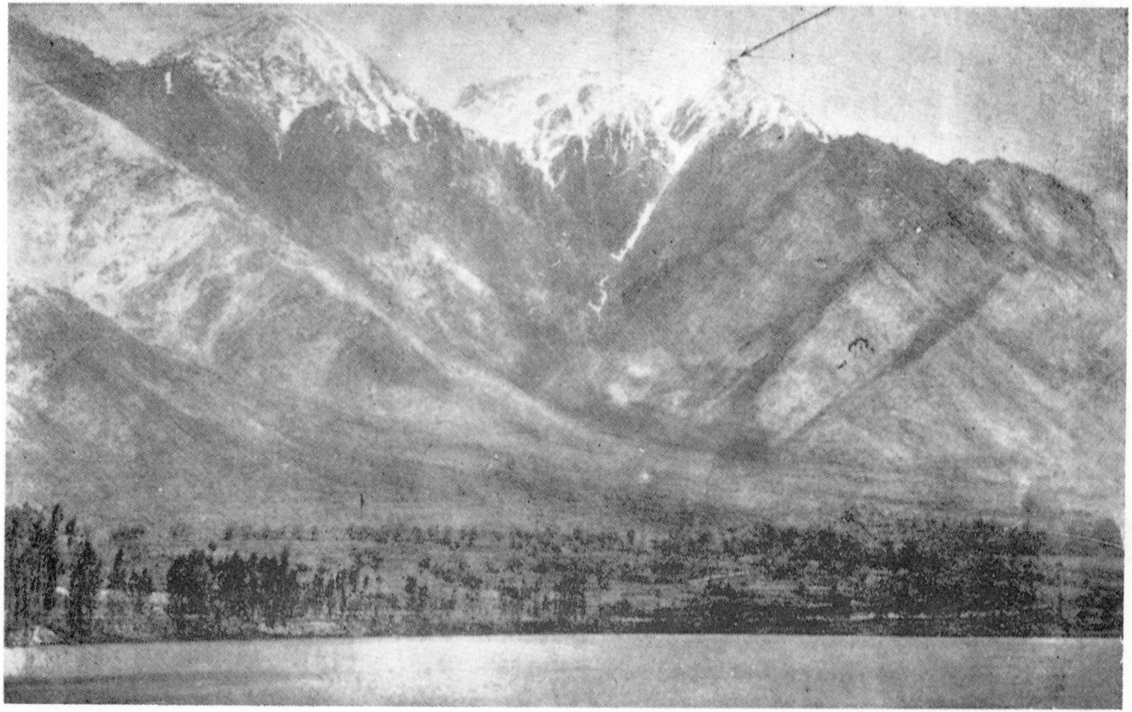

Plate 1

Date of the Discovery of the Sūtras :

We know from Rājataraṅgiṇī that Kallaṭa flourished in the reign of king Avanti-Varman of Kashmir, Avanti-Varman reigned in the 9th Century A.D. Vasugupta who had discovered the Śiva-Sūtras was the *guru* (teacher) of Kallaṭa. He must have flourished either in the last part of the 8th Century or the beginning of the 9th Century A.D. This must have been therefore, the date of the discovery of the Sūtras.

Commentaries on the Śiva-Sūtras :

Kṣemarāja says in his commentary Vimarśinī that he noticed discrepancies in the various commentaries prevalent in his time. Therefore, he undertook to write a new commentary. He has not named the commentaries in which he noticed discrepancies. Only four commentaries have survived.

1. The Vṛtti.
2. The Vārttika by Bhāskara.
3. The Vimarśinī by Kṣemarāja.
4. The Śiva-Sūtra-vārttikam by Varadarāja alias Kṛṣṇadāsa.

The author of the *Vṛtti* is not known. The commentary *vṛtti* tallies with Vimarśinī not only in interpretation but also mostly in words. It appears that either the *Vṛtti* was written at first and was used by Kṣemarāja as a framework for elaboration or that Vimarśinī was written at first and either Kṣemarāja himself or some one else prepared an abstract of it in the *Vṛtti*.

Bhāskara says in the introductory portion of his Vārttika that Vasugupta taught the Śiva-Sūtras to Kallaṭa who taught them to Pradyumnabhaṭṭa, the son of his maternal uncle. Pradyumnabhaṭṭa taught them to his son Prajñārjuna. Prajñārjuna taught them to a pupil, Mahādevabhaṭṭa who in turn taught them to his son, Śrīkāṇṭhabhaṭṭa. Bhāskara himself learned the *sūtras* from Śrīkāṇṭhabhaṭṭa. Bhāskara flourished in the 11th century A.D. So his Vārttika was written during that period.

The *Vṛtti* gives the main ideas of the Sūtras in a very succinct form in prose. Bhāskara in his Vārttika interprets each *sūtra* in verse.

The Vimarśinī commentary of Kṣemarāja gives a lucid and detailed exposition of each *sūtra* in prose. He substantiates his interpretation by giving parallel and valuable quotations from other books some of which are now completely lost to us.

It is well-known that Kṣemarāja was a pupil of Abhinavagupta who flourished in the 10th Century. The Vimarśinī Commentary must have been written by Kṣemarāja in the 10th Century. Kṣemarāja was a prolific writer. He wrote the following works :

Pratyabhijñāhṛdayam, Spandasandoha, Spandanirṇaya, Svacchandoddyota, Netroddyota, Vijñānabhairavoddyota, Śivasūtra-vimarśinī, Stavacintāmaṇiṭīkā, Parāprāveśikā, Tattvasandoha, Utpala's Stotrāvalīṭīkā.

The fourth commentary on the Śiva-Sūtras is the Śiva-Sūtravārttikam by Varadarāja alias Kṛṣṇadāsa. The Vārttika of Varadarāja is only a rehash of the Vimarśinī in Verse. Varadarāja has no interpretation of his own to give. He lived towards the end of the 15th Century A.D.

Of all the commentaries that have survived, Vimarśinī by Kṣemarāja is the oldest and the most learned.

2. *Spanda Śāstra*

This elaborates the principles laid down in the Śiva-Sūtras. It works out the details of the Śiva-Sūtras mainly from the point of view of Śakti.

The main work of this Śāstra is the Spanda-sūtras or Spanda Kārikā as generally known. On this, there are the following commentaries :

Pradīpa by Utpala Vaiṣṇava, Vivṛti by Rāmakaṇṭha, Spandasandoha and Spandanirṇaya by Kṣemarāja. Spandasandoha contains a commentary only on the first Kārikā.

Kṣemarāja thinks that the Spanda-Sūtras were written by Vasugupta. Others maintain that they were written by Kallaṭa, the pupil of Vasugupta.

3. *The Pratyabhijñā Śāstra* :

This contains the philosophy proper of the system. It expounds the Trika philosophy by arguments and discussions.

The first philosophical work was Śiva-dṛṣṭi composed by Somānanda. He was the pupil of Vasugupta. He flourished in the 9th Century A.D. Śiva-dṛṣṭi is a very important philosophical work. Unfortunately the full text is not yet available.

Somānanda composed a vṛtti on Śiva-dṛṣṭi, but it has not been traced as yet.

The most important available work of this Śāstra is the Pratyabhijñā-sūtras or Īśvara-pratyabhijñā by Utpala who was a pupil of Somānanda. The Pratyabhijñā-sūtras acquired so much importance that the whole philosophy of Kashmir is generally known as Pratyabhijñā-darśana. There are the following commentaries on the Pratyabhijñā-sūtras.

1. The Vṛtti by Utpala himself available only in an incomplete form.
2. The Pratyabhijñāvimarśinī by Abhinavagupta.
3. The Pratyabhijñā-vivṛti-vimarśinī by Abhinavagupta. This is a commentary on the lost *ṭikā* known as *Vivṛti* by Utpala himself.

Besides the above, there is the great work known as Tantrāloka by Abhinavagupta. It is in 12 volumes and contains the Śaiva philosophy and practice in all their aspects. There is also the digest of the twelve volumes known as Tantrasāra. Jayaratha has written the commentary Viveka on Tantrāloka.

The Philosophical Background of the Śiva-Sūtras :

Śiva-sūtras are a treatise on Yoga, but this Yoga is based on a definite system of Philosophy. It will not be possible to understand this yoga unless there is a clear grasp of the philosophy on which it is based.

We may consider the philosophical background of this Yoga under the following heads : 1. Ultimate Reality. 2. Manifestation or the world-process. 3. Bondage. 4. Liberation.

1. *Ultimate Reality* :

Ultimate Reality is *cit* or *Parāsaṁvit*. It is non-relational consciousness. It is the changeless principle of all changes. In it, there is no distinction of subject and object, of I and This. It is the Supreme Self surveying Itself. In the words of Pratyabhijñā Śāstra, it is *prakāśa-vimarśamaya*. *Prakāśa* is the Eternal Light without which nothing can appear. It is Śiva. *Vimarśa* is Śakti, the *svabhāva* of Śiva. It is, so to speak, the mirror in which Śiva realizes His own grandeur, power and beauty. Vimarśa is the *Kartṛtva Śakti* (the power of doership) of Śiva.

Mere *Prakāśa* cannot be the nature of Reality. Even diamond is *prakāśa*, but the diamond does not know itself as *prakāśa*. *Vimarśa* is that aspect of *prakāśa* by which it knows itself. That self-knowledge is an activity.

Vimarśa betokens that activity. As Kṣemarāja says in his Parāprāveśikā (p. 2), Vimarśa is "akṛtrimāham iti visphuraṇam." It is the *non-relational*, *immediate* awareness of I. Kṣemarāja rightly says, "Yadi nirvimarśaḥ syāt anīśvaro jaḍaśca prasajyeta" (Parāprāveśikā, p. 2) i.e. "If Ultimate Reality were merely prakāśa and not also vimarśa, it would be entirely powerless and inert." It is this I-consciousness of Ultimate Reality that is responsible for the manifestation, maintenance, and re-absorption of the universe.

Cit is conscious of itself as *Cidrūpiṇī śakti*. This consciousness of itself as Cidrūpiṇī śakti is *Vimarśa*. *Vimarśa* has been named variously as *parāśakti*, *svātantrya*, *aiśvarya*, *Kartṛtva*, *sphurattā*, *sāra*, *hṛdaya*, *spanda*. (Parāprāveśikā, p. 2).

It is because Śāṅkara Vedānta considers Brahman to be only *prakāśa* or *jñāna* (light or illumination) without any *vimarśa* or activity that it has to invoke the help of Māyā for the manifestation of the universe. Brahman is devoid of any activity; it is, therefore, impotent to create. It is, only Īśvara or *māyopahita caitanya* that can manifest the universe. But whence does this Māyā drop in ? If it is some power extraneous to Brahman or Īśvara, then Śāṅkara Vedānta is reduced to dualism. If Māyā is only an expression of the power of Brahman, then Brahman cannot be divested of activity. Both Sāṅkhya and Vedānta consider the Puruṣa or Ātmā to be *niṣkriya* or inactive, because they take the word 'activity' in a very crude sense. Surely, Brahman or Ātmā does not work like a potter or watch-maker. The very Vimarśa, the very *Icchā* (will) of the Divine is spiritual energy of incalculable force that can proliferate into any form from the subtlest to the grossest.

Svātantrya or unimpeded Sovereignty is the characteristic *par excellence* of Śiva. It expresses itself into *Ichhā* (will) which immediately translates itself into *jñāna* (knowledge) and *kriyā* (action).

Ultimate Reality is not only Universal Consciousness but also Supreme spiritual energy or Power. This All-inclusive

Universal Consciousness is also called Anuttara, the Highest Reality, the Absolute. It is both transcendental (*viśvottīrṇa*) and immanent (*viśvamaya*).

2. *Manifestation or the World Process :*

It is the *svabhāva* or very nature of Ultimate Reality to manifest. Creativity is of the very essence of Divinity. If Ultimate Reality did not manifest, it would not be Self or consciousness, but not-Self, something like a jar.

As Abhinavagupta puts it :

"अस्थास्यदेकरूपेण वपुषा चेन्महेश्वरः ।
महेश्वरत्वं संवित्त्वं तदत्यक्षद् घटादिवत् ॥"

Tantrāloka, III, 100.

"If the Highest Reality did not manifest in infinite variety, but remained cooped up within its solid, singleness, it would neither be the Highest Power nor Consciousness, but something like a jar."

Ultimate Reality or Parama Śiva is *prakāśavimarśamaya*. In that state, the 'I' and the 'This' are in an undivided unity. The 'I' is the *prakāśa* aspect. 'This' or its consciousness of itself is the *vimarśa* aspect. This *Vimarśa* is *svātantrya* or unimpeded sovereign power or *Śakti*. This *Vimarśa* is not contentless. It contains all that is to be.

"यथा न्यग्रोधबीजस्थः शक्तिरूपो महाद्रुमः ।
तथा हृदयबीजस्थं विश्वमेतच्चराचरम् ॥"

Parātriṁśikā, 34.

"As the great banyan tree lies only in the form of potency in the seed, even so the entire universe with all the mobile and immobile beings lies as a potency in the heart of the Supreme."

The Śakti of the Supreme is called *Citi* or *parāśakti* or *parāvāk*. We shall see in the sequel what part *parāśakti* or *parāvāk* plays in the manifestation of word and its object.

Parama Śiva has infinite powers, but the following may be considered to be the main ones :

1. *Cit* — the power of Self-revelation, the changeless principle of all changes. In this aspect, the Supreme is known as Śiva.

2. Ānanda or Absolute bliss. This is also called *svātantrya*, In this aspect, the Supreme is known as Śakti. *Cit* and *ānanda* are the very *svarūpa* or nature of Parama Śiva. The rest may be considered to be His Śaktis.

3. *Icchā* or Will. In this aspect, He is known as Sadāśiva or Sādākhya.

4. *Jñāna* or knowledge. In this aspect, He is known as Īśvara.

5. Kriyā — the power of assuming any and every form. In this aspect, He is known as *Sadvidyā* or *Śuddha Vidyā*.

The Universe is simply an opening out (*unmeṣa*) or expansion (*prasara*) of the Supreme as Śakti.

The following appear in the course of manifestation.

I. THE TATTVAS OF THE UNIVERSAL EXPERIENCE 1-5

As has already been said Parama Śiva has two aspects, viz., transcendental (*viśvottīrṇa*) and immanent or creative. This creative aspect of Parama Śiva is known as Śiva tattva.

1. Śiva tattva is the initial creative movement (*prathama spanda*) of Parama Śiva.

2. Śakti tattva is the Energy of Śiva. She polarizes Consciousness into *Aham* and *Idam* (I and This) — Subject and object.

Śakti, however, is nothing separate from Śiva. Śiva in his creative aspect is known as Śakti. She is His *ahaṁvimarśa* (I-consciousness), His *unmukhatā* or intentness to create.

Just as an artist cannot contain his delight within himself, but pours it out into a song, or a poem, even so Parama Śiva pours out the delightful wonder of His splendour into manifestation.

In *Śakti tattva*, *ānanda* aspect of the Supreme is predominant.

Śiva and *Śakti tattvas* can never be separated.

3. *Sadāśiva or Sādākhya Tattva :*

The will (*Icchā*) to affirm the 'This' side of the Universal Experience is known as *sadāśiva* or *Sādākhya tattva.* In Sadāśiva, *Icchā* (Will) is predominant.

The experience of this stage is 'I am this', but the 'this' is only a hazy (*asphuṭa*) experience. The predominant side is still 'I'. The Ideal Universe is experienced as an indistinct something in the depth of consciousness.

Sadāśiva tattva is the first manifestation (*ābhāsa*). In this Universal Experience, both the subject and object are consciousness. Consciousness in this aspect becomes perceptible to Itself; hence a subject and an object.

4. *Īśvara or Aiśvarya Tattva*

The next stage of the Divine experience is that where *Idam* or the *This* side of the total experience becomes a little more defined (*sphuṭa*). This is known as *Īśvara tattva.* It is *unmeṣa* or distinct blossoming of the Universe. At this stage, *jñāna* or knowledge is predominant.

The experience of *Sadāśiva* is 'I am this'. The experience of *Īśvara* is : 'This am I.'

5. *Sadvidyā or Śuddhavidyā Tattva :*

In the *Sadvidyā tattva*, the 'I' and the 'This' side of experience are equally balanced like the two pans of an evenly held balance (*samadhṛtatulāpuṭanyāyena*). At this stage, *kriyā śakti* is predominant. The 'I' and 'This' are recognized in this state with such equal clarity that while both 'I' and 'This' are still identified, they can be clearly distinguished in thought. The experience of this stage may be called diversity-in-unity (*bhedābheda-vimarśanātmā*) i.e. while the 'This' is clearly distinguished from 'I', it is still felt to be a part of the 'I' or Self. What is 'I' is 'This', what is 'This' is 'I' i.e. they have *samānādhikaraṇa*.

The experience of this stage is known as *parāpara daśā.* It is intermediate between the *para* or higher and *apara* or the lower.

Upto this stage, all experience is ideal i.e. in the form of an idea. Hence it is called the perfect or pure order (*Śuddhādhvā*) i.e. a manifestation in which the *svarūpa* or the real nature of the Divine is not yet veiled.

II. THE TATTVAS (PRINCIPLES) OF THE LIMITED INDIVIDUAL EXPERIENCE

6-11 *Māyā and the Five Kañcukas*

Now begins the play of *Māyā tattva.* From this stage onward, there is *Aśuddhādhvā* or impure order in which the higher, ideal nature of the Divine is veiled. All this happens because of

Māyā and her kañcukas, Māyā is derived from the root 'mā', to measure out. That which makes experience measurable i.e. limited, and severs the 'This' from 'I' and 'I' from 'This' and excludes things from one another is Māyā.

Upto *Sadvidyā*, the experience is universal; the 'This means 'all this', the total universe. Under the operation of Māyā, 'this' means merely 'this', different from every thing else. From now on starts *saṅkoca* or contraction, limitation. Māyā draws a veil (*āvaraṇa*) on the Self owing to which he forgets his real nature, and thus Māyā generates a sense of difference.

The products of Māyā are the five *Kañcukas* or coverings. Their functions are given below :

(i) *Kalā*. This reduces the *sarvakartṛatva* (universal authorship) of the universal Consciousness and brings about limitation in respect of authorship or efficacy.

(ii) *Vidyā*. This reduces the omniscience (*sarvajñatva*) of the Universal Consciousness and brings about limitation in respect of knowledge.

(iii) *Rāga*. This reduces the all-satisfaction (*pūrṇatva*) of the Universal Consciousness and brings about desire for particular things.

(iv) *Kāla*. This reduces the eternity (*nityatva*) of the Universal Consciousness and brings about limitation in respect of time i.e. division of past, present and future.

(v) *Niyati*. This reduces the freedom and pervasiveness (*svatantratā* and *vyāpakatva*) of the Universal consciousness and brings about limitation in respect of cause, space, and form.

It is interesting to note that the Trika Philosophy of Kashmir had anticipated the German philosopher Kant a thousand years before in the analysis of experience.

Hume had reduced experience to a passing phantasmagoria of ideas among which there was no binding principle whatsoever. Kant brought about a Copernican revolution in Philosophy by proving that real experience consists of synthetic judgements which are characterized by necessity and universality. Necessity and Universality are not products of experience. They are *á priori* i.e. prior to experience. Senses only provide the data of experience, but Understanding imposes its own laws on the data of experience to transform them into synthetic, harmonious whole of knowledge. Kant called these laws categories. These are inherent in the very constitution of mind.

Trika or Pratyabhijñā philosophy maintains that the experience of the empirical individual is constituted by *Māyā* together with her *Kañcukas* of *Kalā*, *vidyā*, *rāga*, *kāla* and *niyati*.

Kant takes time and space to be forms of intuition. All our experiences are delimited by space and time — Pratyabhijñā philosophy also teaches that all our experiences are delimited by *Kāla* and *Niyạti*. Kant believes that man's experience occurs only in a spatio-temporal frame. Pratyabhijñā philosophy also believes that man is so constituted by Māyā that his experiences are bound to be circumscribed by *Kāla* and *Niyati*.

The very word Māyā means that power by which experience is measured in a particular way (*mīyate anayā iti Māyā*. In Pratyabhijñā philosophy, *māyā-pramātā*, *citta-pramātā*, *sakala*, *aṇu* and *jīva* are all synonyms for the empirical individual.

There are three functions of Niyati in Pratyabhijñā — limitation in space, causality and the measure of a form of things. The first two are covered by Kant's idea of space and the category of causality. There is nothing in Kant's philosophy similar to the third function of Niyati. Kant's category of relation is included in Niyati. His categories of quantity, quality and modality come under the Kañcuka Vidyā.

Kant's theory is confined only to epistemology. Kant has formulated his theory only with reference to knowledge. Pratyabhijñā has formulated its theory both with referene to knowledge and activity. In Pratyabhijñā philosophy, there are two Kañcukas, viz., Kalā and Rāga which have no parallel in Kant's system. Both of these are connected with activity. Man is not only a bundle of knowledge. He is also an active being. Kalā denotes limitation in respect of action. No man is all-powerful like Śiva. Rāga denotes his valuation, his craving for various things. Just as Kalā expresses loss of full sovereignty in the case of the *māyā-pramātā*, the empirical individual, even so *Rāga* expresses loss of perfection.

Kant maintained that there are two sources of knowledge — matter and form. Matter is provided by Nature and form is imposed on it by mind. Thus there is dualism in Kant's philosophy. According to Pratyabhijñā philosophy, both matter and form are provided by Māyā. Form is provided by Vidyā, Kāla and Niyati and matter is provided by Kalā. Māyā gives rise to Pradhāna or Prakṛti by her power of Kalā.* From Prakṛti are derived *buddhi*, *ahaṁkāra* and *manas*. From *ahaṁkāra* arise five sense-organs, and five organs of action and the five *tanmātrās*, and from the five *tanmātrās* arise the five gross elements. So both matter and form of knowledge arise from Māyā and Māyā arises from Śiva-Śakti. Thus there is unmitigated non-dualism in Pratyabhijñā.

Kant says that we cannot know the world, Self, and God by the understanding and the categories. Pratyabhijñā philosophy also maintains that Māyā and the phenomena built by her are in *ásuddha adhvā* and the knowledge derived in *aśuddha adhvā* is through *vikalpas* or distinction-making mental constructs whereas knowledge of the cosmos, Self and God is *nirvikalpa* — non-distinctive, non-discursive.

Kant maintains that the knowledge of the cosmos, self and God can be obtained only through moral and spiritual discipline. Pratyabhijñā philosophy also maintains that the knowledge of the highest Reality can be obtained only through *sādhanā* (spiritual praxis) — through *āṇava*, *śākta* and *śāmbhava upāya*.

III. THE TATTVAS OF THE LIMITED INDIVIDUAL

12 *Puruṣa*

Śiva through Māyāśakti which limits His universal knowledge and power becomes Puruṣa or the individual subject. *Puruṣa* in this context means every sentient being.

Puruṣa is also known as *aṇu* in this system. The word *aṇu* is used in the sense of limitation of the divine perfection.

13 *Prakṛti*

While *Puruṣa* is the subjective manifestation of *Śiva*, *Prakṛti* is the objective manifestation.

There is a difference between the Sāṅkhya conception of *Prakṛti* and that of Trika. Sāṅkhya believes that *Prakṛti* is

*"वेद्यमात्रं स्फुटं भिन्नं प्रधानं सूयते कला"

(Tantrāloka, 2)

one and universal for all the *Puruṣas*. Trika believes that each *Puruṣa* has a different *Prakṛti*. *Prakṛti* is the matrix of all Objectivity.

Prakṛti has three *guṇas* or genetic constituents, viz., *sattva*, *rajas* and *tamas*. In her unmanifested state *Prakṛti* holds these *guṇas* in perfect equipoise. In the order of being, *sattva* is characterized by brightness and lightness, in the psychological order, it is characterized by transparency, joy and peace; in the ethical order, it is the principle of goodness. In the order of being, *tamas* is the principle of darkness, inertness; in the psychological order, it is characterized by dullness, delusion and dejection, and in the ethical order, it is the principle of degradation, debasement. In the order of being, *rajas* is characterized by activity; in the psychological order, it is characterized by craving and passion; in the ethical order, it is the principle of ambition and avarice.

According to Pratyabhijñā, *Prakṛti* is the Śāntā Śakti of Śiva, and the *guṇas sattva*, *rajas* and *tamas* are only the polarization of His *śaktis* of *jñāna*, *icchā* and *kriyā* respectively. Thus in the Pratyabhijñā system, there is perfect non-dualism, not dualism of Prakṛti and Puruṣa, as in Sāṅkhya.

Puruṣa is the experient (*bhoktā*) and Prakṛti is the experienced (*bhogyā*).

IV. THE TATTVAS OF MENTAL OPERATION
14-16 Buddhi, Ahaṁkāra, and Manas

Prakṛti differentiates into *antaḥkaraṇa* (the psychic apparatus), *indriyas* (senses) and *bhūtas* (matter).

Antaḥkaraṇa means the inner instrument, the psychic apparatus of the individual. It consists of the *tattvas—buddhi*, *ahaṁkāra*, and *manas*.

1. Buddhi is the ascertaining intelligence (vyavasāyātmikā). The objects that are reflected in *buddhi* are of two kinds — (a) external, e.g., a jar which is perceived through the eye, (b) internal — the images built out of the *saṁskāras* (the impressions left behind on the mind).

2. *Ahaṁkāra*. This is the product of *buddhi*. It is the I-making principle and the power of self-appropriation.

3. *Manas.* It is the product of *ahaṁkāra.* It co-operates with the senses in building up perceptions, and by itself, it builds images and concepts.

V-VII. THE TATTVAS OF SENSIBLE EXPERIENCE 17-31

1. The five powers of sense-perception. *Jñānendriyas* or *Buddhīndriyas* which are products of *ahaṁkāra* are the tattvas of sensible experience. The five powers are those of (i) smelling (*ghrāṇendriya*), (ii) tasting (*rasanendriya*), (iii) seeing (*cakṣur-indriya*), (iv) feeling by touch (*sparśendriya*), (v) hearing (*śravaṇen-driya*).

2. The five *Karmendriyas* or powers of action. These are also products of *ahaṁkāra.* These are powers of (i) speaking (*vāgindriya*), (ii) handling (*hastendriya*), (iii) locomotion (*pāden-driya*), (iv) excreting (*pāyvindriya*), (v) sexual action and restful-ness (*upasthendriya*).

The *indriyas* are not sense-organs but powers which operate through the sense-organs.

3. The five *tanmātras* or primary elements of perception. These are also products of *ahaṁkāra.* Literally *tanmātra* means 'that only'. These are the general elements of the par-ticulars of sense-perception. They are :

(i) sound-as-such (*śabda-tanmātra*) (ii) touch-as-such (*sparśa-tanmātra*), (iii) colour-as-such (*rūpa-tanmātra*), (iv) flavour-as-such (*rasa-tanmātra*), (v) odour-as-such (*gandha-tanmātra*).

VIII. THE TATTVAS OF MATERIALITY
32-36 The Five Bhūtas

The five gross elements or the *pañca-mahābhūtas* are the products of the five *tanmātras.*

(i) Ākāśa is produced from *śabda-tanmātra.*
(ii) Vāyu is produced from *sparśa-tanmātra.*
(iii) Teja (Agni) is produced from *rūpa-tanmātra.*
(iv) Āpas is produced from *rasatanmātra.*
(v) Pṛthivī is produced from gandhatanmātra.

The Individual Self or Jīva

Caitanya or *Śiva* forms the very core of the being of every individual. It is his real Self.

The physical aspect of the individual Self consists of the *pañca mahābhūtas*, the five gross elements highly organized, known as *sthūla śarīra* or the physical body.

There is also *prāṇa śakti* working in him. It is by this *prāṇa śakti* — that he is sustained and maintained.

His psychic apparatus is known as *antaḥkaraṇa* (the inner apparatus) consisting of *manas*, *buddhi* and *ahaṁkāra*. These three together with the five *tanmātras* form a group of eight known as *puryaṣṭaka*. This, according to Trika, forms the subtle body (*sūkṣma-śarīra*) in which the soul leaves the body at the time of death.

In each individual, there is *Kuṇḍalinī* which is a form of Śakti and lies dormant at the base of the spine.

Each individual has normally an experience of three states of consciousness waking, dream and deep sleep. There is, however, a fourth state of consciousness, known as *turīya*. This is the consciousness of the central Self or *Śiva* in each individual, This is a witnessing consciousness of which the individual is normally not aware. The turīya is pure *cidānanda*-consciousness and bliss. The individual's mind is conditioned by habit energy (Vāsanā) of previous lives. When by *yogic* practices, his mind becomes deconditioned, then he attains the *turīya* consciousness, and becomes a *jīvan-mukta* i.e. liberated while still alive.

3. *Bondage*

The bondage of the individual is due to innate ignorance or *āṇava mala*. It is this primary limiting condition which reduces the universal consciousness to an *aṇu* or a limited creature. It comes about by the limitation of the *Icchā Śakti* of the Supreme. It is owing to this that the *jīva* considers himself to be a separate entity cut off from the universal stream of consciousness. It is consciousness of self-limitation and imperfection.

Coming in association with *aśuddhaadhvā*, he becomes further limited by *māyīya mala* and *kārma mala*. *Māyīya mala* is the limited condition brought about by *māyā*. It is *bhinna vedya prathā* — that which brings about the consciousness of difference owing to the differing limiting adjuncts of the body etc. This comes about by the limitation of the *jñāna śakti* of the Supreme. *Kārma mala* is the limiting condition brought about by the *vāsanās* or residual traces of actions done under the influence of desire. It is the force of these *vāsanās* that carries the *jīva* from one life to another.

4. *Liberation* :

Liberation, according to the system, means the recognition (*pratyabhijñā*) of one's true nature which means *akṛtrima-ahaṁ-vimarśa* — the original, innate, pure I-consciousness.

The normal psychological I-consciousness is relational i.e. the Self-consciousness is in contrast with the not-Self. The pure I-consciousness is immediate awareness. When one has this consciousness, one knows one's real nature. This is what is meant by liberation.

As Abhinavagupta puts it :

"मोक्षो हि नाम नैवान्यः स्वरूपप्रथनं हि तत्" Tantra I, p. 192.

Mokṣa or liberation is nothing else but the awareness of one's true nature.

The highest attainment, however, is that of Śiva-consciousness in which the entire universe appears as I or Śiva and this comes by Śaktipāta — the descent of Divine *Śakti* or *anugraha* (Divine grace).

Upāyas :

In order to earn grace, one has to undergo spiritual discipline. This is known as *upāya* or *yoga*. The *upāyas* are divided under four broad heads, viz., (1) Anupāya, (2) Śāmbhavopāya (3) Śāktopāya and (4) Āṇavopāya.

The prefix 'an' in *anupāya* in this context means 'little'. When through extreme *Śaktipāta*, only by once hearing a word from the *guru* (the spiritual director), the aspirant realizes the real Self and gets absorbed in the divine consciousness without any particular effort, one is said to have attained Self-realization through *anupāya*.

Śiva-sūtra is a text on Yoga. It leaves anupāya, for it refers to a stage in which Self-realization is achieved without any specific Yoga. It has been rightly said by Abhinavagupta:

उपायजालं न शिवं प्रकाशयेद्
घटेन किं भाति सहस्रदीधितिः ।
विवेचयन्नित्थमुदारदर्शनः
स्वयंप्रकाशं शिवमाविशेत्क्षणात् ॥

"Even innumerable means cannot reveal Śiva. Can a jar reveal the Sun ? Pondering thus, one with a lofty vision gets absorbed immediately in Śiva who is Self-luminous."

Since this stage transcends all yogic activity, no description of it can be given.

The book has three sections — In the first Section, it gives a description of Śāmbhavopāya, in the second of Śāktopāya, and in the third of Āṇavopāya.

We shall now consider these *upāyas* in detail in the following pages.

Śiva-Sūtras :

FIRST SECTION

The first *sūtra* of this section gives the philosophical background of this system as well as the experience of *Śāmbhava Yoga*. It says that *caitanya* or consciousness is Self or nature of reality. Caitanya in this system does not mean merely consciousness. It means consciousness which has the absolute freedom of will, knowledge and action. Its essential nature is *cit* (consciousness) and *ānanda* (bliss). It expresses itself in *icchā* (will), *jñāna* (knowledge) and *kriyā* (action).

The question arises 'If the essential nature of *jīva* and *jagat*, of all experients and the world is Śiva, how is it then that all beings in the world do not enjoy the bliss of Śiva, but experience bondage — limitation in respect of willing, knowledge, and action ?

The answer is that the bondage of the empirical individual is due to *āṇava*, *māyīya*, and *kārma malas* or limiting conditions. *Āṇava mala* is an innate, limiting condition which is the primal ignorance of our essential nature as Śiva. *Māyīya mala* is due to

Māyā which gives to the soul its gross and subtle body, and brings about sense of difference and *kārma mala* is due to *vāsanās* or impressions left behind on the mind due to *karma* or motivated action. The primal ignorance which brings about *āṇava mala* is described in *sūtra* 2, and the *māyīya* and *kārma mala* have been described in *sūtra* 3.

Sūtra 2 says that the bondage of the *jīva* or the empirical individual is due to *saṅkucita jñāna* or limited knowledge. *Ajñāna* or primal ignorance does not mean total absence of knowledge but limited and vitiated knowledge.

Śiva has *svātantrya śakti*, unimpeded power of bringing into being the cosmic drama. Through this, he brings into play His *Mahāmāyā-śakti* by means of which he veils his essential nature (*sva-svātantrya-śaktyābhāsita-svarūpa-gopanā-rūpayā mahāmāyā-śaktyā*) and assumes limited knowledge and limited forms. Thus begins the world drama. The first stage is *svarūpa-nimeṣa* or *svarūpa-gopanā* or veiling of His essential nature. This is the stage of the involution of the Divine into inconscient gross matter. This is the arc of descent. After that starts the slow and gradual process of *svarūpa-unmeṣa* or *svarūpa prakāśana* or gradual revelation of His essential nature. This is the arc of ascent. Now begins the process of evolution, of the play of life and mind. It is only at the stage of man that the question of recognizing one's essential Divine nature arises. And it is for this recognition (*pratyabhijñā*) that there is provision for *yoga* or spiritual praxis.

Ajñāna or *āṇava mala* is only vitiated knowledge by which one considers the vehicles—gross, subtle bodies etc. as the Self.

The three kinds of *malas* or limited, vitiated knowledge are rooted in words which have a tremendous influence on our lives. These are formed of letters which are known as Mātṛkā. The Mātṛkā becomes the basis of all limited knowledge. This is explained in *Sūtra* 4.

Mātṛkā means unknown, unrealized mother. So long as the mystery of Mātṛkā is not realized, she is a source of bondage or limitation. When her mystery is realized, she becomes the source of liberation.

Śāmbhava Yoga :

Sūtra 5. *Udyamo Bhairavaḥ* gives in a nut-shell the description of *Śāmbhava yoga.*

Udyamaḥ in this context does not mean exertion. There can be no question of exertion in Śāmbhava Yoga. It is known as *icchopāya* or *icchā-yoga.* It occurs by a mere orientation of the Will. It is also known as *abhedopāya*, a *yoga* in which there is complete identification of 'I' and Śiva, in which the idea of the so-called 'I' which is only a psycho-physical complex, a mere *nāma-rūpa* disappears and Śiva alone is experienced as the real I, as the real Self. It is also known as *avikalpaka* or *nirvikalpaka yoga* or *upāya,* for this experience occurs when there is complete cessation of all thought-constructs.

This is a *yoga* in which there is no active process either of body or *prāṇa* or *manas* or *buddhi*. Obviously *udyama* cannot mean exertion or discipline in this context. Kṣemarāja rightly interprets *udyama* here as *unmajjanarūpaḥ* — as a form of emergence of Śiva-consciousness. Śāmbhava Yoga is that (1) in which there is a sudden flash of the I-consciousness of Śiva (2) in which all ideation ceases completely (*sakala-kalpanākulālaṅkavalana*) (3) which occurs to those whose entire consciousness is absorbed in the inner Bhairava principle (*antarmukha-etat-tattvāvadhāna-dhanānāṁ jāyate*).

Mālinīvijaya puts Śāmbhava upāya in the following words :

अकिंचिच्चिन्तकस्यैव गुरुणा प्रतिबोधतः ।
जायते यः समावेशः शाम्भवोऽसावुदाहृतः ॥

"That is said to be Śāmbhava-samāveśa (absorption in Śiva-consciousness) which occurs to one who has freed himself of all ideation by an awakening imparted by the guru (the spiritual director) or by an intensive awakening (of his own)."

When there is identification with Śiva without any mentation or thought-process, merely by an intensive orientation of Will power (icchā Śakti) towards the inner Reality, then is there Śāmbhava-Yoga or Śāmbhava Samāveśa.

In the *jīva* or empirical individual, Reality or Śiva or the Divine transcendental Self is Light—Bliss that is ever shining within in its glory but is hidden from our gaze on account of our thought-constructs. Reality is an Eternal Presence within ourselves. It is *Siddha*, an everpresent Fact, not *sādhya*, not something to be brought into being by our efforts. It cannot be caught by our *vikalpa-jāla*, by the net of our thought constructs, however cleverly we may cast it. The more we try to catch it, the more we try to grasp it, the more does it recede from us. We are prisoners of our own mind. Thought has to commit suicide in order to know our real Self, the Śiva within ourselves. *Vikalpa*, the dichotomizing activity of our mind has to cease, the wheel of imagination has to stop. The ghost of our discursive intellect has to be laid to rest, before we are allowed to realize our essential Self. *Vikalpa* 'like a dome of coloured class stains the white radiance of eternity'. When *vikalpa* ceases, the transcendental Self within us shines of itself. It is an Experience in which the distinction of seer, seen and sight is completely annulled. That is why it is called *abhedopāya*, a yoga in which the above distinction has disappeared.

Thus when the mind neither accepts nor rejectes any idea, its activity ceases and one abides in one's essential Reality. As Abhinavagupta puts it beautifully :

मा किञ्चित् त्यज, या गृहाण, विरम स्वस्थो यथावस्थितः ।

(Anuttarāṣṭikā, 2)

"Neither reject anything, nor accept, abide in your essential Self which is an Eternal presence."

Mr. J. Krishnamurti, a modern Yogī uses these very words (neither accept, nor reject) and calls it choiceless awareness, an awareness which is not of thought. Awareness is not thought. Awareness is not discipline, not habit. It cannot be practised. It is alertness from moment to moment.

There is an inner dimension of Reality in which we are always living but which we do not know. Śāmbhava Yoga exhorts us to rediscover and realize it. This comes about, not by seeking, not by choice, not by discipline, but spontaneously when the mind has ceased cogitating and surrenders itself completely to the effulgence of the Divine Presence within.

We find parallel attitudes to Śāmbhava Yoga in 'wu-wei (non-interference) of Taoism, 'let-go' of Zen, and choiceless awareness of Krishnamurti.

In the third section of his Tantrasāra, Abhinavagupta says that in Śāmbhavopāya, *icchā śakti* may be re-inforced by *jñānaśakti*, by realizing that the entire universe of objective and subjective entities abides in the essential Self as its reflection. My own *Śaktis* (powers) being reflected within me appear as the thirty-six *tattvas.* The *śaktis* appear as *Mātṛkā*, i.e. group of letter-sounds from 'ka' to 'ha' whose reflection appears in the form of the *tattvas* (constitutive principles) from Śiva to earth. (For details, see the exposition of the 7th *Sūtra* of the 2nd section).

Kṣemarāja adds at the end of his commentary on the 5th *sūtra* of the first section that *Śāmbhavopāya* may be helped by the following *Śāktopāya* :

"एकचिन्ताप्रसक्तस्य यतः स्यादपरोदयः ।
उन्मेषः स तु विज्ञेयः स्वयं तमुपलक्षयेत्" ॥ (III, 9)

"While one is engaged in one thought, and another arises, the junction-point between the two is the *unmeṣa*, i.e. revelation of the true nature of the Self which is the background of both the two thoughts. This may be experienced by every one for oneself."

Krishnamurti, a modern mystic who has not read any Sanskrit book speaks of this experience in almost these very words on page 211 of his book, "The First and Last Freedom." He calls *unmeṣa* the creative moment. It is not thought, but a flash of Understanding. *Unmeṣa* literally means opening of the eye-lid i.e. uncovering, Self-revelation.

The sixth *sūtra* says that when the experience of the essential Self, of Śiva-consciousness continues in the normal course of life, then the entire universe appears only as an expansion of the collection of the *Śaktis* (powers) of the Self and by an intensive awareness of this collective whole of *śaktis*, the universe as something separate from Śiva or the divine Self disappears. There is complete unity-consciousness.

Sūtra 7 says that the experience of the inner Divine Self is the experience of the fourth (*turīya*) or transcendental consciousness and its bliss continues even when there is appearance of difference in the three states of waking, dream and deep sleep consciousness.

Sutras 8, 9 and 10 tell us that from the spiritual point of view, he alone should be called awake who has realized Self. He who is subject to all kinds of uncontrolled fancies and thoughts is really in the state of dream although apparently he may be wide awake. He who has not obtained the discerning insight into Reality is in the state of deep sleep. The activities of those who have not awakened to the transcendental consciousness within are like those of a somnambulist, a sleep-walker.

Sūtra 11 tells us that he who retains the experience of the 4th or transcendental consciousness even in the other three states of deep sleep, dream and waking is alone the real *bhoktā* or enjoyer and is the perfect master of his senses.

Sūtra 12 says in a general way that the *Yogī* who realizes his essential Self develops wonderful supernormal powers. *Sūtra* 13 says that he develops *Icchā śakti*, the divine Will power and through this, he can bring about many marvellous changes.

Sūtras 14 and 15 maintain that to such a *yogī*, every objective observable phenomenon, whether external or internal appears as a form of his own consciousness. *Sūtra* 16 says that he is now able to trace the origin of everything to *Parama Śiva* and is completely absolved of all limiting conditions.

Sūtra 17 says that he is now fully convinced that his Self is none else but Śiva, the Self of the universe. *Sūtra* 18 tells us that the awareness of the Yogī that he is the subject of every experience continues unabated. *Sūtra* 19 says that by being united with *Icchā śakti*, the *yogī* can create any sort of body according to his desire. *Sūtra* 20 tells us that such a *yogī* develops the power of joining the elements of all existence, the power of separating elements and the power of bringing together everything removed by space and time.

Sūtra 21 says that such a *yogī*, however, does not desire limited powers. Through the appearance of *Śuddha Vidyā* i.e. *Unmanā śakti* in this context, he acquires cosmic consciousness and lordship over all the *śaktis*. His highest experience is not simply self-realization (*ātmavyāpti*) but *śivatva-yojanā* complete identification with *Śiva* (*Śiva-vyāpti*) — a state in which the universe is experienced as the Self-expression of *Śiva*.

Sūtra 22 says that such a *yogī* being united with the infinite reservoir of Divine Power (*mahāhrada*) has the experience of the Supreme I-consciousness which is the generative source of all the *mantras*.

Concluding Remarks :

We have seen that *Śāmbhava upāya* does not advocate any particular effort or discipline for Self-realization.

When we neither accept, nor reject, when there is simple awareness freed of all ideation, then there is a sudden, spontaneous flash of experience of our essential Self : This is *Śāmbhava Samāveśa.* This is direct, immediate realization.

Āṇava and Śākta upāyas are only pāramparika i.e. leading to realization through successive stages — *āṇava upāya* leading to *Śākta* and *Śākta* leading to *Śāmbhava upāya.* The ultimate goal is *Śāmbhava Samāveśa* — a spontaneous flash of Understanding. Āṇava and Śākta upāyas are only intermediate means to *Śāmbhava Yoga.*

As has already been said, help in Śāmbhava Yoga may be taken from a proper understanding of *Mātṛkā.* We shall discuss in detail about the proper application of *Mātṛkā* in connection with *Śākta upāya. Śāmbhava upāya* is a special feature of *Śaivāgama.* There is no such *yoga* either in *Vedānta* or *Pātañjala yoga.* The *jñāna-yoga* of *Vedānta* corresponds somewhat to *Śākta upāya* and *Pātañjala yoga* corresponds to a part of *āṇava-upāya. Śāmbhava yoga* is unknown to these systems.

Anupāya is, really speaking, *Śāmbhava yoga* itself in its highest maturity **स (शाम्भवोपायः) एव परां काष्ठां प्राप्तश्चानुपाय इत्युच्यते ।** (Ta.K1-142)." The *Śāmbhava upāya* itself, in its highest maturity is known as *anupāya.* "Later on, the word Sāhasa was employed by Vātūlanātha of Kashmir to express the idea of *Śāmbhava yoga* and *anupāya.* The word Śāhasa means sudden, unexpected happening. It beautifully expresses the idea of sudden spontaneous flash of the Experience of the Divine Self.

The ultimate aim of both *Sāṁkhya-yoga* and *Vedānta* is *mukti* (liberation). By *mukti,* both of them understand *Kaivalya,* perfect isolation or Soleness, the only difference being that Sāṁkhya-yoga aims at isolation from *Prakṛti* while *Vedānta* aims at isolation from *Māyā.* There is, however, one difference between the two in the concept of Self. According to Sāṁkhya-Yoga, Self or *Puruṣa* is *saccit* (existence-consciousness) and there is nothing higher than *Puruṣa.* According to *Vedānta,* Self or *Ātmā* is *Saccidānanda* (existence-consciousness-bliss) and is identical with Brahman.

The ultimate aim of Śaivāgama is not simply *mukti* or Self-realization but *Śivatva-yojanā* acquiring the status of Śiva. In the words of Śaivāgama, the ultimate ideal is not merely *Ātma-vyāpti* but *Śiva-vyāpti*. In *Ātma-vyāpti*, there is Self-realization, but the concept of Self-realization in *Śaivāgama* is different from that of *Vedānta*. In *Vedānta*, Self is merely *jñāna* devoid of any activity whatsoever. In *Śaivāgama*, Self is characterized by both *jñāna* and *kriyā*. But *Ātma-vyāpti* in *Śaivāgama* is a lower ideal. The highest ideal is *Śiva-vyāpti*. In *Śiva-vyāpti*, there is *Śiva-Śakti-sāmarasya*, fusion and union of *Śiva-śakti*. In *Ātma-vyāpti*, there is limited *jñāna-kriyā* (knowledge and activity); in *Śiva-vyāpti*, there is universal, all-pervasive *jñāna-kriyā*. This *Śiva-vyāpti* is the status of *Parama Śiva* who is *simultaneously* transcendent to and immanent in the universe. This comes about only when *unmanā śakti* is developed.

In *Vedāntic* liberation, *Māyā* disappears and along with it goes the wretched universe which was only a fiction conjured up by her. In *Śiva-vyāpti*, the universe appears as a magnificent expression of *Śiva's* — one's own—*Śakti*.

The liberated Self in Sāṁkhya-yoga is only *Saccit* (existence-consciousness). The Self or *Puruṣa* is freed of all pain and suffering, but he has no positive bliss. In Vedānta, the characteristic of Self is *saccidānanda* (existence-consciousness-bliss). There is positive bliss in liberation. But it is only *ātmānanda*, the delight of Self. In *Śiva-vyāpti*, the entire universe gleams as the wondrous delight of I-consciousness.

Both in *Sāṁkhya-Yoga* and *Vedānta*, the *citta* or mind reverts to its causal matrix, the Prakṛti at the time of liberation. Pātañjala yoga has a special word for this reversion, viz; *pratiprasava* which means reabsorption, remergence (into *Prakṛti*). The defiling *buddhi* or *citta* has to withdraw into its primal cause. It is only then that *Puruṣa* can shine in his pristine, inherent glory. The *citta* can never be allowed to enter the sacred precincts of *Puruṣa*. It is an alien and has to be repatriated to its original home.

Śaivāgama which is undiluted *advaita* (non-dualism) has, however, a word of cheer even for the poor *citta*. According to it, the *citta* of the self-realized person becomes regenerated, transformed, transfigured into *Cit* (the Universal Divine

Consciousness). *Sūtra* 13 of Pratyabhijñāhṛdayam announces the reassuring tidings of its higher destiny in unmistakable terms :

"तत्परिज्ञाने चित्तमेव अन्तर्मुखीभावेन चेतनपदाध्यारोहात् चितिः" ।

On the realization of the five-fold act of the Self *citta* (the individual consciousness), by inward movement becomes *citi* (universal consciousness) by rising to the status of *cetana* (the knowing subject).

The following lucid commentary of Kṣemarāja on this *sūtra* deserves to be carefully pondered over :

"चित्तं संकोचिनीं बहिर्मुखतां जहत् अन्तर्मुखीभावेन चेतनपदाध्यारोहात् ग्राहकभूमिकाक्रमणक्रमेण संकोचकलाया अपि विगलनेन स्वरूपापत्त्या चितिर् भवति—स्वां चिन्मयीं परां भूमिमाविशति इत्यर्थः।"

"The *citta* giving up the limiting tendency of extroversion, becoming introverted, rises to the status of cetana i.e. to the status of the knowing subject, when by the dissolution of the aspect of limitation and attaining its real nature, it becomes *citi*. That is to say, it now enters its highest stage of cit."

Citta is not an alien in this system. Sūtra 5 of Pratyabhijñāhṛdayam says clearly :

"चितिरेव चेतनपदादवरूढा चेत्यसंकोचिनी चित्तम्" ।

"*Citi* (universal consciousness) itself, descending from the stage of *Cetana* (knower) becomes *citta* (individual consciousness), inasmuch as it becomes contracted in conformity with the objects of consciousness."

In involution (*avaroha, nimeṣa*) *citi* becomes *citta*; in the highest stage of evolution (*adhyāroha, unmeṣa*) *citta* attains its real nature and becomes *citi* again.

Section II.

In section I, *Śāmbhava upāya* has been explained. It has been pointed out that the essential Self within is the Divine Self or Śiva, but mind whose main characteristic is *vikalpa* (thought-construct) acts as a barrier and does not allow us to have a view of the Reality shining within ourselves. It is only when there is *laya* or dissolution of *vikalpa* that the screen that hides the essential Reality, the essential Divine Self from ourselves is removed and we have a view of that Reality which has always been scintillating within in all its glory. That Reality is not something to be *achieved*, but *uncovered*. But the crux of the problem is how to make the *vikalpaful* mind retire. Abhinavagupta says, "When there is *vikalpa*, neither accept, nor reject, it will retire of itself and you will find yourself to be what you are." This is an artless art. It is effortless, spontaneous. This Śāmbhava upāya is, in one sense, the simplest, in another, the most difficult. It is simplest, because no particular effort or discipline is needed for it. It is most difficult, because *vikalpa-making* is the habit, the very life of *citta* or mind. In attempting to be *vikalpa-free*, the mind begins to make all kinds of *Vikalpa*. To try to become *vikalpa*-or thought-free is like trying to jump out of our own skin. It is given to very few mortals to be *vikalpa-free*.

The second section, therefore, recommends another *upāya*, viz., *Śāktopāya*. The last i.e. the 22nd *sūtra* of the first section serves as a propaedeutic to the second section. It has three important words, viz., *mahāhrada*, *anusandhāna* and *mantravīryānubhavaḥ*.

Mahāhrada denotes *mahāśakti*, *anusandhāna* means close (mental) examination with a view to union, *mantravīryānubhavaḥ* means experience of the virility of *mantra*. One has to resort to *mahāśakti* mentally in order to have an experience of the potency of *mantra* that will prove to be his saviour. In *Śāmbhava upāya*, one has to resort to Śiva or Śambhu as *prakāśa*. That is why it is called *Śāmbhavopāya*.

In *Śāktopāya*, one has to resort to *cit-śakti* or *Vimarśa-śakti* (the Divine I-consciousness) for realization. Therefore, this is called *Śāktopāya*. *Śāktopāya* is also known as *Śākta yoga*, *jñānopāya*, *jñānayoga*, *bhāvanopāya*, *mantropāya*.

It is not possible for most people to become *vikalpafree*. Is there no way out for them ? There is, says *Śāktopāya*. Catch hold of one *śuddha vikalpa*. That will prove to be a veritable boat by which we can cross the turbulent waters of phenomenal existence and safely land on the certain ground of our noumenal Reality. In the following passages, Abhinavagupta clearly explains the nature of *aśuddha* and *śuddha vikalpa*. Regarding *aśuddha vikalpa*, he says :

"विकल्पबलात् एव जन्तवो बद्धम् आत्मानम् अभिमन्यन्ते । स अभिमानः संसारप्रतिबन्धहेतुः । अतः प्रतिद्वन्द्विरूपो विकल्प उदितः संसारहेतुं विकल्पं दलयति इति अभ्युदयहेतुः" ॥

(Tantrasāra, p. 21)

"People consider themselves bound on account of (*aśuddha*) *vikalpa.* This wrong conception of theirs about themselves becomes the cause of their being bound in transmigratory existence. Therefore when an opposite *vikalpa* arises, it dispels the *vikalpa* that is the cause of transmigratory existence and thus becomes the cause of their elevation." *Aśuddha* (vitiated, wrong) *vikalpas* are those ideas and beliefs on account of which one considers his psycho-physical organism, his mind-body complex to be the Self. "I am thin, weak, ignorant etc." are examples of *aśuddha vikalpas*. *Aśuddha vikalpa* means the idea about the usual, psychological, empirical self.

What then is *śuddha vikalpa* (correct mental attitude and belief) ? This is what Abhinavagupta has to say about it.

"स च एवंरूपः समस्तेभ्यः परिच्छिन्न-स्वभावेभ्यः शिवान्तेभ्यः तत्त्वेभ्योयत् उत्तीर्णम् अपरिच्छिन्न-संविन्मात्ररूपं तदेव च परमार्थः तदेव च अहम् । अतो विश्वोत्तीर्णो विश्वात्मा च अहम् इति ।"

(Tantrasāra, p. 21)

"That which is unlimited consciousness transcending all limited expressions of Reality from earth right up to Śiva, that alone is the highest Reality; that am I. Therefore I am both transcendent to and immanent in the universe." The *śuddha vikalpa* is the idea and belief that I am the met-empirical, transcendental Self; that the universe is an expression of my power, etc.

The practice of this *śuddha vikalpa* is *Śāktopāya*, A question that arises here is "Can the highest Reality or *parama Śiva* be ever brought within the range of *vikalpa* ? If one enters it (the highest Reality) by means of *vikalpa*, however well-refined and purified, that would mean that the highest Reality can be brought within the province of thought. If not, what is the utility of even this *śuddha vikalpa* ?

With regard to the first question, Śaiva philosophy says categorically that the highest Reality cannot be brought within the province of *vikalpa*. Says Abhinavagupta :

"परं तत्त्वं तु सर्वत्र सर्वरूपतया प्रकाशमेव इति न तत्र विकल्पः कस्यैचित् उपक्रियायै खण्डनायै वा"।
(Tantrasāra, p. 23)

"The highest reality is everywhere and in every way Self-luminous. Vikalpa can neither help nor hinder it." In fact the highest reality cannot be brought under any practice or discipline.
"अभ्यासश्च परे तत्त्वे शिवात्मनि स्वस्वभावे न संभवत्येव।...संविद्रूपे तु न किंचित् आदातव्यं न अपसरणीयम् इति कथम् अभ्यासः।"
(Tantrasāra, p. 24) "No discipline or practice can be possible with regard to the highest Reality or Śiva that is also one's essential nature. Nothing can be added to or removed from the highest Reality; of what avail can practice be here ?"

What then is the utility even of *śuddha vikalpa* ? The utility of *śuddha vikalpa* is in removing the sense of duality. What is this sense of duality? Abhinavagupta says, "द्वैताधिवासो नाम न कश्चन पृथक् वस्तुभूतः, अपितु स्वरूपाख्यातिमात्रं तत्। अतो द्वैतापासनं विकल्पेन क्रियते। (Tantrasāra p. 24)" The sense of duality is nothing else. It is only the ignorance of one's essential nature. Therefore, this sense of duality is annulled by *śuddha vikalpa*. This is the negative function of *śuddha vikalpa*.

There is also a positive function of *Śuddha vikalpa*. It works in three ways (1) by *mantra-śakti* (2) by *sat-tarka* leading to bhāvanā and finally by (3) *śuddha vidyā*. These are distinct but not different. All these are inter-connected. We may consider each of these separately for the convenience of exposition.

1. *Mantra-Śakti* :

As has already been said the last *sūtra* of the first section leads to Śāktopāya. In the introductory portion to the first *sūtra* of the second section, Kṣemarāja says : "तत्र शक्तिः मंत्रवीर्यस्फाररूपा...इति मंत्रस्वरूपं तावत् निरूपयति" "Śakti signifies the expansion of the potency of *mantra*. Therefore the nature of *mantra* is being examined first." So the first *sūtra* of *Śāktopāya* is *Cittam mantraḥ*. *Cittam* in this *sūtra* does not mean any and every mind. In this context, *cittam* means the mind that is seriously bent on reflecting over and finding out the highest reality. चेत्यते विमृश्यते अनेन परं तत्त्वम् इति चित्तम् That which ponders over the highest Reality is *cittam.*

And what is *mantra* ? The word *mantra* consists of two syllables — *man* and *tra.* The syllable *man* means to reflect, to be aware; the syllable *tra* means that which saves. "परस्फुरत्तात्मकमननधर्मात्मता, भेदमयसंसार-प्रशमात्मकत्राणधर्मता च अस्य निरुच्यते" । "*Mantra* means that mental awareness by which one feels one's identity with the highest Reality enshrined in a *mantra* and thus saves oneself from a sense of separateness and difference characteristic of the world."

It has already been said that *śāktopāya* is that in which consciousness as *śakti* or power is the guiding principle. *Śakti* assumes the form of *mantra* or mystic syllable or syllables. The mind of the aspirant is so intensely identified with the deity of the *mantra* that it becomes that *mantra* itself. *Citta* in this context means the condensed aspect of Self as consciousness. In the first *sūtra* of the first section Self was described as pure universal consciousness having *svātantrya śakti* and *jñāna* and *kriyā* as its characteristics. Here *citta* is that condensed aspect of Self in which *mantra* is realized.

Every *mantra* consists of certain syllables. Muttering of the syllables mechanically is of no avail. The aspirant must identify himself with the deity invoked in the *mantra.* Pūrṇāhantā or the full I-consciousness of Śiva which is His *Vimarśa śakti* — the creative pulsation of the Divine is the source of all the *mantras.* Every *mantra* leads back to that divine I-consciousness which is the creative *śakti* of the Supreme. That I-consciousness is no speech, but the source of all speech and thought and objectivity. *Śuddha vikalpa* means pondering over that full, divine I-consciousness as our real Self. Since that I-consciousness is the Śakti of Śiva, pondering over that *śakti* is *śāktopāya* which brings about the absorption of the individual self in the divine Self of *Śiva.* This is why Mālinīvijaya gives the following definition of Śāktopāya.

उच्चाररहितं वस्तु चेतसैव विचिन्तयन् ।
यं समावेशमाप्नोति शाक्तः सोऽत्राभिधीयते (II, 22)

"When an aspirant with one-pointedness of mind, apprehends that Reality which is not within the range of utterance (gross or subtle), and thus obtains *samāveśa* (absorption in divine consciousness), then that *samāveśa* is known as *śākta.* (i.e. obtained through *śakti*)."

What is that *uccāra-rahitaṁ vastu,* the Reality which is not within the range of utterance ? It is *parāvāk* also known as *parāśakti, parāhantā, vimarśa-śakti, pūrṇāhaṁ-vimarśātmikā-saṁvit-śakti, mātṛkā* etc. It is the I-consciousness of the Divine which is above all thought and speech, which is the primal creative pulsation that brings the universe into being, the origin of all words and objects and yet above words. In the order of manifestation the next stage after parāvāk is that of *paśyantī.* At this stage, word and object are an undivided, indistinguishable whole. The next stage is that of *madhyamā.* Though the division between word and object has started, at this stage it is not pronounced yet. It is implicit. The division is only at the level of thought. This is an intermediate stage between *paśyantī* and *vaikharī.* There is a sort of subtle speech only at this level. It has not taken shape into words yet. At the *Vaikharī* stage, there is gross speech, The word and the object are completely divided. The word *vikhara* means body. So *vaikhari* is the stage when the bodily organs are employed in utterance. Thus there are three stages in the manifestation of the universe *para, sūkṣma* and *sthūla,* higher, subtle, and gross.

The *parāvāk* or the I-consciousness of the Supreme is the *raison d'etre* of all the *mantras.* As Tantrasadbhāva puts it :

"मंत्राणां जीवभूता तु या स्मृता शक्तिरूपया ।
तथा हीना वरारोहे निष्फलाः शरदभ्रवत्" ॥

"She who is considered to be imperishable *śakti* is the soul of all the *mantras.* Without her, O fair one, all the *mantras* are as useless as autumnal clouds." This imperishable *Śakti* is the *śakti* of the supreme I-consciousness.

This idea is further re-inforced by the third *sūtra* of this section. विद्याशरीरसत्ता मंत्ररहस्यम्—which means "the luminous being of the perfect I-consciousness inherent in the multitude of words whose essence consists in the knowledge of the highest non-dualism is the secret of the *mantras*".

Mantras consist of letters. These letters are not meaningless jargon. They are symbols of the creative *śaktis* of the Divine. These *śaktis* inherent in the letters are collectively known as *Mātṛkā*. This *Mātṛkā* is the secret of all the *mantras*. As has been said in Tantrasadbhāva :

"सर्वे वर्णात्मका मंत्रास्ते च शक्त्यात्मकाः प्रिये ।
शक्तिस्तु मातृका ज्ञेया सा च ज्ञेया शिवात्मिका" ॥

"O dear one, *mantras* consist of letters. These are a form of *śakti*. *Śakti* as such should be known as Mātṛkā and Mātṛkā should be known as the nature of Śiva". The same book says further on :

"या सा तु मातृका देवि परतेजः-समन्विता ।
तया व्याप्तमिदं विश्वं सब्रह्मभुवनान्तकम्" ॥

"O goddess, the universe right from Brahmā down to earth is pervaded by *Mātṛka* who is full of the lustre of *parāhantā* — the I-consciousness of the Supreme". This *parāhantā* or I-consciousness is the creative power of *Parama Śiva*. Parāhantā is also known as *parāśakti* or *parāvāk* or *parā* or *mahāmātṛkā* or simply *matṛkā*. In order to acquire *mantra-śakti*, one has to approach a *guru* or spiritual director who imparts a *mantra* with his grace and instils *caitanya śakti* or power of consciousness into it, and teaches him the mystery of *Mātṛkā*. As has already been said *Mātṛkā* means the collective whole of all letters and also the I-consciousness which is the *fons et origo* of all letters and thus of the entire universe of subjects and objects. The word for 'I' in Sanskrit is 'अहं' (aham). 'A' (अ) and 'ha' (ह) between themselves include all the letters of the Sanskrit language. As each one of these letters is symbolic of the creation of either an objective or subjective element, this means that *aham* or consciousness of Parama Śiva is creative of the entire universe of subjects and objects. *Sūtra* seven of this section says that the disciple gets enlightenment from the *guru* regarding *Mātṛkā*. The translation of this *sūtra* together with the detailed note on it should be carefully read in order to understand the creativity of *Mātṛkā*.

The I-consciousness of the Supreme holds within itself the entire universe in an ideal state. As *Kṣemarāja* puts it in Pratyabhijñāhṛdayam :

"अत एव अनुत्तराकुलस्वरूपात् अकारात् आरभ्य शक्तिस्फाररूपहकलापर्यन्तं यत् विश्वं प्रसृतं...तत् अकारहकाराभ्यामेव संपुटीकारयुक्त्या प्रत्याहारन्यायेन अन्तःस्वीकृतं सत् अविभागवेदनात्मकबिन्दुरूपतया स्फुरितम् अनुत्तर एव विश्राम्यति—इति शब्दराशिस्वरूप एव अयम् अकृतको विमर्शः" । (pp. 108-190)

"Therefore the extended universe beginning with the letter 'a' (अ) which is of the nature of the body of *anuttara* or the highest Reality and upto the letter 'ha' (ह) indicative of the expansion of Śakti, flashing forth by virtue of the combination of 'a' and 'ha' and being accepted inwardly in the manner of *pratyāhāra* rests in the Highest Reality in the form of *bindu* indicative of the consciousness of non-differentiation. Thus this natural *vimarśa* or I-consciousness is of the nature of the congregation of words."

'A' (अ) represents *prakāśa* or *Śiva*; 'ha' (ह) represents *vimarśa* or *Śakti*; the *bindu* or dot on 'ha' represents the fact that though Śiva is manifested right up to the earth through Śakti, he is not divided thereby; he remains integrally the same.

Mātṛkā when unknown or unrealized leads to all kinds of worldly experience. When she is realized, she leads to liberation. When the aspirant through *śuddha vikalpa* reflects over a *mantra* and feels his identity with *Śiva*, the *Mātṛkā* which is the *mantra-śakti* inherent in the *mantra* transforms the *citta* or mind of the aspirant; his *śuddha vikalpa* which was only an ideation is dissolved; his *citta* is transformed into *citi* (divine consciousness); he now feels the throb of the true I-consciousness of the Supreme, and he realizes that the entire universe is only a proliferation of *Mātṛkā śakti* or the divine I-consciousness. This aspect of I-consciousness which reveals the universe as only an expression of the Self is brought about finally by *unmanā* or *unmanī śakti* which is the highest development of the *mantra śakti* inherent in Mātṛkā. *Unmanā* is also known as *parā vidyā*, the highest gnosis. Kṣemarāja refers to it in *sūtra* 21 of the first section where it has been called *śuddha vidyā* and sūtra 5 of the second section where it has been called *khecarī Śivāvasthā*.

2. *Sat-tarka* helps the aspirant in his onward march. The aspirant learns from a great *guru* or from the *āgama* (the traditional text-book of the system) that his essential Self is *Śiva*

and not the physico-bio. psychical complex. Abhinvagupta says : आगमस्य समुचितविकल्पोदये व्यापारः (Tantrasāra p. 3) "The function of the āgama is to awaken in the mind *śuddha vikalpa* i.e. pure and correct thought about Self." Regarding *sat-tarka,* he says, तथाविधविकल्पप्रबन्ध एव सत्तर्क इति उक्तः (ibid, p. 23) "Sat-tarka is the reflection that re-inforces continuity of ideas similar to the *śuddha vikalpa.* This leads to *bhāvanā. Bhāvanā* is a word well-nigh untranslatable in English. 'Creative contemplation' is the best word for *bhāvanā.*" It is a power of spiritual attention. Abhinavagupta defines *bhāvanā* in the following words, "अस्फुटत्वात् भूतमिव अर्थम् अभूतमिव स्फुटत्वापादनेन भाव्यते यया" । (ibid, p.23) "Bhāvanā is that contemplation by which a thing which though real and existent appeared as non-existent and unreal previously owing to obscurity reappears as manifest reality by sheer clarity". Constructive imagination plays an important role in *bhāvanā.* It is a sort of auto-suggestion which sinks into the unconscious and fishes out surprizing reality from its mysterious depth. It leads to (3) *Śuddha vidyā* which slowly and gradually makes manifest the light of I-consciousness. Through the influence of *śuddha vidyā, jñeya,* the knowable appears as a form of *jñāna* or knowledge. Then the *jñāna* terminates in the *jñātā,* the knower. Finally this is displaced by the transcendental I-consciousness in which the distinction between the *jñātā, jñāna* and *jñeya* totally disappears.

There is another *śāktopāya* by *spanda* principle. By means of this, *vikalpas* or thoughts can be liquidated if one can develop the art of grasping mentally the *spanda* or dynamic reality which reveals itself in the interval of two thoughts. This revelation is known as *unmeṣa.*

The total life of the aspirant who has received full enlightenment about *mātṛkā-cakra* is changed. He is oriented Godward. His whole life becomes *yoga.* His formal rituals are changed into spiritual practices. *Sūtra* 8 of this section says that instead of pouring oblation of clarified butter, barley etc. into fire, he pours his thought of the gross and subtle bodies as the self into the fires of *cit.* (universal consciousness) by means of *bhāvanā.*

Sūtra 9 says that instead of rice, wheat etc. being his food, his thought of the essential Self becomes the food that nourishes and satisfies him.

Abhinavagupta adds a few more examples of this kind. "All objects actually abide in God" — with this purifying thought such an aspirant offers everything unto God by *bhāvanā*. This is his *yāga* or sacrifice. "The perfect, infinite God is my real Self" — constant repetition of this idea is his *japa*. Viewing objects like the body, jar etc. as simply an aspect of God is his *vrata* (vowed observance). The quest of the Divine that is not an object of thought is his *yoga*.

The main *Śākta-upāya*, however, consists in *mantra śakti* which is inherent in Mātṛkā and arises out of the contemplation of the Divine I-consciousness. A door gently swings open; a force arises from within which embraces our so-called 'I' to death. The limited 'I' dies to live in the universal 'I'.

SECTION III

Āṇavopāya

The third section of the *Śiva-sūtras* deals with *āṇavopāya*. The word *upāya* connotes 'means of approach'. In *Śāmbhavopāya*, the means of approach to the Divine is, if it can be called means at all, alert passivity or choiceless awareness. In this, there is no object or support on which the *citta* is to be steadied or fixed. Rather, the *citta* has to withdraw, to cease playing an active role. Therefore, this is also known as *nirālamba yoga* (supportless *yoga*).

In *Śāktopāya*, *citta* is the means of approach to the Divine. Here again the *citta* is not fixed or steadied on any object; there is no concentration or meditation on any thing. In this, the *citta* is used for seeking the source of its being, for seriously thinking out what exactly is meant by 'I' or Self. It is used to understand the deeper significance of *mantra* and the supreme I-consciousness which is the source of all *mantras*. By constantly dwelling on the significance of the real 'I', the *citta* gets sanctified and is ultimately transformed by the Śakti of the *mantra* and the aspirant has thus *prātibha jñāna* or intuitive realization of the real divine Self. The *Citta* is lifted up by *bhāvanā* and *śuddha vidyā*, and as pointed out above, is ultimately transformed. It should be borne in mind that Śāktopāya is also not possible for every individual. It is meant for those whose *citta* is already oriented spiritually. As Kṣemarāja says in his commentary on the first *sūtra* of the second section *cetyate vimṛśyate anena paraṁ tattvam iti cittam* — *Citta* (in this context) is that which earnestly seeks to apprehend the highest Reality. *Sākta-yoga* is a process of self-inquiry. Of modern yogis, Ramaṇa Maharṣi may be said to have set the best example of *Śākta yoga*. The *ālambana* or support of the *citta* in Śākta yoga is the essential Self.

In *āṇavopāya*, the case is different. Here *aṇu*, the limited, conditioned individual takes up same limited aspect as *buddhi*, *prāṇa*, *body*, some object in space from which he starts his yogic practice.

In *Śāmbhavopāya*, the first *sūtra* is *caitanyam ātmā*. It is the universal consciousness characterized by absolute freedom, *jñāna* (knowledge) and *kriyā* (activity) which is the Self. In *Śāktopāya*, the first sūtra is *cittam mantraḥ*. It is the spiritually oriented *citta* which by *mantra śakti* realizes the essential divine Self. In *āṇavopāya*, the first *sūtra* is *cittam ātmā*. In this, it is the *citta* (the complex of *buddhi*, *ahaṁkāra* and *manas*) that moves about from one form of existence to another which is the *ātmā* (atati-*sañcarati iti ātmā* — that which moves about is *ātmā*). Here the word *ātmā* is used in the sense of the psychological complex that is mostly considered to be the Self. This psychological or empirical self is known as *aṇu*. It is because this yoga starts from the standpoint of *aṇu* or the limited psychological, empirical self that it is called *āṇava yoga*. In this, the *citta* has to fix itself on something different from the essential Self. Therefore, it is called *bhedopāya* i.e. a technique of approach by means of something different from the essential Self. In *Śāktopāya*, it is *jñāna* which is most predominant. In *āṇavopāya*, it is *kriyā* (activity) which is most predominant. Even meditation which this technique uses is also *kriyā* (*mānasī kriyā*). It also uses *kriyā* (activity) in a grosser form, e.g. repetition of a *mantra*, worship of a chosen deity, an idol etc. Therefore, this is called *Kriyopāya*.

It should be carefully borne in mind that the three *upāyas* are not water-tight compartments. *Āṇavopāya* has to lead to *śāktopāya* and finally to *śāmbhavopāya*. The realization of *śāmbhavopāya* is the highest, and that is the goal of all the *upāyas*. One *upāya* passes into another. Even when something different from Self is worshipped as an aspect or expression of the divine, it finally terminates into *Śāktopāya*. The practice of *śāktopāya* in which I-consciousness is considered to be the *fons et origo* of everything terminates in *śāmbhavopāya* in which the I-consciousness is not simply an expression of Śiva but is also inclusive of the universe, which is simply an expansion of His *Śakti*. That is why the *Śiva-Sūtras* in describing each *upāya* or technique do not confine themselves solely to that *upāya* but also refer to other *upāyas* as aids.

Special Features of Āṇavopāya :

Mālinīvijaya thus describes *āṇavopāya* :

"उच्चारकरणध्यानवर्णस्थानप्रकल्पनैः ।
यो भवेत्तु समावेशः सम्यगाणव उच्यते ॥" (II, 21).

"A perfect absorption into the essential divine Self that is achieved through *uccāra*, *karaṇa*, *dhyāna*, *varṇa*, and *sthāna-kalpanā* is known as āṇava."

As said above, the support of the *citta* of the aspirant following *āṇavopāya* is something different from his essential divine Self. Either it is his (1) *buddhi* (2) gross *prāṇa* (3) subtle *prāṇa* known as *varṇa* (4) the body and the disposition of its organs in particular ways, known as *karaṇa* (5) some external object known as *sthāna-kalpanā*. Mālinīvijaya has summed these up in the above verse. We shall now take these up in detail.

1: *Dhyāna* :

Abhinavagupta says in his Tantrasāra (p. 36) that in this, the aspirant should meditate on the *pramātā* (knower or subject), *pramāṇa* (knowledge) and *prameya* (known or object) in a unified way (devoid of these distinctions). In consequence, the fire of the deeper, inner consciousness will be sharply lit up. Then grasping all external objects through the collective whole of the powers (*śaktis*) moving out through his sense-organs, he should, by *bhāvanā*, pour them into the fire of inner consciousness that has already been lit up. Then the difference between the inner and outer, between consciousness and its object will disappear and there will be unity-consciousness. Thus one will have *āṇava samāveśa* in the divine.

Another way of *dhyāna* (meditation) has been described in *Sūtra* 4 of the third section of Śiva-Sūtras. The *tattvas* from earth right up to *Śiva* should be considered by *bhāvanā* to be dissolved in the gross, then in the subtle, and finally in the causal body by the aspirant. This is known as *layabhāvanā.* Or one should think that Kālāgni Rudra is arising from the toe of the right foot and burning the whole body. This is known as *dāhabhāvanā*. This is really a kind of Śākta technique.

By these means, the *citta* (mind) of the aspirant acquires *samāveśa* or absorption into the divine consciousness. The exposition of the 4th *sūtra* should be read for details.

2. *Uccāra :*

Uccāra is connected with *prāṇa* which means life-energy or bioplasma. Its main characteristic is *uccāra* which means 'rising upward and appearing as sound'. The word *prāṇa* is used in two senses — general or subtle and specific. In general sense, it is simply known as *prāṇanā*. In the specific sense it acquires different names as *prāṇa, apāna, samāna, udāna, vyāna* according to the various functions of the *prāṇa śakti*. The characteristic of the specific *prāṇas* is *uccāra*. The subtle prāṇa is characterized as *varṇa* which will be considered separately.

The technique of *uccāra* is concerned with *prāṇa-dhāraṇā* or fixing the attention on the various aspects of *prāṇa* in the specific sense.

Various kinds of *ānanda* or delight are experienced by fixing the attention on the various *prāṇas*. When the mind rests only on the *pramātā* or the subject of experience, then the *ānanda* experienced is known as (1) *nijānanda*. When the mind contemplates over the absence of all objects of experience, then the delight experienced is known as (2) *nirānanda*. When there is contemplation on *prāṇa* and *apāna* jointly, then the delight experienced is known as (3) *parānanda*. When the mind rests on *samāna* which unifies the various objects of experience, then the delight experienced is known as (4) *brahmānanda*. When the mind of the aspirant rests on *udāna* after dissolving all knowledge and objects of knowledge in the Self, then the delight experienced is known as (5) *mahānanda*. When the mind rests on *vyāna*, then the *ānanda* experienced is known as (6) *cidānanda*.

After the experience of these six kinds of *ānanda*, when the aspirant realizes his *prāṇa-śakti* in its fulness, he has the experience of (7) *jagadānanda* in which there is no division or limitation, for it flashes forth all round, in which it is consciousness alone which expresses itself as knower, means of knowledge or known, which expands by the nectar of divine joy of absolute sovereignty, in which there is no need for contemplation.

This entire practice is briefly known as *uccāra yoga* or *prāṇa yoga*. When it is fully developed, the following characteristics appear as a consequence: (1) Experience of delight (2) *Udbhava*—a kind of inner leap (3) *Kampa* or tremour (4) *Nidrā* in which the aspirant is asleep to all outward objects (5) *Ghūrṇi* or reeling with delight.

It will be seen that this *prāṇa yoga* is entirely different from *prāṇāyāma* which is only an exercise of breath control.

3. *Varṇa* :

It has already been mentioned that the word *prāṇa* is used in two senses, viz., (1) general or subtle (2) specific. We have seen that *uccāra* is the natural characteristic of *prāṇa*. We have also seen how *āṇava yoga* is practised by fixing the mind on the various specific *prāṇas*. We have now to see what *āṇava yoga* is to be practised in connexion with the *uccāra* of the general *prāṇa*. Abhinavagupta says :

उक्तो य एष उच्चार-
स्तत्र यो ऽसौ स्फुरन् स्थितः ।
अव्यक्तानुकृतिप्रायो
ध्वनिर्वर्णः स कथ्यते ॥

(Tantrāloka V. 131)

"From the *uccāra* of this general *prāṇa*, there vibrates an imperceptible, inarticulate sound which is known as *varṇa*." This goes on *naturally* and *continuously* in every living creature.

Svacchanda Tantra says :

नास्योच्चारयिता कश्चित्प्रतिहन्ता न विद्यते ।
स्वयमुच्चरते देवः प्राणिनामुरसि स्थितः ॥

"No one sounds it voluntarily, nor can any one prevent its

being sounded. The deity abiding in the heart of living creatures sounds it himself." Abhinavagupta says about it :

"एको नादात्मको वर्णः सर्ववर्णविभागवान् ।
सोऽनस्तमितरूपत्वादनाहत होदितः ।।" (Tan. 61216)

"There is one *varṇa* in the form of *nāda* in which lie all the *varṇas* (letters) latently in an undivided form. As it is ceaseless, it is called *anāhata*, i.e. unstruck, natural, uncaused.

Jayaratha's commentary on this runs as follows :

"सर्ववर्णाविभागस्वभावत्वादव्यक्तप्रायो योऽसावनाहतरूपो नादः स वर्णोत्पत्तिनिमित्तत्वाद्वर्ण उच्यते वर्णशब्दाभिधेयो भवेदित्यर्थः"

"In this imperceptible, inarticulate *anāhata nāda*, all the *varṇas* (letters) lie latently in an undivided way. As all the *varṇas* (letters) originate from this *nāda*, therefore, is it called *varṇa* proleptically."

The *anusandhāna* or intensive awareness of this *nāda* is called *varṇa yoga* or *dhvani yoga*. It is a very ancient form of yoga. Śaṅkarācārya in his *yoga-tārāvalī* calls it *nādānusandhāna*. It goes by this name in some of the *tantras* and in the yoga tradition of Gorakhanātha. Among the mediaeval saints of north India, such as Kabir and others, it is called *surati-śabda yoga*. In Rādhāsvamī sect also, it is known as *surati-śabda yoga*.

How are we to know about this *nādātmaka varṇa* ? Abhinavagupta points out in the following verse how we can form an idea of it.

"सृष्टिसंहारबीजं च
तस्य मुख्यं वपुर्विदुः"
(Tantr. V, 132)

The *sṛṣṭi bīja* and the *saṁhāra bīja* are its main forms.

Jayaratha explains the main forms in the following words. 'प्रधानमभिव्यक्तिस्थानमित्यर्थः' The *sṛṣṭi bīja* and *saṁhāra bīja* are the main spots of its revelation.

What is meant by *sṛṣṭi bīja* and *saṁhāra bīja* ? *Sa* is *sṛṣṭi bīja* or the mystic letter denoting expiration and *ha* is *saṁhāra bīja* or the mystic letter denoting inspiration.

In the following verse, quoted by Kṣemarāja in his commentary on the 27th *sūtra* of the third section is given the process by which this *nāda* expresses itself in the breath of every living creature :

"सकारेण बहिर्याति हकारेण विशेत्पुनः ।
हंसहंसेत्यतो मंत्रं जीवो जपति नित्यशः ॥
षट्शतानि दिवारात्रौ सहस्राण्येकविंशतिः ।
जपो देव्या विनिर्दिष्टः सुलभो, दुर्लभो जडैः ॥

"The breath is exhaled with the sound *sa* and inhaled with the sound *ha*. Therefore the empirical individual always repeats the *mantra haṁsaḥ*. Throughout the day and night, he repeats this *mantra* 21,600 times, Such a *japa* (repetition of the *mantra*) of the goddess (Gāyatrī) has been prescribed which is quite easy for the wise, and difficult for the ignorant."

The *mantra haṁsaḥ* is repeated by every *jīva* (living being) automatically in every round of expiration-inspiration. Normally it is repeated 21,600 times a day. Since the outgoing and incoming breaths repeat this naturally, automatically without any effort on any body's part, it is known as *ajapā-japa* i.e. a repetition of the *mantra* that is going on naturally without any body's repeating it. Since the sounds of expiration and inspiration resemble *haṁ* and *saḥ*, therefore it is called *haṁsa mantra*. It is also known as *ajapā gāyatrī*. By *anusandhāna* or mental observation or awareness of this automatic process, *prāṇa* (exhalation) and *apāna* (inhalation) become equilibrated and then the dormant *kuṇḍalinī* that lies in three and a half folds at the base of the spine rises upwards. At that time, a number of pleasant sounds is heard. But the aspirant should not dwell on these sounds. He should neglect these and dwell on the *para nāda* which is *anāhata nāda* in the strictest sense of the word. By dwelling on this *nāda*, the *citta* gets dissolved and then one can have the experience of *viśuddha caitanya* — the highest aspect of consciousness.

The awakened *Kuṇḍalinī* pierces the *brahmagranthi*. Then she pierces the *mūlādhāra cakra*. Rising further, she pierces the *svādhiṣṭhāna* and *maṇipūra cakras*. Then she pierces the *viṣṇugranthi* and the *anāhata and viśuddha cakras*. Now she pierces the *rudragranthi* and then *ājñācakra* and finally enters the *sahasrāra*. The aspirant can now experience the ambrosia raining down from *sahasrāra*. (Vide plates 2 and 3).

The *nāḍīs* and *cakras* are not physical constituents. They are in the *prāṇamaya kośa*, the vital sheath in the subtle body.

KUṆḌALINĪ

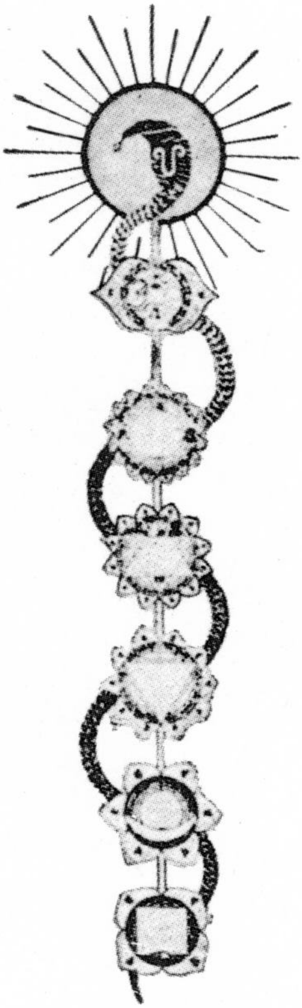

Plate 2

CAKRAS

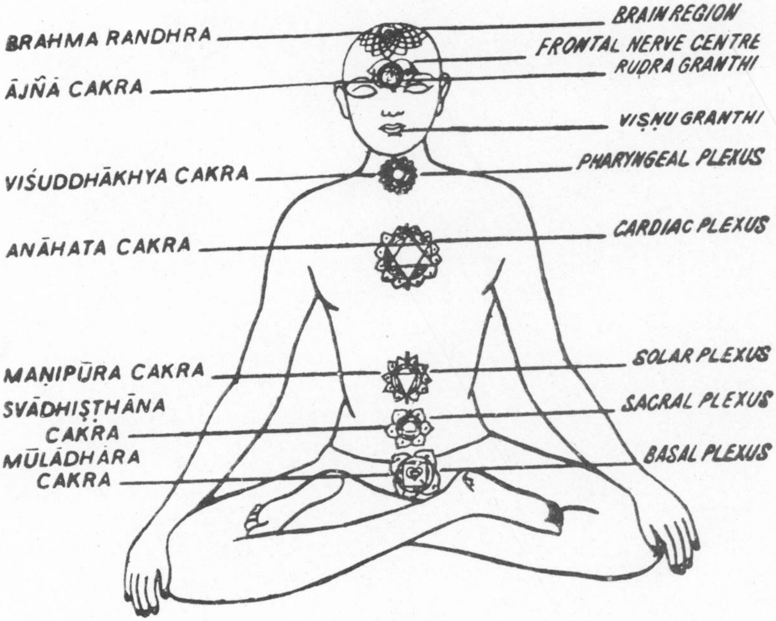
BRAHMA RANDHRA
ĀJÑĀ CAKRA
VIŚUDDHĀKHYA CAKRA
ANĀHATA CAKRA
MAṆIPŪRA CAKRA
SVĀDHIṢṬHĀNA CAKRA
MŪLĀDHĀRA CAKRA
BRAIN REGION
FRONTAL NERVE CENTRE
RUDRA GRANTHI
VIṢṆU GRANTHI
PHARYNGEAL PLEXUS
CARDIAC PLEXUS
SOLAR PLEXUS
SACRAL PLEXUS
BASAL PLEXUS

Plate 3

Only their impact is felt through the nerves and the ganglia. The *cakras* are the seats of vital energy. They are called *cakras* because they are like a wheel in appearance, They absorb and distribute *prāṇa* to the *prāṇamaya kośa* and through it to the physical body.

The *nāda* is subtle in *madhyamā* stage and finally when it reaches the *paśyanti* stage, it is no longer audible. The aspirant has now an experience of *jyoti* (light). All the *vikalpas* are now calmed and one can have the experience of *pūrṇāhantā* or the supreme I-consciousness.

Haṁsaḥ is that manifestation of *nāda* which is symbolic of life. The *anāhata nāda* in its inner significance is symbolic of *praṇava* (Om). By the intensive awareness of this *praṇava* there arise nine stages of *yoga* which are subtle forms of *nāda*, known as nine *nādas*. The first stage is (1) *bindu* which is known as *ardha mātrā*. The next stage is (2) *ardha candra* which is subtler than the previous. Each succeeding stage goes on getting subtler than the preceding (3) *rodhinī* (4) *nāda* (5) *nādānta* (6) *śakti* (7) *vyāpinī* (8) *samanā* and (9) *unmanā or unmanī* are the other stages that follow. *Unmanā* is the highest aspect of consciousness. Upto *samanā*, there can be only *ātma-vyāpti*, realization of the essential Self. It is only at the stage of *unmanā* that there can be *Śiva-vyāpti* which includes not only the realization of the metaphysical Self but also the realization of the world as an aspect of the Self.

In *sūtra* seven of the third section of the *Śiva-Sūtras* Kṣemarāja refers to *unmanā*. He says that upto *samanā*, there is the play of *māyā*. It is only at the stage of *unmanā* that *māyā* ceases completely. Another name of *unmanā* is *sahaja vidyā*.

Kṣemarāja makes the following remark :

"आत्मव्याप्त्यन्तस्य मोहस्य जयात् उन्मनाशिवव्याप्त्यात्मनः सहजविद्यायाः प्राप्तिरुक्ता"

Svacchanda Tantra speaks of the achievement of *Sahaja vidyā* which is *unmanā* enabling one to gain Śiva-consciousness after the conquest of *moha* (māyā) which lasts till the realization of the essential Self.

Kṣemarāja adds that though the process of reaching the *unmanā* stage is *śāktopāya*, yet it has been included in *āṇavopāya*, because the *āṇavopāya* has to lead to *śāktopāya.* Of this section the *sūtras* 15, 21, 26, 44 and 45 also refer to *śāktopāya.*

4. *Karaṇa* :

We have seen how *āṇavopāya* utilizes (1) *buddhi,* (2) gross *prāṇa* and (3) subtle *prāṇa* (*varṇa*). *Karaṇa* is the technique which utilizes the body (*deha*). By body is here meant all the bodies — gross, subtle and causal. In *Karaṇa, mudrās* (dispositions of certain parts of the body in particular ways) are also utilized.

There are seven varieties of *karaṇa* technique, viz. (1) *grāhya* (2) *grāhaka* (3) *cit* or *saṁvitti* (4) *niveśa* or *sanniveśa* (5) *vyāpti* (6) *tyāga* and (7) *ākṣepa.* (Tantr. V, 129). Jayaratha in his commentary gives the main purpose of these *karaṇas* in the following words :

"इह ग्राह्यादिभिः सप्तभिः प्रकारैर्भिन्नं करणं नाम बोधपूर्वकमभ्यासं प्राहुः बोध्यन्यग्भावेन स्वात्मैकताततामापन्नं बोधमेव कथितवन्तः"

"Here the seven varieties of *karaṇa,* viz. *grāhya* etc. are meant to subordinate and ultimately assimilate all objective phenomena to the consciousness of the essential Self".

The first four varieties come purely under *āṇavopāya.* Assimilating the entire world of objects first into the empirical self and then all these into *saṁvitti* or *cit,* the highest consciousness, and finally establishing them into the essential divine consciousness constitute the first four *karaṇas.* The first practice consists of assimilating *grāhya* or all objects of perception into *grāhaka* or the sense organs; the next practice consists of assimilating all these into *cit* or *saṁvitti*; the third practice consists of being completely established in *cit* or *saṁvitti.* Being completely established in *saṁvitti* is known as *sanniveśa.* In *sanniveśa,* there is no trace of the object as something extraneous.

When the aspirant pervades every object with universal consciousness, he is said to have achieved *vyāpti, Vyāpti* is achieved by means of *bhāvanā. Tyāga* is the stage where all effort is abandoned. The universal consciousness now abides spontaneously. *Vyāpti* and *tyāga* reach the stage of *śāktopāya. Ākṣepa* means projection of the universal consciousness in the entire universe. This is the stage of *śāmbhava yoga.*

The sūtras 16 and 25 also of this section refer to *śāmbhava yoga*.

Sthāna-kalpanā :

For those who cannot fix their *citta* even on *buddhi*, the inner *prāṇa* or *nāda*, there are other *āṇavopāyas* which deal with the fixing of the mind on externals. These are known as *sthāna-kalpanā*.

As Abhinavagupta puts it :

"अथ बाह्यविधिः स एव स्थानप्रकल्पनशब्देन उक्तः। तत्र त्रिधा स्थानं प्राणवायुः, शरीरं, बाह्यं च।

(Tantrasāra, p. 45)

The external process (of *āṇava upāya*) is known as *sthāna-prakalpanā*. There are three *sthānas* or places on which mind can be fixed, viz., *prāṇavāyu*, body, and something outside the body.

The *prāṇavāyu* in this context is used in a sense different from that in which it is used in connexion with *uccāra*. In *uccāra*, one has to fix the mind on *prāṇa*, *apāna*, *samāna*, *udāna* and *vyāna* which are internal aspects of *prāṇa śakti*.

In *sthāna kalpanā*, one has to fix the mind on *prāṇa* in the sense of exhalation and inhalation through the nose. From the centre of the body *prāṇa* (exhalation) covers a distance of twelve fingers in the outer space and again from that point *apāna* (inhalation) covers the same distance up to the centre. These two points or places are known as external *dvādaśānta* and internal *dvādaśānta*. By the practice of fixing the mind on these two points, the *vikalpas* of the mind begin to dissolve, and finally one has *āṇava samāveśa*, or absorption in the essential Self through the *āṇava* technique.

By body in this context is meant the gross body. The things external to the body include idol, picture etc. Those who are unable to fix the mind even on *prāṇa* may fix it on these external things.

As has been said above, the ultimate goal is the attainment of Śiva-consciousness which includes the world as its aspect.

Āṇava yoga has to lead to *śākta yoga* and *śākta yoga* has to lead finally to *śāmbhava yoga*.

———

A SUMMARY OF THE CONTENTS OF THE SŪTRAS

I SECTION :

ŚĀMBHAVOPĀYA

Sūtras

1. Characteristic of Ātman; *Ātmā* is foundational consciousness characterized by absolute freedom of knowledge and action.

2. The bondage of the empirical individual is due to an innate limiting condition, known as *āṇavamala* which, in fact, is the ignorance of our essential nature.

3. There are two other limiting conditions, viz., *Māyīya* and *kārma mala* which contribute to the bondage of the individual.

4. The three limiting conditions are a kind of limited, vitiated knowledge rooted in words which have a tremendous influence on our lives. These words are formed of letters known as *Mātṛkā*. The *Mātṛkā*, therefore, forms the basis of all limited knowledge.

5. *Śāmbhava-upāya* or emergence of the *Bhairava* or transcendental consciousness shatters the shackles of ignorance and sets the individual free.

6. When *Bhairava*-consciousness arises, the entire universe appears as an expression of Śiva's *Śakti* and when the mind of the aspirant is united with that *Śakti* with intensive awareness, the world as something separate from consciousness disappears. The sixth *sūtra* shows both the effect of *Śāmbhava* consciousness and a re-inforcement of that consciousness by *Śāktopāya*.

7. When through grace there is the emergence of *Bhairava*-consciousness and through *Śakti-Sandhāna*, it is re-inforced then the rapturous delight of the fourth or transcendental consciousness becomes a constant feature even of the three states of waking, dream and profound sleep. It is not only in meditation but also in the usual, normal course of

life that one experiences the delight of the transcendental consciousness.

8. Waking state consists of knowledge gained by the external senses and common to all subjects.
9. The dream state consists of experience generated only by the mind in the form of fancies and reveries which are confined only to the dreamer.
10. Deep sleep is a state of complete unawareness. It is a state of delusion brought about by Māyā. All the above three states may be considered both from the point of view of the common man and the *yogī*.
11. One who experiences the delight of Supreme I-consciousness in all the states of consciousness becomes the master of his senses.
12. Such a *yogī*, in his ascent to the Highest Reality passes through many stations of experience which are full of pleasant surprises.
13. The *Icchā* or Will of a *Yogī* who has realized *Bhairava*-consciousness is *Svātantrya-Śakti* (Absolute Will power of *Śiva*) that can manifest and withdraw the world.
14. To such a *Yogī*, all that is observed as an object—whether externally or internally, is an expression of consciousness.
15. Such experience is possible by the absorption of the individual mind into the Universal Consciousness which is the centre and foundation of all reality.
16. When one is mentally united with the pure *Śiva*-principle, he becomes, like *Sadāśiva*, completely free from the limitations of the empirical individual.
17. Full conviction of one's identity with *Śiva* is what is meant by knowledge of Self.
18. In every bit of knowledge, the *Yogī* feels the delight of I-consciousness. There is the transmission of this delight among those who come in contact with him.
19. Being united with *Icchā-Śakti* (the Divine Will power) the Yogī can create any kind of body that he desires.
20. By uniting his consciousness with *Śakti*, the *yogī* can acquire the power of joining together components in a whole or separating components or joining together events, etc. far removed in space and time.

21. Being united with *Icchā Śakti*, when the *Yogī* desires to acquire universal consciousness, he gets established in *Śuddha vidyā*, i.e. *unmanā śakti*, and feels as if he is the lord of the whole universe.
22. The Highest Śakti (*Parā Śakti*) is, on account of its depth, transparency etc, like a lake. When an aspirant is united with it, i.e., when he is constantly aware of his identity with it, he has an experience of the potency of the great *mantra*. Having an experience of it means the feeling of the throb of the supreme I-consciousness as his own inmost Self. This I-consciousness is the generative source of all the *mantras* i.e., all *mantras* derive their power from it.

II SECTION

ŚĀKTOPĀYA

Sūtras

1. When the mind broods constantly over the *mantra* of the Highest Reality i.e., over the Supreme-I consciousness, it gets identified with it. Thus the mind itself becomes the *mantra*. There is no longer any difference between the practiser of the *mantra* and the *mantra* itself. *Śāktopāya* is the technique of *jñāna*. By constant awareness of the *jñāna* of the real I-consciousness, the mind (*Cittam*) of the aspirant is transformed into that Supreme I-consciousness itself. Thus he has full realization.
2. It is zealous, spontaneous effort on the part of the aspirant that brings about the communion of his mind with the deity inherent in the *mantra*.
3. *Vidyāśarīra* is a compound word, meaning *śabda-rāśi*—a multitude of words or *mantra*. The *sattā* or luminous being of the multitude of words consists in supreme I-consciousness which is non-different from the world. So the secret of all *mantras* is the communion of the individual mind with the Supreme divine I-consciousness that includes within itself the universe. If the aspirant's mind is satisfied with *māyic* limited powers, he has fallen from the high ideal of *mantra*, for these *māyic* limited powers are only a form

of common inferior knowledge and are illusory like a dream. The ideal of *mantra* and therefore of *Śāktopāya* is not the acquisition of inferior power, but rather of the Supreme I-consciousness of *Śiva*—a consciousness which includes the universe within itself.

5. On the emergence of spontaneous Supreme knowledge, the aspirant acquires *Khecarī Mudrā* which is the state of *Śiva.*
6. *Guru* is a help in attaining the potency of *mudrā* and *mantra,* for he expounds the means to the goal. Or the divine grace acts as a *guru* in affording a favourable opportunity (in acquiring the potency of *mantra*).
7. All words (*vācaka*) and objects (*vācya*) are the outcome of words which consist of letters (*mātṛkā*). The collective whole of *Mātṛkā* (मातृकाचक्र) arises in the last analysis from the Supreme I-consciousness of Śiva. This is the secret of *Mātṛkā-cakra.* Knowing that this Supreme I-consciousness is our real Self, one is liberated.
8. All the bodies, gross, subtle etc. which were previously identified with faked I-consciousness are now thrown into the fire of real I-consciousness as oblation.
9. If *jñāna* is interpreted as limited knowledge, then the *sūtra* would mean 'limited knowledge is *annam* i.e. is devoured by the *Yogī.*'

   If *jñāna* is interpreted as *svarūpa-jñāna* or knowledge of Self, then *annam* would mean food that gives satisfaction, and the whole *sūtra* would mean "Self-realization becomes his food i.e. fills him with the highest satisfaction." Bhāskara also gives the above interpretation in his *vārttikas.*
10. On the submergence of *śuddha vidyā*, all kinds of *vikalpas* (thought-constructs) full of a sense of difference arise in the mind.

    According to Bhāskara, this *sūtra* means to say that when the knowledge common to the ordinary folk of the world dissolves on the realization of one's real Self, the previously apprehended delusive knowledge of the objects of the world is remembered only like a dream.

III SECTION

ĀṆAVOPĀYA

Sūtras

1. That which is deeply affected with desire for objects of sense is *citta*. The constituents of *citta* are *buddhi*, *ahaṁkāra* and *manas*. In the context of the individuals, it is this *citta* or the conditioned mind that is knower or *ātmā*. The *citta* is called *ātmā*, because by means of *sattva*, *rajas* and *tamas*, it moves on from one form of existence to another. (*Atati iti ātmā*, that which moves on is *ātmā*).
2. The knowledge of this *aṇu* or limited individual self is confined to the modes of his psychic apparatus, and his desires are associated with the pleasure of sense objects. Under their influence, he wanders about from one form of existence to another.
3. Man's bondage is due mainly to *māyā*. *Māyā*, in this context, means non-discrimination between the real Self and the pseudo-self constituted by the *kañcukas* like *kalā* (limited efficiency), *Vidyā* (limited knowledge), *rāga* (egoistic desires) etc. and subtle and gross body.
4. One should meditate on the dissolution of all the *tattvas* successively in their preceding source right up to *Śiva*, i.e. of the gross body into the subtle, and of the subtle into the causal and thus realize the highest *tattva*, viz., *Śiva*.
5. By means of *prāṇāyāma*, *pratyāhāra*, *dhāraṇā* etc. one can acquire the power of dissolving *prāṇa* and *apāna* in *suṣumnā*, control over the elements like earth, water etc. withdrawal of the mind from the elements, and isolation from the elements.
6. By *prāṇāyāma*, *dhāraṇā* etc. one acquires Supernormal powers over the elements, but such powers are the outcome of *moha* (delusion about the essential nature of the self) which draws a veil over the Highest Reality. By these means, one cannot realize the Highest Reality.
7. When there is complete conquest of *māyā*, there is acquisition of *Sahaja Vidyā* which makes for complete identification with *Śiva*.

8. In one who is at-onement with *unmanā*, the world appears only as a ray of his light. Dualism has completely disappeared in his case.
9. The essential Self is like an actor on the world-stage. He is unaffected by the parts he plays.
10. The inner self, i.e. the subtle body, constitutes the stage of the actor of the world-drama.
11. The senses of the *yogī* are introverted and thus behold the drama of the inmost Self who delights in exhibiting the world drama.
12. Just as an actor can act out the *sattva*—the inner mental state only through great talent, even so the *yogī* can give expression to *sattva* (inner Light) only through the higher spiritual intelligence.
13. Such a *yogī* attains full freedom to know and control the whole universe.
14. As the Yogi can manifest Freedom in his own body, so can he manifest it elsewhere also.
15. The *Yogī* should constantly direct his attention to *parā śakti* (the primal power of the Divine) which is the source of the universe.
16. If the *Yogī* is firmly established in *parāśakti*, he will be easily steeped in the highest bliss of Self without any practice of concentration, meditation, etc.
17. Being established in *Śuddha vidyā*, the *Yogī* can create forms in accordance with the measure of the creative power of his consciousness.
18. So long as *Śuddha vidyā* is emergent, there is no further birth of the *yogī*.
19. The *yogī* who has attained *Sahaja Vidyā* (*Śuddha Vidyā*) should not become heedless. If he is not on the alert, he may be deluded by the deities presiding over letters like other ordinary folk.
20. The *Yogī* should take care that the fourth state permeates the three states of waking, dream and deep sleep and not only at their initial and even final stage even as oil permeates its receptacle completely.
21. Rejecting the notion of body, etc. as the Self, one should plunge into the fourth state without any thought-construct.

22. When the *prāṇa* of the *yogī* who is united with the fourth, i.e. the transcendental consciousness, spreads outside, i.e. when he is actively aware of external objects, he (the *yogī*) experiences everything as identical with *cidānanda*, with the bliss of Śiva-consciousness.
23. In the case of the *Yogī* experiencing the delight of the fourth state at the initial and final stages of waking, etc. inferior states of mind may arise in the intervening stage. He should, therefore, be on guard and see to it that the intervening stages are also permeated by the transcendental consciousness.
24. When the *Yogī* joins his real I-consciousness to everything, i.e. when everything appears to him as the expression of Śiva, then the transcendental consciousness which had been obscured is revived.
25. When by the continuous practice of the *turya* state (the fourth state) the *Yogī* attains the *turyātīta* state, he becomes similar to *Śiva*.
26. Remaining in the body till the *prārabdha karma* is exhausted is all the pious act (*vrata*) that such a *yogī* observes.
27. Since the I-consciousness of the *Yogī* is the awareness of the pure, spiritual I, every speech of the *yogī* amounts to a *japa* of the divine I.
28. He disseminates knowledge of Self all round. This is his *dānam* or gift.
29. Such a *Yogī* acquiring mastery over the *śakti-cakra* that controls the limited empirical individuals is alone competent to enlighten others regarding Reality.
30. Because this *Yogī* is similar to *Śiva*, so the universe is the unfoldment of his consciousness-power just as it is the expression of the *Śakti* of *Śiva*.
31. The maintenance and reabsorption of the universe are also an unfoldment of his consciousness-power.
32. Even when there is change in the objective appearance, there is no change in the subject of experiences, for even the experience of change requires an experient.
33. Such a *yogī* considers pleasure and pain as something external like blue jar, etc., not as an aspect of his I-consciousness. So he is not affected by them.

34. The *Yogī* that is untouched by any trace of pleasure and pain is known as *Kevalī* i.e. one who is a knower only as pure consciousness.
35. When, however, an aspirant is under the influence of primal ignorance and does not know his real Self, he is subject to *karma* and is thus bound to *saṁsāra*.
36. When the *Yogī* discards all difference due to the identification of Self with body, *prāṇa* etc. and there emerges in him the realization of Self as pure consciousness, he can create another form of world according to his desire.
37. The Yogī's power of creativity can be inferred from one's own experience of imaginative creation in dream, etc.
38. In all the three states of waking, dreaming, and deep sleep, one should enliven oneself with the creative bliss of the transcendental consciousness which is the primal condition of all the three states.
39. Just as the internal mental states should be vitalized with the bliss of the fourth or transcendental consciousness, even so the external objects also should be vitalized with the bliss of the transcendental consciousness.
40. Those ordinary empirical individuals whose Self is not identified with the fourth or transcendental consciousness but is rather identified with the subtle and gross bodies, are, on account of *āṇavamala*, prompted by desire for various objects. They are extroverted and carried from one form of existence to another.
41. Of the *yogī*, however, who is established in the fourth or transcendental consciousness, all egoistic desires disappear and then ends his state of a limited empirical individual tied down to the subtle and gross bodies and he now becomes a *citpramātā*, a knower as pure consciousness.
42. With the disappearance of desire, his life of a limited, empirical individual identified with his subtle body comes to an end. He retains the gross body only as an outer covering with which he is not identified in the least. Being completely possessed of the divine I-consciousness he is now like *Śiva*.
43. Even after Self-realization, the *yogī* has to retain his gross body, because the body is linked with *prāṇa*, the universal Life Force which is generated from *Svātantrya Śakti*—the

Absolute Free Will of the Divine. So long as this natural link of *prāṇa* with the body lasts, the *Yogī* cannot dispense with the body.

44. *Nāsikā* or *prāṇa-śakti* flows in the right, (*piṅgalā*), left (*iḍā*) and middle (*suṣumnā*) *nāḍīs*. The internal aspect of *prāṇa śakti* is *saṁvid* (or consciousness), the *madhya* or the central aspect of this consciousness is the awareness of the divine, transcendental 'I'. By constant mindfulness of this I-consciousness, there is *nirvyutthāna samādhi* in all conditions.

45. The soul that had forgotten its essential nature now recognizes its divine nature again. The *Yogī* who has realized his essential, divine nature, shedding all sense of difference, inwardly feels the universe as dissolved in *Śiva* and outwardly experiences it only as an expression of I-consciousness which is identified with Śiva.

FIRST SECTION

The first verse

Prayer to Śaṁkara, the Supreme Awareness.

TEXT

रुद्रक्षेत्रज्ञवर्गः समुदयति यतो यत्र विश्रान्तिमृच्छेद्
यत्तत्त्वं यस्य विश्वं स्फुरितमयमियद्यन्मयं विश्वमेतत् ।
स्वाच्छन्द्यानन्दवृन्दोच्छलदमृतमयानुत्तरस्पन्दतत्त्वं
चैतन्यं शाङ्करं तज्जयति यदखिलं द्वैतभासाद्वयात्म ॥

TRANSLATION

That consciousness of *śaṁkara*[1] is (ever) victorious[2] which in its wholeness is non-dual in reality though having an appearance of duality, from which the class of *Rudra* and *kṣetrajña*[3] springs and in which it comes to rest, which is the fundamental Reality (*yat tattvam*), from which bursts forth into view the universe, whose form is this universe, from whose unimpeded Free Will ever leaps forth his divine power which is a mass of bliss, bringing about the unsurpassed, immortal spanda[4] principle (the primal creative pulsation).

NOTES

1. *Śāṁkaraṁ caitanyam* : *Śam* (the bliss of the revelation of the supreme non-dualism) *Karoti* (brings about) iti *Śaṁkaraḥ*, i.e., *Śaṁkara* is one who brings about the bliss of the revelation of the supreme non-dualism.

Caitanya is the *svātantrya-svabhāva* (unimpeded Free Will and knowledge and action). *Śāṁkara* = of *Śaṁkara*. *Śāṁkaraṁ Caitanyam*, therefore, means *Śaṁkara's* autonomous, unimpeded Free Will in Knowledge and action (jñāna and kriyā).

2. *Tajjayati*: Lit., that is (ever) victorious. The idea is 'that surpasses every thing', that, in spite of its varied manifestation as subject, object etc. ever abides in its autonomy and bliss.

3. *Kṣetrajña* : is the soul in bondage, known as *paśu*, full of

āṇava mala (inherent limitation) from Brahmā down to the tiniest creature.

Rudras are the free souls whose *āṇava mala* has completely vanished. They are in the category of *pati.* They bring about *Sṛṣṭi* (emergence) *Sthiti* (maintenance) and *Saṁhāra* (withdrawal) of the world system according to the *karmas* of individuals. Śiva is directly concerned only with *vilaya* (veiling of the essential nature of the soul) and *anugraha* (grace or unveiling of the essential nature). Ananta Bhaṭṭāraka, Aghoreśa and Rudra are synonyms. Rudra corresponds to Īśvara of Śāṁkara Vedānta.

4. *Anuttara Spanda tattva* : The *svātantrya* or *svācchandya* (unimpeded Free Will) of Parama Śiva appears in its primal cosmic creative pulsation (spanda) as Śiva. Śiva is the highest (*anuttara*) *Spanda* (cosmic creative pulsation) of Parama Śiva. This comes into being on account of *ānanda* (supernal creative joy) that wells up (ucchalat) from Parama Śiva or the Absolute.

The word 'spanda' which literally means 'throb' or 'vibration' is difficult to translate, since it has a technical meaning in this system. It is the cosmic creative pulsation of the Absolute, throbbing with life, quickening to manifest.

EXPOSITION

This verse is a prayer to the foundational Divine Consciousness. It also indicates the subject-matter of the *sūtras* which is the non-dual Reality, from which arises every thing, and to which every thing is withdrawn. This is also a *maṅgala-śloka* or an auspicious verse written with the idea that the book may end successfully, without any difficulty or impediment.

This also brings out the main powers of *Śiva*. *Rudra-Kṣetrajña-vargaḥ samudayati yato* indicates *kriyā* (activity) and *icchā* (will), Śiva's innate nature of creativity. *yat tattvam* hints at His power of *jñāna* (knowledge), *yasya viśvaṁ sphuritamayam-iyat* indicates his *ānanda* (bliss); *caitanyam* indicates His power of *Cit* (consciousness). The five fundamental characteristics, viz., *cit*, *ānanda*, *icchā*, *jñāna*, and *kriyā* of the Highest Reality are hinted at in this verse.

The Reason for Writing his Commentary

TEXT

आसमञ्जस्यमालोच्य वृत्तीनामिह तत्त्वतः ।
शिवसूत्रं व्याकरोमि गुर्वाम्नायविगानतः ॥

TRANSLATION

Having noticed confusion in the *Śiva-sūtra-vrttis* owing to inconsistency with the sacred tradition (*āmnāya*) of the teachers, I am expounding the *śiva-sūtras* according to their real meaning.

EXPOSITION

Kṣemarāja says that he noticed confusion in the *Śiva-sūtra vṛttis*. That is why he is writing his *vimarśinī* commentary. Vimarśinī means a commentary based on sound investigation and critical examination. It is not clear which *Śiva sūtra vṛttis* Kṣemarāja is referring to.

In his introductory verse, Kṣemarāja says that the interpretation of the *sūtras* given by the prevalent *vṛttis* is, at places, inconsistent inasmuch as it is opposed to the traditional teaching of the great teachers of the system (*gurvāmnāya-vigānataḥ*); hence he is writing a commentary on the *sūtras* in order to dispel the wrong notion caused by the *vṛttis* written on the *Śiva-sūtras*.

Kṣemarāja belonged to the tradition of Abhinavagupta who was his teacher.

There is a *double entendre* in the word *vigānataḥ*. The prefix vi in the word may mean *virodhena* (*virodhena gānataḥ*) i.e., as opposed to the original meaning of the *sūtras* or it may mean *viśeṣeṇa* (*viśeṣeṇa gānataḥ*) i.e., with a definite, clear understanding of the *sūtras*. In the former case, the prose order will be *vṛttīnāṁ gurvāmnāya-vigānataḥ āsmañjasyam ālokya* i.e.; noticing inconsistency in the interpretation of the *sūtras* as given by the *vṛttis* inasmuch as it is opposed to the sacred tradition of the ancient teachers; in the latter case, the prose order will be, *śiva-sūtraṁ gurvāmnāya-vigānataḥ vyākaromi* i.e., I am expounding the *Śiva-sūtras* in accordance with the particular interpretation given by my *guru*, an interpretation which is wholly consistent with the ancient sacred tradition.

COMMENTARY

TEXT

इह कश्चित् शक्तिपातवशोन्मिषन्माहेश्वरभक्त्यतिशयात् अनङ्गीकृताधर-दर्शनस्थ-नाग-बोध्यादि-सिद्धादेशनः शिवाराधनपरः पारमेश्वर-नानायोगिनी-सिद्धसत्संप्रदाय-पवित्रितहृदयः श्रीमहादेवगिरौ महामाहेश्वरः श्रीमान् वसु-गुप्तनामा गुरुरभवत् ।

TRANSLATION

In this world, there was on the mountain, *Mahādeva* one *Guru* (a Self-realized teacher) by the name *Vasugupta* who was a great personage[1] and a devotee of *Maheśvara* (great Lord, the Supreme Divine), who, owing to excess of devotion to *Maheśvara*, which (devotion) blossomed forth by divine grace (*Śakti-pātonmiṣat*), did not accept the teaching of *Nāgabodhi*[2] and other Siddhas[3] obtaining in the inferior philosophical systems, who was given to the devotion to *Śiva*, and whose heart had become pure by the correct and noble traditional teaching (*sat-sampradāya-pavitrita-hṛdayaḥ*) of the various *Yoginīs*[4] and *siddhas*[5] pertaining to the supreme Lord.

NOTES

1. A great personage—Vasugupta has been called *mahān* or a great personage, because he had realized his identity with the Lord.

2. Nāgabodhi : He was a Buddhist teacher. He has written "Śrī Guhyasamāja-maṇḍalopāyikāviṁśavidhi" which is based on 'Guhya-samāja'—a Buddhist Tantra. According to Alex Wayman, 'Guhyasamāja' was written in about the 4th century A.D. Nāgabodhi may have utilized this book in about 500-700 A.D.

3. Other Siddhas : refers to other accomplished Buddhist Yogīs.

4. *Yoginīs* : Self-realized female Yogīs—representations of Śakti.

5. *Siddhas* here refers to the perfect male yogīs who had realized the non-dualistic Truth as taught by the *Śaiva Āgamas*.

Discovery of the Śiva-Sūtras

TEXT

कदाचिच्च असौ 'द्वैतदर्शनाधिवासितप्राये जीवलोके रहस्यसंप्रदायो मा विच्छेदि' इत्याशयतः अनुजिघृक्षापरेण परमशिवेन स्वप्ने अनुगृह्य उन्मिषित-प्रतिभः कृतः यथा "अत्र महीभृति महति शिलातले रहस्यम् अस्ति तत् अधिगम्य अनुग्रहयोग्येषु प्रकाशय" इति । प्रबुद्धश्च असौ अन्विष्यन् तां महतीं शिलां करस्पर्शनमात्रपरिवर्तनतः संवादीकृतस्वप्नां प्रत्यक्षीकृत्य, इमानि शिवोपनिषत्संग्रहरूपाणि शिवसूत्राणि ततः समाससाद । एतानि च सम्यक् अधिगम्य भट्टश्रीकल्लटाद्येषु सच्छिष्येषु प्रकाशितवान् स्पन्दकारिकाभिश्च संगृहीतवान् । तत्पारम्पर्य-प्राप्तानि स्पन्दसूत्राणि अस्माभिः स्पन्दनिर्णये सम्यक् निर्णीतानि । शिवसूत्राणि तु निर्णीयन्ते ॥

तत्र प्रथमं नरेश्वरभेदवादि-प्रातिपक्ष्येण चैतन्यपरमार्थतः शिव एव विश्वस्य आत्मा इति आदिशति—

TRANSLATION

Once upon a time his (Vasugupta's) genius was graciously unfolded in dream by the great *Śiva* disposed to impart grace, who with the intention that the esoteric traditional teaching may not be lost in the world of the living which was mostly influenced with dualistic philosophical view, imparted the following message. "On the yonder mountain, there is the esoteric doctrine under a big stone-piece. Having obtained it, reveal it to those who are fit for grace."

Having awakened, while searching about, he saw that big stone-piece, which turning round by a mere touch of the hand, confirmed his dream. He thus obtained the *Śiva-sūtras* which are a compendium of the secret doctrine of Śiva.

Having fully understood these, he revealed them to his excellent pupils like venerable *Śrī Kallaṭa* and others, collected and expounded them in the *Spandakārikās*.

The exact meaning of those *Spandasūtras* received by way of tradition has been fully explained by me in *Spandanirṇaya*.

The Śiva-sūtras are now being expounded in their exact significance.

In this book, it (the *sūtra*) at first teaches, in opposition to those who hold that there is a difference between *man* (*nara* i.e., the human self)[1] and *Īśvara* (the Supreme Lord), that Consciousness of *Śiva* alone is, in the highest sense, the Self of the entire manifestation.

NOTES

1. Nareśvara-bheda-vādi. This may also refer to a book 'Nareśvara-parīkṣā' by Sadyojyoti, which teaches *bheda* (difference) between *nara* or the human self and Īśvara.

Sūtra[1] — 1

चैतन्यमात्मा[2] ॥१॥

Caitanyamātmā

चैतन्यम —:Awareness which has absolute freedom of knowledge and activity. आ मा—Self or nature of Reality. Awareness which has absolute freedom of all knowledge and activity is the Self or nature of Reality.

COMMENTARY

TEXT

इह अचेतितस्य कस्यापि सत्त्वाभावात्, चितिक्रिया सर्वसामान्यरूपा इति, चेतयते इति चेतनः सर्वज्ञानक्रियास्वतन्त्रः, तस्य भावः चैतन्यं सर्वज्ञानक्रियासंबन्धमयं परिपूर्णं स्वातन्त्र्यम् उच्यते । तच्च परमशिवस्यैव भगवतः अस्ति; अनाश्रितान्तानां तत्परतन्त्रवृत्तित्वात् । स च यद्यपि नित्यत्व-व्यापकत्वामूर्तत्वाद्यनन्तधर्मात्मा, तथापि नित्यत्वादीनाम् अन्यत्रापि संभाव्यत्वात्, अन्यासंभविनः स्वातन्त्र्यस्यैव उद्धुरीकारप्रदर्शनमिदम् । इत्थं धर्मान्तरप्रतिक्षेपतश्च, चैतन्यमिति भावप्रत्ययेन दर्शितम् । तदेतत् आत्मा, न पुनरन्यः कोऽपि भेदवाद्यभ्युपगतो भिन्नभिन्नस्वभावः । तस्य अचैतन्ये जडतया अनात्मत्वात् । चिदात्मत्वे भेदानुपपत्तेः; चितो देशकालाकारैः चिद्व्यतिरेकात् अचेत्यमानत्वेन असद्भिः चेत्यमानत्वेन तु चिदात्मभिः, भेदस्य आधातुम् अशक्यत्वात्; चिन्मात्रत्वे तु आत्मनां स्वभावभेदस्य अघटनात्; वक्ष्यमाण-नीत्या अव्यतिरिक्तमलसंबन्धयोगेनापि भेदस्य अनुपपत्तेः; प्राक् मलस्य सत्त्वेऽपि मुक्तिदशायां तदुपशमनात् नानात्मवादस्य वक्तुम् अशक्यत्वात्, मलसंस्कार-संभवे वा, अनादिशिवात् कथंचित् अपकर्षे वा, मुक्तशिवाः संसारिण एव स्युरिति । यथोक्तम् 'चैतन्यमेक एवात्मा' इति नानात्मवादस्य अनुपपत्तिः सूचिता ।

TRANSLATION

In this world, nothing exists which is outside the range of

consciousness (*acetitasya*[3]). The activity of consciousness is universal throughout. A conscious being (*cetana*) is one who conscires (i.e. thinks), who is absolutely free in all knowledge and activity. *Caitanya* or consciousness is the state of one who is *cetana* or conscious. (The ṣyañ-suffix in) *caitanya* shows relationship. *Caitanya*[4], therefore, connotes absolute freedom in respect of all knowledge and activity (*paripūrṇaṁ svātantryam*).[5] The great Lord, Highest Śiva alone has that (absolute freedom). Others (i.e., from the *sakalas* or individual souls) up to *anāśrita-śiva*[6] depending as they do on Highest Śiva (tat *paratantravṛttitvāt*), do not have this absolute freedom.

Though Highest Śiva has infinite number of other attributes, such as eternity,[7] all-pervasiveness, formlessness etc., yet because eternity etc. are possible elsewhere also, here it is intended to show the predominance of absolute freedom which is not possible in any other being. Thus his (highest *Śiva's*) characteristic has been indicated in the form of an abstract noun, viz., *caitanya* (the state of being conscious) by excluding other attributes (inasmuch as an abstract noun excludes all other attributes). Therefore this (i.e., *caitanya* or consciousness which is Absolute Freedom) is Ātmā or Self, not anything else of varied nature as assumed by pluralists (those who propound the doctrine of *bheda* or difference among Selves) (Are these different Selves conscious beings or non-conscious beings ?) If Ātmā or varied nature is assumed to be non-conscious, then it would be inconscient matter and thus not Self. If it be considered to be of the very essence of consciousness, then there can be no valid reason for considering one *ātman* or Self as different from another Self. Difference in the case of *cit* or consciousness cannot be established either by means of space or time or form, for if these (space, time and form) are different from *cit* or consciousness, then being deprived of the light of consciousness, they cannot appear at all and thus are unreal; if they appear, then they are consciousness itself (for it is only consciousness that can appear). Thus it is not possible to attribute difference to consciousness (i.e., Self) on the basis of difference in space, time and form. As it is now clear that Selves are only consciousness (and nothing else), then difference[8] in the nature of the various selves cannot be established (since consciousness is the only nature of all

Selves, therefore they are the same); nor can difference be maintained on account of their contact with *mala*[9] or limiting condition, since the limiting condition is not something outside consciousness as will be explained in the sequel. Even though *mala*-or limiting condition may exist before (liberation), (it will be admitted on all hands that) it ceases to exist in the state of liberations. It is, therefore, impossible to maintain the theory of the plurality of Self. If it be maintained (that even in the state of liberation), there is a possibility of the residual traces of the limiting condition remaining behind or one is even then far below the beginningless Śiva, (anādi Śiva)[10] then those (so-called) liberated souls would still be in the state of transmigratory existence (and not really liberated). As has been said, "Consciousness (as consciousness) is only one Self". Thus is indicated the invalidity of the theory of plurality of Self.

NOTES

1. Sūtra : Lit., 'thread', hence, it has come to mean that which like a thread holds together certain ideas, a rule, a formula, Cf. Latin, sutura, English suture. A *sūtra* must contain the fewest possible words, must be free from ambiguity, must be meaningful and comprehensive, must not contain useless words and pauses and must be faultless.

2. The word 'ātmā' in the *sūtra* means both Self and *svabhāva* or nature of Reality. Hence the *sūtra* is interpreted in two ways —(1) Being-Awareness (Sat-cit) is Self. (2) Being-Awareness is the nature of Reality i.e., Reality is nothing but Awareness.

There is no word for *caitanya* in English. The word 'consciousness' has a relational colour. (of subject-object duality), but *caitanya* is non-relational. Perhaps the word awareness or Being-Awareness may be better. With this caution, the word 'consciousness' may be used. Our discursive mind, inseparable from the conditioned, relational state cannot conceive of mere *caitanya*—a self, without a predicate relation between it and its attribute or nature, but all the major systems of Indian Philosophy maintain that the Self is pure awareness, non-relational (i.e. without subject-object relation) and without a predicate relaion in its essential form.

3. *Acetitasya* : means *aprakāśitasya* (not appearing by the light which is consciousness). *Prakāśa* in Indian Philosophy

is a most significant word which is not translatable into English, The word *prakāśa* 'means 'light', but it is not in the sense of physical light in which this word is used in Indian Philosophy. Prakāśa is the light of consciousness by which even physical light is visible. Hence wherever there is any appearance, there is *prakāśa* or presence of consciousness. Without *prakāśa* or light of consciousness, nothing can appear, just as without physical light, nothing is visible. Every appearance is nothing but expression of consciousness. Cf. Kaṭha Upaniṣad, II 2, 15. "Consciousness is the supreme light. No physical light such as the sun, moon or stars or lightning shines there, to say nothing of fire. Consciousness is its own light. It shining, everything else shines in its wake. It is by its light alone that every thing else appears." Every appearance bespeaks consciousness.

4. *Caitanya* : This is grammatically formed from *cetana* (conscious being) by the *taddhita* affix 'ṣyañ' which indicates *sambandha* or relationship. *Caitanya*, therefore, means the state of consciousness and being formed by a *taddhita* affix points out its relationship to one who has absolute freedom of all knowledge and activity. That is why Kṣemarāja qualifies *caitanyam* with the expression *sarvajñānakriyāsambandhamayam*, and adds *paripūrṇam—svātantryam ucyate* i.e., *caitanya* indicates absolute freedom of all knowledge and activity.

5. *Svātantrya* : This word literally means self-dependence. It is a technical word of this system. It includes three important ideas—(1) absolute freedom to create, complete autonomy of Will, not depending on any external material or means for its activity, absolute sovereignty or lordship (*aiśvarya*), (2) *Vimarśa* or ever present Self-consciousness, a Self which is all-inclusive (knower, known and means of knowing) (3) *Jñāna* and *kriyā*. The absolute freedom to create includes jñāna and kriyā (knowledge and activity).

Śiva in this system is not like the inactive Brahman of Śaṁkara Vedānta. He has *svātantrya*, unimpeded Will, absolute knowledge, absolute power of creativity, and absolute Self-consciousness.

6. *Anāśrita Śiva* : This is a state below *Śakti tattva* and above *Sadāśiva tattva*. This is only an *avasthā* or state, not a *tattva*. This refers to that phase of reality where *Śakti* begins

temporarily to veil the Self and thus to isolate the universe from itself, producing *akhyāti* or ignorance of its real nature.

7. Eternity, all-pervasiveness etc. are possible in the case of *ākāśa* (ether), *paramāṇus* (atoms) also according to certain schools, but *svātantrya* or absolute freedom is possible only in the case of *Parama Śiva* or Absolute Reality whose nature is *Caitanya* (consciousness).

8. Consciousness *qua* consciousness is one and the same. So there cannot be difference in its essential state. Since all Selves are only consciousness, there cannot be any difference among them.

9. *Mala* : This literally means dross, taint or impurity. *Mala* is what covers and conceals the pure gold of divine consciousness. It is a limiting condition which hampers the free expression of the spirit. It is of three forms, *āṇava mala*, *māyīya mala* and *kārma mala*.

Āṇava mala : It is the primal limiting condition which reduces the universal consciousness to that of an empirical being. It is a cosmic limiting condition over which the individual has no control. It is owing to this that the *jīva* or individual soul considers itself *apūrṇa* or imperfect, a separate entity cut off from the universal consciousness. The greatness of *Śiva* in this condition is concealed, and the individual forgets his real nature. The *āṇava mala* is brought about in two ways. There may be *bodha* or knowledge, but the perfect I-consciousness whose nature is freedom of all cognition and activity may be missing (as in Vijñānakala) or there may be I-consciousness with *abodha* or ignorance (as in common folk).

Māyīya mala is the limiting condition brought about by *Māyā* that gives to the soul its gross and subtle body. It is also cosmic. It is *bhinna-vedya-prathā*--that which brings about the consciousness of difference owing to the differing limiting adjuncts of the bodies.

Kārma mala. It is the *vāsanās* or impressions of actions done by the *jñānendriyas* and *Karmendriyas* under the influence of *antaḥ-karaṇa*. It is a limiting condition brought about by the individual by his *karma* and its *vāsanās*.

10. *Anādiśiva* : Some theorists hold that there are two kinds of Śiva—one, *Anādiśiva* who never assumes *mala* and thus never

descends into bondage; the other kind of *Śiva* assumes *mala* and descends into bondage. Hence, *Śivas* when liberated are after all inferior to *Anādiśiva*. Kṣemarāja controverts this view and says that such so-called liberated Śivas are no better than transmigratory souls, as is the case of the empirical self who considers the body etc. (not-Self) to be the Self.

TEXT

अथ च 'आत्मा क' इति जिज्ञासून् उपदेश्यान् प्रति बोधयितुं, न शरीर-प्राण-बुद्धि-शून्यानि लौकिक-चार्वाक-वैदिक-योगाचार-माध्यमिकाद्यभ्युपगतानि आत्मा; अपि तु यथोक्तं चैतन्यमेव । तस्यैव शरीरादि-कल्पितप्रमातृपदेऽपि अकल्पिताहंविमर्शमय-सत्यप्रमातृत्वेन स्फुरणात् । तदुक्तं श्रीमृत्युजिद्भट्टारके

'परमात्मस्वरूपं तु सर्वोपाधिविवर्जितम् ।
चैतन्यमात्मनो रूपं सर्वशास्त्रेषु पठ्यते ।'

इति । श्रीविज्ञानभैरवेऽपि

'चिद्धर्मा सर्वदेहेषु विशेषो नास्ति कुत्रचित् ।
अतश्च तन्मयं सर्वं भावयन् भवजिज्जनः ॥'

इति । एतदेव

'यतः करणवर्गोऽयं··············· ·।'

इति कारिकाद्वयेन संगृह्य उपदेश्यान् प्रति साभिज्ञानं गुरुणा उपदिष्टं श्रीस्पन्दे ।

TRANSLATION

And so in order to explain to the inquisitive disciples 'what is Self', the author says, "It is not the body, as maintained by the common folk and the materialists (Cārvaka), not the vital principle (*prāṇa*) as maintained by the followers of the Vedas, not the ascertaining power of the mind as maintained by the *Yogācāra Buddhists*, nor the Void as maintained by the *Mādhyamika Buddhists*, but as has already been said, it is the foundational consciousness (absolute Will characterized by knowledge and activity). Even in the case of those subjects who imagine the body etc. to be the Self, the *caitanya* (foundational, pure consciousness) shines forth as the true subject or Self characterized by natural original I-consciousness. As has been said in *Mṛtyuñjit*.[1] "Consciousness is the nature of Self which verily is the Divine Self freed of all limiting conditions. This is what has been described in all the Śāsıras (Sacred Texts)" (VIII, 28).

It has been said in *Vijñāna-bhairava* also "The same Self characterized by consciousness is present in all the bodies; there is no difference in it anywhere. Therefore, a person contemplating on every thing as full of that (consciousness) can conquer transmigratory existence." (Verse 100).

The same idea has been summarized in the following two *Kārikās* in the *Spandakārikas* and explained to the disciples with an illustration by the great teacher (*Vasugupta*).[2]

"The principle (i.e. the divine autonomy) of that source should be investigated with persevering effort, zeal and faith from which the group of outer senses together with the inner *Karaṇeśvarī cakra*,[3] though apparently inconscient, acting like a conscious being, acquires the power to move forward towards an object (*pravṛtti*), to take pleasure in maintaining it after having obtained it (*sthiti*), and to withdraw within the peace of oneself (*Saṁhṛti*).[4] The absolute freedom of that source is natural and spontaneous[5] in all beings and conditions". (sp. k.I. 6,7).

NOTES

1. *Mṛtyuñjit* : This is only another name of Netra Tantra which has been published in the Kashmir Śaiva Text Series.
2. *Vasugupta* was the teacher who for the first time expounded the *Śaiva* philosophy in a systematic form. He lived towards the end of the 8th or beginning of the 9th century A.D.
3. The senses are the five organs of sense, and the five organs of action. The *Karaṇeśvarī Cakra* is the group of divine powers functioning in the various senses.
4. The powers of *pravṛtti*, *sthiti*, and *saṁhṛti* of the empirical selves are derived from those of the absolute Self or Śiva.
5. The Freedom of the Absolute Self to do any thing and everything is spontaneous i.e., it does not depend on any extraneous material or instrumental cause.

TEXT

किंच यदेतत् चैतन्यम् उक्तं स एव आत्मा, स्वभावः, विशेषाचोदनात् भावाभावरूपस्य विश्वस्य जगतः। नहि अचेत्यमानः कोऽपि कस्यापि कदाचिदपि स्वभावो भवति। चेत्यमानस्तु स्वप्रकाशचिवेकीभूतत्वात् चैतन्यात्मैव। तदुक्तं श्रीमदुच्छुष्मभैरवे

'यावन्न वेदका एते तावद्वेद्याः कथं प्रिये ।
वेदकं वेद्यमेकं तु तत्त्वं नास्त्यशुचिस्ततः ॥'

इति । एतदेव

'यस्मात्सर्वमयो जीवः .... ।'

इति कारिकाद्वयेन संगृहीतम् ।

यतः चैतन्यं विश्वस्य स्वभावः तत एव तत्साधनाय प्रमाणादि वराकम् अनुपयुक्तम्; तस्यापि स्वप्रकाशचैतन्याधीनसिद्धिकत्वात्, चैतन्यस्य च प्रोक्तयुक्त्या केनापि आवरीतुम् अशक्यत्वात् सदा प्रकाशमानत्वात् । यदुक्तं श्रीत्रिकहृदये

'स्वपदा स्वशिरश्छायां यद्वल्लङ्घितुमीहते ।
पादोद्देशे शिरो न स्यात्तथेयं बैन्दवी कला ॥'

इति । यो लङ्घितुम् ईहते तस्य यथा पादोद्देशे शिरो न स्यात् तथा इयमिति अत्र संबन्धः । अनेनैव आशयेन स्पन्दे

'यत्र स्थितम् .... ।'

इत्यादि उपक्रम्य

'............ तदस्ति परमार्थतः ॥'

इत्यन्तेन महता ग्रन्थेन शङ्करात्मक-स्पन्द-तत्त्वरूपं चैतन्यं सर्वदा स्वप्रकाशं परमार्थसत् अस्ति इति प्रमाणीकृतम् ॥ १ ॥

TRANSLATION

Moreover the aforesaid consciousness is the *ātmā* or nature of the entire universe consisting of both existent objects (like 'jar' or cloth) or non-existent but imagined objects (like sky-flower). This interpretation is possible, because there is no mention in the *sūtra* of the self of any particular being.

Every appearance owes its existence to the light of consciousness. Nothing can ever have its own being without the light of consciousness. Being experienced, it is of the nature of consciousness itself, because of its being identical with that light. The same idea has been expressed in Ucchuṣmabhairava in the following way.

"Oh dear one, so long as there are no knowers, how can there be anything known. The knower and the known are really the same principle. Therefore, there is nothing which is inherently impure."

The same idea has been expressed succinctly in the following two verses in *Spandakārikā.*

"The Self is the whole of reality, because all existents derive their existence from the Self, and because in the process of knowing, the known gets identified with the Self."[29]

Hence whether in the world or object or mental apprehension of it, there is no state which is not *Śiva.* It is only the experient who always and everywhere exists in the form of the experienced." (II, 3,4).

Since consciousness is the nature of the universe, therefore in order to prove it, the means of right knowledge etc. (*pramāṇas*) are inadequate, for these means of right knowledge are themselves dependent for their proof on the Self-luminous consciousness, and consciousness being ever luminous, it is impossible for anything whatever to veil it, as it is ever luminously present.

As has been said in *Śrī Trikahṛdaya* "Just as (when) one tries to jump over the shadow of one's head with one's own feet, the head will never be at the place of one's feet, so also is it with *Baindavī kalā.*" Just as the head is never at the place of the feet of one who attempts to jump over (the shadow of one's head), so is this (viz. *baiṁdavī* Kalā), this is the syntactical connexion here. With this intent, it has been authoritatively proved by a great many verses (in the *Spandakārikā*) that *caitanya* or consciousness is Divine (*Śaṁkarātmaka*) and the principle of *spanda* (the creative pulsation of delight) and that *caitanya* is ever self-luminous and the highest reality in the verse beginning with,

"That from which everything arises, because it is already existing in it (and arising still exists in it), can never be veiled by anything, there is no check to it anywhere" (I, 2)

and ending with,

"That in which there is neither pain nor pleasure, nor object, nor subject (empirical subject), nor is it insensible (i.e. incapable of experiencing any thing), that indeed abides as Absolute Reality."

NOTES

Baindavī or Vaindavī Kalā

Baindavī Kalā : means the *śakti* of *para-pramātā* or highest knower. *Vetti iti vinduḥ.* The Highest Self or consciousness which is the knower is known as *Vindu* or *Bindu. Bindoriyam iti baindavī*. Baindavī means pertaining to *Bindu. Kalā* means śakti. *Baindavī Kalā*, therefore, means 'the power of knowership of the Highest Self or consciousness'. Here it means the power of the Self by which it is always the knower and never the known.

EXPOSITION

The most important point to note in the first Sūtra is that *caitanyam* in this system does not mean merely consciousness. Since it is the abstract noun derived from *cetana* i.e. one who conscires, one who cognizes, it connotes the idea of both knowledge and activity. *Caitanyam*, therefore, in this system means *Sarvajñānakriyāmayaṁ paripūrṇaṁ svātantryam*, the perfect, absolute freedom of cognizing and doing everything.

The next important point to note is that *ātmā* may mean not simply Self but also *svabhāva* (nature). From this point of view, the *sūtra* means that *caitanya* or consciousness is the nature of Reality. The knower, knowledge, and known are all various forms of consciousness.

The third important point to note is that *caitanya* is not simply *prakāśa* but is also imbued with Universal I-consciousness which is the source of all manifestation.

The fourth important point is that *caitanya* cannot be proved by any logical means, for all means of proof owe their existence to it, and so cannot prove their own source.

Lastly this system is against the theory of the plurality of Self. The nature of all Selves is consciousness. Consciousness *qua* consciousness is the same in all Selves. Therefore the theory of the plurality of Self is not satisfactory.

INTRODUCTION TO THE 2nd SŪTRA

TEXT

यदि जीवजडात्मनो विश्वस्य परमशिवरूपं चैतन्यमेव स्वभावः तत् कथम् अयं बन्ध इत्याशङ्काशान्तये संहितया इतरथा च अकारप्रश्लेषाप्रश्लेष-पाठतः सूत्रम् आह—

TRANSLATION

If the nature of the entire universe consisting of empirical selves and inert matter is only consciousness or in other words *Parama Śiva* (Highest Śiva), then how is this (apparent) bondage to be explained. In order to remove this doubt, the second *sūtra* has been formulated. Kṣemarāja cautions—that this *sūtra* is to be read in two ways (1) according to the rules of *Sandhi* (euphonic coalescence of the final and initial letters) with the coalescence of the final and initial letters in which case this sūtra combined with the previous one would stand thus : चैतन्यमात्माज्ञानं बन्धः (*Caitanyamātmājñānam bandhaḥ*) i.e. the form of the *sūtra* would be *caitanyamātmā+ajñānam bandhaḥ*, (2) without the coalescence of the final letter of the previous *sūtra* and the initial letter of the second *sūtra* in which case the second *sūtra* would stand separately simply as *jñānam bandhaḥ*.

Sūtra-2

ज्ञानं बन्धः ॥ २ ॥

Jñānam Bandhaḥ.

ज्ञानम् vitiated or limited knowledge; बन्धः bondage;

Sūtra—Ajñāna or ignorance of one's real nature which is a kind of shrunken or limited knowledge is the cause of bondage (of the empirical Self).

COMMENTARY

TEXT

इह उक्तयुक्त्या चित्प्रकाशव्यतिरिक्तं न किञ्चिद् उपपद्यत इति मलस्यापि का सत्ता कीदृग् वा तन्निरोधकत्वं स्यादिति भेदवादोक्तप्रक्रियापरिहारेण

'मलमज्ञानमिच्छन्ति संसाराङ्कुरकारणम् ॥'

इति ।

'अज्ञानाद्बध्यते लोकस्ततः सृष्टिश्च संहृतिः ॥'

इति श्रीमालिनीविजय-श्रीसर्वाचारोक्तस्थित्या यः परमेश्वरेण स्वस्वातन्त्र्यशक्त्या-भासितस्वरूप-गोपनारूपया महामायाशक्त्या स्वात्मन्याकाशकल्पेऽनाश्रितात्प्र-भृति मायाप्रमात्रन्तं संकोचोऽवभासितः स एव शिवाभेदाख्यात्यात्मका-ज्ञानस्वभावोऽपूर्णम्मन्यतात्मकाणवमलसतत्त्वसंकुचितज्ञानात्मा बन्धः ।

TRANSLATION

By the argument advanced before, it has been established that there can be nothing which can be proved to be separate from the light of consciousness.

The dualists maintain that there are two separate realities, viz. *Śiva* and *mala*. (Since it has already been proved that there is nothing separate from consciousness), how can there be separate existence of *mala* and how can this *mala* veil consciousness of a Self ? Therefore, Mālinīvijaya by rejecting the way of the dualists says.

"*Mala*, it is said, is nothing but *ajñāna* or ignorance of one's real nature. This ajñāna is the *āṇava mala*[1] which is the cause of *saṁsāra* or *māyīya mala* which again serves as the cause of *Kārmamala*".

According to *Sarvācāra* also—

"People are bound by *ajñāna* and on account of this (*ajñāna*) they undergo birth and death."

A limitation is made to appear by the Highest Lord in His own being which is pure like the sky in the form of *anāśrita śiva* etc. down to *māyāpramātā*.[2] This limitation is due to His power of *Mahāmāyā*[3] which is simply a form of Self-veiling brought about by His power of absolute freedom. That limitation alone is bondage which is (1) of the nature of *ajñāna* (ignorance) i.e. non-awareness of one's non-difference from Śiva and (2) of the nature of limited knowledge in the form of *āṇavamala* which makes one consider oneself as thoroughly reduced in respect of knowledge and action and thus imperfect.

NOTES

1. *Āṇava mala* is of two kinds—(1) *Pauruṣa*—ignorance innate in the very being of the individual Self, and *bauddha*—ignorance inherent in the *buddhi*. Here the *ajñāna* referred to is the *pauruṣa ajñāna* i.e. ignorance of his real nature innate in the individual.

2. *Māyāpramātā* is the self under the influence of *māyā*. This includes the *pralayākalas* and the *sakalas*.

3. *Mahāmāyā*. There are two states of *mahāmāyā*—*aparā* and *parā*. *Aparā* is that which flourishes below *Śuddhavidyā* and above *māyā*. In this are stationed the *Vijñānākalas*. It also denotes that mentality of the experients by which they have *śuddha prakāśa* or clear knowledge but are devoid of pure, full I-consciousness.

Parā mahāmāyā is that lower level of *Śuddha Vidyā* in which are stationed the *Vidyeśvaras* who, though they consider themselves to be pure consciousness, still consider the objects to be different from themselves.

TEXT

यथा च व्यतिरिक्तस्य मलस्यानुपपन्नत्वं तथा अस्माभिः श्रीस्वच्छन्दोद्द्योते पञ्चमपटलान्ते दीक्षाविचारे वितत्य दर्शितम् । एष च सूत्रार्थः

'निजाशुद्ध्यासमर्थस्य . . . . ।'

इति कारिकाभागेन संगृहीतः । एवमात्मनि अनात्मताभिमानरूपाख्याति-लक्षणाज्ञानात्मकं ज्ञानं न केवलं बन्धो यावद् अनात्मनि शरीरादौ आत्मता-भिमानात्मकम् अज्ञानमूलं ज्ञानमपि बन्ध एव । एतच्च

'परामृतरसापाय . . . . ।'

इति कारिकया संगृहीतम् ।

TRANSLATION

I have shown at great length while discussing *dīkṣā* (initiation) in my commentary *Udyota* on Svacchanda Tantra at the end of the 5th *paṭala* that *mala* as something separate from consciousness cannot be proved logically.

The same purport of the above *sūtra* has been epitomised in the following verse (in Spandakārikā).

"The empirical self is reduced to inefficiency on account of his innate impure limiting conditions (*āṇava*, *māyīya* and *kārma mala*) He is driven to desire various objects, but owing to his inefficiency is never fully satisfied. When the restless condition of his mind brought about by his identification of himself with his conditioned selfhood fully ceases, then he experiences the highest state" (sp. k. I.9)

Thus it is not only the limited knowledge due to that ignorance on account of which the conditioned self considers his real Self as not-Self which is the cause of bondage but also the limited knowledge due to that ignorance on account of which the conditioned self considers the not-Self i.e., the body etc. to be his Self.

This idea has been expressed in the following verse of Spandakārikā:

"The *paśu* (conditioned individual) has all his knowledge born of sense and ideation. It is because of this sense and ideation-born knowledge that he loses the enjoyment of the ambrosia of the Highest Self and his innate freedom, Such sense and ideation-born knowledge is confined to the sphere of the *tanmātrās* i.e. sound, colour and form, taste, touch, and odour and the pleasures derived from them". (Sp. K. III, 14)

NOTES

1. Ajñāna or primal ignorance appears in two forms—

(1) *ātmani anātmābhimāna* i.e. considering the real Self as not Self (not knowing the real Self as Self), and (2) *anātmani ātmābhimāna* i.e. considering the not-Self i.e. body etc. as the Self.

Ajñāna in this system does not mean complete absence of knowledge, but *saṅkucitajñāna*. i.e. imperfect knowledge, limited knowledge, incomplete knowledge, not knowledge in its wholeness.

TEXT

एवं चैतन्यशब्देनोक्तं यत्किञ्चित् स्वातन्त्र्यात्मकं रूपं; तत्र चिदात्मन्यपि स्वातन्त्र्याप्रथात्मविज्ञानाकलवद् अपूर्णम्मन्यतामात्रात्मना रूपेण; स्वातन्त्र्येऽपि देहादौ अबोधरूपेण अनात्मन्यात्मताभिमानात्मना रूपेण; द्विप्रकारमाणवमलम् अनेन सूत्रेण सूत्रितम् । तदुक्तं श्रीप्रत्यभिज्ञायाम् ।

'स्वातन्त्र्यहानिर्बोधस्य स्वातन्त्र्यस्याप्यबोधता ।
द्विधाणवं मलमिदं स्वस्वरूपापहानितः ॥'

इति ॥ २ ॥

TRANSLATION

It has been indicated in the previous *sūtra* i.e. the first *sūtra* that the word *caitanya* connotes *svātantrya* i.e. absolute freedom to know everything and absolute freedom to do everything (*jñāna-kriyā-svātantrya*). Now in respect of this (double-faced) *svātantrya*, even if there be only *prakāśa* or *jñāna* (*cidātmani api*), but without *kartṛtva-svātantrya*, in other words, without I-consciousness, which leads one to consider onself incomplete or deficient as in the case of Vijñānākala[1], there is *āṇava mala*; or even if there is *svātantrya* in the form of *kartṛtva* (doership indicating I-consciousness) but full of *abodha* or ignorance leading to consider the not-Self like the body etc. as the Self (as in the case of *sakala*), then again there is *āṇava mala*. Thus this *sūtra* points out that there is *āṇava mala* in two ways. As has been said in *Īśvara-pratyabhijñā*. There may be *bodha* or *jñāna* without the sense of doership or I-consciousness (which is the loss of *kartṛtva-svātantrya*); or there may be the sense of doership without *bodha* or *jñāna* (which is the loss of *jñāna-svātantrya*). So there is *āṇava mala* in two ways both of which are due to one's loss of the grip of one's essential nature"[2] (III, 2,4)

NOTES

1. Vijñānākala: the experient below *śuddhavidyā* but above Māyā. He has pure awareness but no agency. He is free of *kārma* and *māyīya mala*, but is not yet free of *āṇava mala*.

2. Essential nature : The essential nature of Self consists in full freedom of both *jñāna* and *kriyā*.

EXPOSITION

The first *Sūtra* says that Self is pure consciousness. The question arises that if Self is pure consciousness, how is it that it is in bondage?

The second Sūtra provides the answer to this question. It says that the bondage of the individual is due to his so-called *jñāna* (limited knowledge) which really speaking is *ajñāna* or ignorance. Ignorance or *ajñāna* is not negative; it is positive, a kind of positive *jñāna*, a shrunken, vitiated knowledge. It is this shrunken, vitiated *jñāna* which is responsible for the individual's bondage. But this kind of *jñāna* or knowledge is, truly speaking, *ajñāna* or ignorance. This ignorance is of two forms (1) not knowing the real Self to be Self at all, completely withdrawn from one's real Self and (2) knowing the not-Self i.e. the body etc. to be the Self.

This *ajñāna* is known as *āṇava mala*, a limitation innate in the individual.

What is this *āṇava mala* due to ? It is due to a wonderful power of *Śiva* (the Supreme). A person may conceal everything, but he cannot conceal his own nature. But *Śiva* has this wonderful power of veiling his real nature. This Self-veiling power of *Śiva* is known as *Mahāmāyā*. In the *aṇu*, (the limited individual), that Self-veiling works as *mala*. This Self-veiling is His technique or stratagem for the play of life in varied, multiple forms. Man is bound to transmigratory existence, to sense-life, to the life of his own vehicles or bodies only so long as heallows himself to be confined to the limited knowledge of his senses and mentation. When he recognises his real nature, he is free.

INTRODUCTION TO THE 3rd SŪTRA

TEXT

किम् ईदृगाणवमलात्मैव बन्धः ? न इत्याह—

TRANSLATION

Is *āṇavamala* as described the only cause of bondage ? The next *sūtra* says, No. (There are other causes also, viz. *māyīya* and *kārma mala*).

Sūtra—3

योनिवर्गः कलाशरीरम् ॥ ३ ॥

Yonivargaḥ kalāśarīram

योनि = the source (of the objective world) i.e. *māyā*. वर्गः = class of *tattvas* (principles and elements). *Yonivargaḥ*, therefore, means *māyā* and her brood i.e. the class of elements to which she gives rise and which thus constitute the source of this world. कला = activity; शरीरम् = form कलाशरीरम् = whose form is activity i.e. activity through which worldly life is carried out. So *yonivargaḥ* is *māyīya mala* and *kalāśarīram* is *kārma mala*.

The word *bandhaḥ* (bondage) is understood in this *sūtra* also. Therefore the *sūtra* means "*Māyīya mala* and *kārma mala* are also the cause of bondage."

This *sūtra* has been slightly differently interpreted by Bhāskara in *Śiva-sūtra-vārttikam*. According to him *Yoni* means the four *Śaktis* of *Ambā*, *Jyeṣṭhā*, *Raudrī* and *Vāmā*. Kalā means letters from 'a' to 'kṣa' which bring about words. The above *śaktis* through the influence of words bring about thought-constructs owing to which the Self is reduced to an empirical being and thus suffers bondage. Kṣemarāja's interpretation is better.

COMMENTARY

TEXT

बन्ध इत्यनुवर्तते, योऽयं योनेर्विश्वकारणस्य मायायाः संबन्धी वर्गः साक्षात्

पारम्पर्येण च; तद्धेतुको देहभुवनाद्यारम्भी किञ्चित्कर्तृताद्यात्मककलादिक्षित्यन्तस्तत्त्वसमूहः; तद्रूपं मायीयम्, तथा कलयति स्वस्वरूपावेशेन तत्तद् वस्तु परिच्छिनत्तीति कला व्यापारः; शरीरं स्वरूपं यस्य तत् कलाशरीरं कार्मंमलमपि बन्ध इत्यर्थः । एतदपि

TRANSLATION

The word *bandhaḥ* or bondage follows from the previous *sūtra*. (The meaning of *yonivargaḥ* is the following).

Yoni means the source of this world i.e. *Māyā*. *Vargaḥ* means (*tattva-samūhaḥ*) the class of elements associated with Māyā directly or through successive stages. This brings about body, worlds, *kalā* (limited agency) etc.[1] down upto earth. So *Yonivargaḥ* means *Māyīya mala*.[2]

Kalā is that which divides the world of entities into separate things as this or that by mental impenetration, in other words, 'activity'. *Śarīra* means form. *Kalāśarīram*, therefore, means 'that whose form is activity', that is to say, *Kārma mala*.[3] (Like the *Māyīya mala*), this *kārma mala* is also the cause of bondage. This is the meaning.

NOTES

1. Etc. indicates the other four *kañcukas* or coverings of māyā, viz., Vidyā, Rāga, Kāla and Niyati.

   (1) Kalā brings about limitation in respect of agency or efficacy.

   (2) Vidyā brings about limitation in respect of knowledge.

   (3) Rāga brings about desire for this or that.

   (4) Kāla brings about limitation in respect of time, viz., past, present, future etc.

   (5) Niyati brings about limitation in respect of cause, space and form.

2. *Māyīyamala* is the *mala* or limitation due to *māyā* which gives to the soul its gross and subtle body and brings about sense of difference. *Kārma mala* is *mala* due to *vāsanās* or impressions left behind on the mind due to *karma* or action.

TEXT

'निजाशुद्ध्यासमर्थस्य कर्तव्येष्वभिलाषिणः ।'

इत्यनेनैव संगृहीतम् । यथा चैतत् तथा अस्मदीयात् स्पन्दनिर्णयादवबोद्ध-

व्यम् । एषां च कलादीनां किञ्चित्कर्तृत्वादिलक्षणं स्वरूपमाणवमलभित्तिलग्नं पुंसामावरकतया मलत्वेन सिद्धमेव । यदुक्तं श्रीमत्स्वच्छन्दे

'मलप्रध्वस्तचैतन्यं कलाविद्यासमाश्रितम् ।
रागेण रञ्जितात्मानं कालेन कलितं तथा ॥
नियत्या यमितं भूयः पुंभावेनोपबृंहितम् ।
प्रधानाशयसंपन्नं गुणत्रयसमन्वितम् ॥
बुद्धितत्त्वसमासीनमहङ्कारसमावृतम् ।
मनसा बुद्धिकर्माक्षैस्तन्मात्रैः स्थूलभूतकैः ॥'

इति । कार्ममलस्याप्यावरकत्वं श्रीमालिनीविजये प्रदर्शितम्

'धर्माधर्मात्मकं कर्म सुखदुःखादिलक्षणम् ।'

इति । तदेतत् मायीयं कार्मं च मलम्

'भिन्नवेद्यप्रथात्रैव मायाख्यं जन्मभोगदम् ।
कर्तर्यबोधे कार्मं च मायाशक्त्यैव तत्त्रयम्........॥"

इति श्रीप्रत्यभिज्ञायाम् आणवमलभित्तिकं संकुचितविशिष्टज्ञानतयैवोक्तम् ॥ ३॥

TRANSLATION

The same idea has been expressed in the following verse (in Spandakārikā) "The empirical self is reduced to inefficiency on account of his innate impure limiting conditions (*āṇava, māyīya,* and *kārma malas*). He is driven to desire various objects, but owing to his inefficiency is never fully satisfied. When this restless condition of his mind brought about by his identification of himself with his conditioned selfhood fully ceases, then he experiences the highest state." (I,9)

That this is so may be understood from my (Kṣemarāja's) commentary *Spandnirṇaya* on *Spandakārikā*. These *kalā* etc. whose characteristic is limited agency etc. are attached to *āṇava mala* as their base and veil the essential nature of *jīvas* (empirical selves). Thus it is fully established that they are *malas* or limiting conditions. As has been said in *Svacchanda.*

"*Caitanya* (Freedom of the Self to know and do every thing) is suppressed by *mala* (i.e., *āṇava mala*) and provided with *kalā* and *vidyā*, is tainted by *rāga,* limited in respect of *kāla* (time), restrained by *niyati*, magnified by the sense of being a *Puruṣa* (an empirical self), furnished with the disposition of *Prakṛti*, endowed with the three *guṇas* (*rajas*, *tamas* and *sattva*), *buddhi*, *ahaṁkāra*, and *manas*. *jñānendriyas* (organs of sense) and *kar-*

mendriyas (organs of action), *tanmātrās*, and the gross elements."[1] (II, 39-41).

Mālinī-vijaya shows in the following line that *Kārma mala* also veils the essential nature of the empirical self. "He (the *jīva*) does good and bad deeds which bring about pleasure and pain.[2] (I, 24). In *Īśvara-pratyabhijñā* also, it has been said in the following verse that *Māyīya* and *kārma mala* are particular kinds of limited knowledge with *āṇava* mala as their base.

"When there is ignorance of real Self, then *Āṇava mala* being present, there arise *māyīya mala* bringing about a sense of difference in respect of every object, and *kārma mala* which brings about birth and experience of pleasure and pain (*bhoga*). All the three *malas* are brought about by the *Māyā Śakti* of Śiva." (III,2.5)

NOTES

1. This gives the details of *māyīya mala.*
2. This indicates *kārma mala*
3. Māyā Śakti is the inherent power of Śiva by which He appears in different forms. Māyā Śakti is different from *Māyā tattva* (the material origin of the various objects in the universe).

EXPOSITION

The second sūtra says that an individual is in a state of bondage, because of his innate *āṇava mala*. The third *sūtra* says that it is not only the *āṇava mala* which is responsible for the individual's bondage. Attached to *āṇava mala* as a base, there are two more *malas*, *māyīya* and *kārma*. They also bring about the bondage of the individual. *Māyīya mala* provides the individual with the physical and psychic vehicles in which he is 'cabined, caged and confined', and *Kārma mala* makes him commit motivated actions. These and their residual traces are not airy nothing. They are kārmika forces that drag the individual to earth-life again and again.

INTRODUCTION TO THE 4th SŪTRA

TEXT

अथ कथमस्याज्ञानात्मकज्ञान-योनिवर्ग-कलाशरीररूपस्य त्रिविधस्य मलस्य बन्धकत्वमित्याह—

TRANSLATION

Now how is it that the three kinds of *mala*, viz. *ajñāna* appearing as limited knowledge (*āṇavamala*), *māyā* and its coverings (*māyīya mala*) and *kārma mala* become the cause of bondage (of the *jīva*) ? In answer to this question, the next *sūtra* says:

Sūtra-4

ज्ञानाधिष्ठानं मातृका ॥ ४ ॥

Jñānādhiṣṭhānam mātṛkā

ज्ञान (limited knowledge), अधिष्ठान basis, seat. ज्ञानाधिष्ठान —the basis of these limited kinds of knowledge (*āṇava, māyīya*, and *kārma*) मातृका = (unknown, ununderstood) Mother or Power of Sound corresponding to the letters of the alphabet. This Power is called Mother, because it produces the entire universe.

It is the un-understood Mother or Power of Sound inherent in the alphabet that is the basis of the limited knowledge (in the form of *āṇava, māyīya* and *Kārma mala*).

COMMENTARY

TEXT

यदेतत् त्रिविधमलस्वरूपम् अपूर्णम्मन्यताभिन्नवेद्यप्रथा-शुभाशुभवासनात्मकं विविधं ज्ञानरूपमुक्तम्, तस्य आदिक्षान्तरूपा अज्ञाता माता मातृका विश्वजननी

TRANSLATION

A threefold form of limited knowledge in the form of threefold *mala* has been described above. Of this threefold limited knowledge, that which makes oneself consider himself as incomplete and imperfect is the *āṇava mala*; that which brings a sense of difference in every thing is *māyīya mala*; that which makes one perform good or bad deeds is *kārma mala*. Of this threefold limited knowledge, *mātṛkā*,[1] or alphabet from *a* to *kṣa* the mother of the entire universe is the presiding deity. She is called *mātṛkā,* because she is unknown, ununderstood.

NOTES

1. *Mātṛkā*: The 'ka' suffix in Saṁskṛta denotes the idea that the thing to which this suffix is added is unknown or un-understood. Hence *Mātṛkā* means the mother who is not properly known or understood. *Mātṛkā* is the subtle form of gross speech. The letters and their ultimate essential nature are known as Mātṛkā. When unknown, the *Mātṛkā* impels people towards all kinds of worldly activities and feelings. When the *Mātṛkā* is known i.e. when her saving power is realized, she leads one to liberation.

TEXT

तत्तत्संकुचितवेद्याभासात्मनो ज्ञानस्य 'अपूर्णोऽस्मि, क्षामः स्थूलो वास्मि, अग्निष्टोमयाज्यस्मि, इत्यादितत्तदविकल्पकसविकल्पकावभासपरामर्शमयस्य तत्तद्वाचकशब्दानुवेधद्वारेण शोक-स्मय-हर्ष-रागादिरूपतामादधाना

TRANSLATION

She (Mātṛkā) brings about knowledge in a limited form, e.g. "I am imperfect" (*āṇavamala*) "I am thin or fat." (*māyīya mala*), "I am a performer of *agniṣṭoma* sacrifice" (*kārma mala*). Such knowledge is subtle or in a concretely expressed form (*avikalpakasavikalpaka—parāmarśa—mayasya*), and by the penetration of different communicative words in the minds of the listener brings about a feeling of sorrow, pride, joy, and passion.

TEXT

'करन्ध्रचितिमध्यस्था ब्रह्मपाशावलम्बिकाः ।
पीठेश्वर्या महाघोरा मोहयन्ति मुहुर्मुहुः ॥'

इति श्रीतिमिरोद्घाटप्रोक्तनीत्या वर्ग-कलाद्यधिष्ठातृब्राह्म्यादिशक्तिश्रेणी-शोभिनी श्रीसर्ववीराद्यागमप्रसिद्धलिपिक्रमसंनिवेशोत्थापिका अम्बा-ज्येष्ठा-रौद्री-वामाख्यशक्तिचक्रचुम्बिता शक्तिरधिष्ठात्री,

TRANSLATION

Mātṛkā is the presiding Power in the form of various deities (*Śaktir adhiṣṭhātrī*), as, for instance, is described by *Timirodghāta* in the following verse:

"The *Mahāghorā*[1] *Śaktis* who are the deities of the *pīṭhas*,[2]

who hover about the consciousness in *Karandhra*[3] i.e. Brahmarandhra with a terrible noose delude people constantly".

She (Mātṛkā) shines in the line of *Śaktis* presiding over *varga* (classes of letters)[4], *kalā*[5] (the subtlest aspect of the objective world) etc.[6] in the form of *Brāhmī* and other *Śaktis*; she rouses people to all kinds of activity and feeling by means of the arrangement of a succession of letters of a script—a fact which is very well made clear in the Sarvavīra and other *āgamas*; she is closely united with the group of *Śaktis* known as Ambā,[7] Jyeṣṭhā, Raudrī and Vāmā.

NOTES

1. There are three *Śaktis, Ghorā, Ghoratarī* or *Mahāghorā* and *Aghorī.* The *Ghorā* (terrible) are the innumerable *Śaktis* (powers) who provide worldly pleasures to men and put obstacles in their path of spiritual progress. The *Ghoratarī* or *Mahāghorā* are those innumerable *śaktis* who delude the worldly-minded people and drive them more and more towards worldliness. The *Aghorā* are those *śaktis* who inspire the *jīvas* (empirical selves) towards the path of liberation.

2. *Pīṭhas*—Seats i.e. the sense-organs which are the seats of these *Śaktis*.

3. 'Ka' in the context means Brahman. *Karandhra,* therefore, means *Brahmarandhra.* This is a psychic centre above the head.

4. The presiding deities over the various classes of letters are the following:

Class of letters.	*Presiding deities.*
1. A varga; (the class of vowels)	Yogīśvari or Mahālakṣmī.
2. Ka varga (ka, kha, ga, gha, ṅa)	Brāhmī.
3. Cavarga (Ca, cha, ja, jha, ña)	Māheśvarī.
4. Ṭavarga (ṭa, ṭha, ḍa, ḍha, ṇa)	Kaumārī.
5. Tavarga (ta, tha, da, dha, na)	Vaiṣṇavī.
6. Pavarga (pa, pha, ba, bha, ma)	Vārāhī.
7. Yavarga (ya, ra, la, va)	Aindrī or Indrāṇī.
8. Śavarga (śa, ṣa, sa, ha, kṣa)	Cāmuṇḍā.

5. *Kalās* are the specific modes of *Śakti.* They are the subtlest aspects of the objective world. There are five *kalās,* viz.

Nivṛtti, Pratiṣṭhā, Vidyā, Śānti, Śāntyatītā. Nivṛtti kalā is so called because here the manifesting energy is stopped and is turned upwards. It is the essential working force in *Pṛthivī tattva* (solidity). There are 16 *bhuvanas* in this.

Pratiṣṭhā Kalā is the subtle force of the *tattvas* from *āp* (fluidity) to *Prakṛti* (in all 23 *tattvas*). It has 56 *bhuvanas*. *Vidyā* is the *kalā* working in the *tattvas* from Puruṣa upto Māyā. It contains seven *tattvas* and 28 *bhuvanas*. The *Śānti* or *Śāntā kalā* is dominant in the *tattvas Sadvidyā, Īśvara* and *Sadā Śiva* and contains 18 *bhuvanas*. The *Śāntyatītā kalā* is the characteristic of Śakti and Śiva *tattvas*. It has no *bhuvana*.

6. Etc. includes Ṣaḍadhvā (*Varṇa, pada, mantra, kalā, tattva* and *bhuvana*).

7. Ambā, Jyeṣṭhā, Raudrī and Vāmā: *Ambā* is the *Śakti* that puts obstacles in all the actions. *Jyeṣṭhā* is *Śivamay*ī the *Śakti* who leads to liberation. *Vāmā* is the *Śakti* who is active in the manifestation of the world. *Raudrī* is the *Śakti* who brings about obstacles for the wicked and destroys them for elevated souls.

TEXT

तदधिष्ठानादेव हि अन्तरभेदानुसंधिवन्ध्यत्वात् क्षणमपि अलब्धविश्रान्तीनि बहिर्मुखान्येव ज्ञानानि, इति युक्तैव एषां बन्धकत्वोक्तिः । एतच्च

'शब्दराशिसमुत्थस्य .... ।'

इति कारिकया,

'स्वरूपावरणे चास्य शक्तयः सततोत्थिताः ।'

इति च कारिकया संगृहीतम् ॥ ४ ॥

TRANSLATION

Because that (Mātṛkā) is the basis (of all limited knowledge), therefore, one is deprived of the investigation of the inner non-difference (from the fullest I-consciousness of Śiva) and all one's knowledge is outward—turned without ceasing for a moment. Therefore, it is rightly maintained that all such knowledge is the cause of bondage.

This idea is also expressed in the following verses in Spanda-kārikā :

"He (the limited, empirical self) being deprived of the knowledge of his essential Self by the Kalās i.e. the letters 'ka' etc. falls a victim to the group of Śaktis like *Brāhmī* etc. arising from a multitude of words. Therefore he is known as *paśu*." (III, 13)

"His *Śaktis* (inherent in letters described before) are always in readiness in veiling his essential real Self, because all his ideas cannot arise without the use of words." (III,15)

EXPOSITION

The basis of all the three *malas* is word-bound ideas. The words are a reflex of the letters and their sound known as *Mātṛkā*, so, ultimately it is *Mātṛkā* which is responsible for the limited knowledge i.e., the three *malas*. Words have a tremendous influence in shaping our ideas which do not allow us to realize the splendour of Śiva-consciousness imprisoned within ourselves.

INTRODUCTION TO THE 5th SŪTRA

TEXT

अथ एतद्बन्धप्रशमोपायमुपेयविश्रान्तिसतत्त्वमादिशति—

TRANSLATION

Now the next *sūtra* teaches that the quintessence of the means for the cessation of the bondage brought about by the limited knowledge consists in resting in *Bhairava*-consciousness.

Sūtra-5

उद्यमो भैरवः ॥ ५ ॥

Udyamao Bhairavaḥ.

उद्यमः in this context means, as Kṣemarāja rightly suggests, उन्मज्जनरूपः sudden emergence of (divine) consciousness; it is an opening out, an efflorescence of consciousness. *Udyamaḥ* in this *sūtra* does not mean exertion or effort. The word is formed from *ut*+ *yam*. *Ut* means 'up', 'upwards' and *yam* means to raise, to hold, (vide Monier-William's Sans-English Dy.) Udyamaḥ, therefore, means 'raising up', 'elevation of consciousness'.

Since this sūtra teaches *Śāmbhavopāya, udyamaḥ* can never mean exertion in this context.

The *Sūtra,* therefore, means that a sudden flash or opening out of transcendental consciousness is *Bhairava* or *Śiva.* That is, since this sudden flash is the means to *Bhairava*-consciousness, it may be called *Bhairava.*

COMMENTARY

TEXT

योऽयं प्रसरद्रूपाया विमर्शमय्याः संविदो झगिति उच्छलनात्मकपरप्रतिभोन्मज्जनरूप उद्यमः स एव संर्वशक्तिसामरस्येन अशेषविश्वभरितत्वात् सकलकल्पनाकुलालंकवलनमयत्वाच्च भैरवो भैरवात्मकस्वस्वरूपाभिव्यक्तिहेतुत्वात् भक्तिभाजाम् अन्तर्मुखैतत्तत्त्वावधानधनानां जायते, इत्युपदिष्टं भवति ।

TRANSLATION

That is *udyama* which is an emergence of an awareness in the form of highest *pratibhā*[1] which is a sudden springing up (i.e. which is a sudden flash) of that I-consciousness of *Śiva* which expands in the form of the entire universe. That *udyama* in itself is Bhairava inasmuch as *Bhairava* holds within Himself the entire universe by reducing all the *śaktis* to sameness with Himself and inasmuch as He completely devours within Himself the entire mass of ideation (which is responsible for sense of difference). That *udyama* may in itself be called *Bhairava* inasmuch as it is the means for revealing *Bhairava* who is one's own essential Self. That *udyama* appears in those who are devoted to Him because of their whole attention being concentrated on that inner Bhairava principle. This is what has been taught in this *sūtra.*

TEXT

उक्तं च श्रीमालिनीविजये

'अकिंचिच्चिन्तकस्यैव गुरुणा प्रतिबोधतः ।
जायते यः समावेशः शाम्भवोऽसावुदीरितः ॥'

इति । अत्र हि 'गुरुणा प्रतिबोधतः' इत्यत्र गुरुतः स्वस्मात् प्रतिबोधतः इत्यस्यार्थो गुरुभिरादिष्टः । श्रीस्वच्छन्देऽपि उक्तम् ।

'आत्मनो भैरवं रूपं भावयेद्यस्तु पूरुषः ।
तस्य मन्त्राः प्रसिद्ध्यन्ति नित्ययुक्तस्य सुन्दरि ॥'

इति । भावनं हि अत्र अन्तर्मुखोद्यन्तृतापदविमर्शनमेव । एतच्च

'एकचिन्ताप्रसक्तस्य यतः स्यादपरोदयः ।
उन्मेषः स तु विज्ञेयः स्वयं तमुपलक्षयेत् ॥'

इत्यनेन संगृहीतम् ॥ ५ ॥

TRANSLATION

It has also been said in *Mālinīvijaya Tantra* : "Absorption of the individual consciousness in the divine (*samāveśa*) results from an awakening (*pratibodhataḥ*) imparted by the *guru* (spiritual director) in one who has freed his mind of all ideation". (II, 23). This *samāveśa* is called *Śambhava*. Another meaning of *guruṇā pratibodhataḥ* has also been taught by the great teachers, viz. (*guru* = great; *pratibodha* = awakening) i.e. 'by one's own great awakening'.

In *Svacchanda Tantra* also, it has been said,

"Oh beautiful one (i.e. *Pārvatī*, consort of *Śiva*), of the man who realizes his Bhairava nature by an apprehension of an inner emergent divine nature and is thus united with the Eternal, all the *mantras* become effective, being charged with power."

The word *bhāvanā* occurring in the above verse means 'an apprehension of an inner emergent divine consciousness' (not meditation or contemplation).

This idea has also been expressed in the following verse of Spandakārikā.

"While one is engaged in one thought, and another arises, the junction-point between the two is the *unmeṣa*[3]-a revelation of the true nature of the Self which is the background of both the two thoughts. This may be experienced by every one for oneself." (III, 9)

NOTES

1. *Pratibhā* is a technical term of this system. It means the *Parāvāka*, the absolutely free creative divine consciousness (vide Parātriṁśikā, p. 102).

2. *Bhairava* is an anacrostic word. The letter *bha* of this word indicates *bharaṇa* or maintenance of the world, *ra* indicates *ravaṇa* or withdrawal of the world, and *va* indicates *vamana* or projection of the world. Thus Bhairava is one who brings about the *sṛṣṭi*, *sthiti* and *saṁhāra* of the universe.

3. *Unmeṣa* means opening out, emergence, revelation of the true nature of Self.

EXPOSITION

This *sūtra* gives in a nutshell *Śāmbhavopāya*—the *Śāmbhava Yoga*. This immersion in divine consciousness occurs to one who is a very advanced aspirant. It is a sudden flash of divine consciousness by an orientation of the will towards the inner creative consciousness which is always present within oneself. It requires no discipline of meditation, *japa* etc.

INTRODUCTION TO THE 6th SŪTRA

TEXT

एवं झगिति परप्रतिभोन्मेषावष्टम्भोपायिकां भैरवसमापत्तिम् अज्ञान-बन्धप्रशमैकहेतुं प्रदर्श्य, एतत्परामर्शप्रकर्षाद् व्युत्थानमपि प्रशान्तभेदावभासं भवतीत्याह—

TRANSLATION

Thus after showing that *Bhairava*-consciousness comes about by taking hold of the emergence of the highest *pratibhā* (sudden flash of the divine I-consciousness) which is the one sure means of putting a stop to bondage that arises on account of spiritual ignorance, the *sūtrakāra* (the formulator of the *sūtras*) now says that when this *Śiva*-consciousness is completely established, there continues the awareness of the cessation of all difference even in the usual normal course of life (when one's attention is not necessarily turned inward).

Sūtra-6

शक्तिचक्रसंधाने विश्वसंहारः ॥ ६ ॥

Śakticakrasandhāne viśvasaṁhāraḥ.

शक्तिचक्रसंध ने =By union with the collective whole of *śaktis* through intensive and fixed awareness. विश्वसंहार: =disappearance of the universe (as something separate from consciousness).

By union with the collective whole of *śaktis* through intensive and fixed awareness, there is the disappearance of the universe as something separate from consciousness.

COMMENTARY

TEXT

योऽयं परप्रतिभोन्मज्जनात्मोद्यन्तृतास्वभावो भैरव उक्तः अस्यैव अन्तर्लक्ष्य-बहिर्दृष्टयात्मतया निःशेषशक्तिचक्रक्रमाक्रमाक्रामिणी अतिक्रान्तक्रमाक्रमाति-रिक्तारिक्ततदुभयात्मतयापि अभिधीयमानापि अनेतद्रूपा अनुत्तरा परा स्वातन्त्र्यशक्तिः काप्यस्ति यया स्वभित्तौ मह्युल्लासात् प्रभृति परप्रमातृविश्रान्त्यन्तं श्रीमत्सृष्टयादिशक्तिचक्रस्फारणात्मा क्रीडेयमादर्शिता । तस्यैतदाभासितस्य शक्तिचक्रस्य रहस्याम्नायाम्नातनीत्या यत्संधानं यथोचितक्रमविमर्शनं तस्मिन् सति कालाग्न्यादेश्चरमकलान्तस्य विश्वस्य संहारो देहात्मतया बाह्यतया च अवस्थितस्यापि सतः परसंविदग्निसाद्भावो भवतीत्यर्थः ।

TRANSLATION

Bhairava who has been described (in the previous *sūtra*) as of the nature of an emergence of awareness which is simply a sudden flash of highest *pratibhā* (i.e. the full I-consciousness of *Śiva*) has the highest *svātantrya śakti* (i.e., the full freedom of knowing and doing any and every thing). This Śakti though fully aware of its inner nature is outwardly engaged in activity and thus seizing the entire host of its *Śaktis* appears in the form of succession (*krama*), non-succession (i.e. simultaneity) (*akrama*)[1], in the transcendence of both succession and simultaneity, in the form of being greatly empty (*atirikta* or *kṛśā*, greatly emaciated), of being not empty at all (*ariktā* or *pūrṇā*—always full) or in the form of both empty and non-empty.[2] Though she (*Śakti*) is described in the various detailed forms as above, she is not any of these forms.

It is this *Svātantrya Śakti* that on her own screen (i.e. in herself) displays this play of manifestation in the form of expansion of the Śakti of emanation etc. from the earth up to rest in the highest Experient (i.e. up to the stage of being established in one's highest nature). When *sandhāna* (i e. union by awareness) of this group of *Śaktis* which has been made manifest is established according to the appropriate manner as described in the secret *śāstras*, then occurs the disappearance of the universe from *Kālāgni*[3] up to the ultimate *kalā*[4]; that is to say, though external existence may continue in the form of the body and other external objects, it is reduced to sameness with the fire of the highest consciousness (i.e. it appears only as a form of consciousness).

NOTES

1. *Krama* (succession) and *akrama* (simultaneity) are concepts used with reference to time. It is only our human way of speaking; the divine Śakti is above the dichotomization of the intellect.
2. This exhausts all the four alternatives, viz., (1) empty (2) non-empty (3) both empty and non-empty (4) neither empty nor non-empty. The idea is that though the divine creative *Śakti* goes on projecting things out of herself (which shows that she is perfectly full and rich), and reabsorbing them into herself (which shows that she is depleted and must take back things to make up her loss), yet in herself she transcends all these alternatives.
3. *Kālāgni*. This is the lowest plane of *Nivṛtti Kalā*.
4. *Carama* (ultimate) *kalā* i.e., Śāntātītā kalā.

TEXT

उक्तं च श्रीभर्गशिखायाम्

‘मृत्युं च कालं च कलाकलापं विकारजालं प्रतिपत्तिसात्म्यम् ।
ऐकात्म्यनानात्म्यविकल्पजातं तदा स सर्वं कवलीकरोति ॥’

इति । श्रीमद्वीरावलावपि

‘यत्र सर्वे लयं यान्ति दह्यन्ते तत्त्वसंचयाः ।
तां चितिं पश्य कायस्थां कालानलसमत्विषम् ॥’

इति. । श्रीमन्मालिनीविजयेऽपि

‘उच्चाररहितं वस्तु चेतसैव विचिन्तयन् ।
यं समावेशमाप्नोति शाक्तः सोऽत्राभिधीयते ॥’

इत्युक्त्या एतदेव भङ्ग्या निरूपितम् । एतच्च सद्गुरुचरणोपासनया अभिव्यक्तिमायातीति नाधिकमुन्मीलितम् ।

एतदेव

‘यस्योन्मेषनिमेषाभ्यां· · · · · · · · · · · · · ।’

इति,

‘यदा त्वेकत्र संरूढः· · · · · · · · · · · · · ।’

इति च प्रथमचरमश्लोकाभ्यां संगृहीतम् ॥ ६ ॥

TRANSLATION

It has also been said in *Bhargaśikhā*:

"Then (on the occasion of *viśvasaṁhāra*), he (the aspirant) devours every thing (i.e. reduces to sameness with consciousness), whether it is death, or *kāla*, the presiding Spirit of death, or the multitude of activity, network of all changes, identification with the knowledge of objects, and the multitude of thought-constructs whether it is a thought-construct of identity with the Highest or thought-construct of varied things."

In *Vīrāvalī* also it is said:

"Observe that divine consciousness present in the body which has the glow like that of *kālāgni Rudra* and in which all things are dissolved and the multitude of the elements is burned."

In *Mālinīvijaya Tantra* also, it is said:

"When an aspirant with one-pointedness of mind apprehends that Reality which is not within the range of utterance (gross or subtle), he obtains *samāveśa* (absorption in divine consciousness); then that *samāveśa* is known as *Śākta* (i.e. obtained by means of Śāktopāya)" (II, 22).

So, the same technique of union with *Śakti* by full awareness has been ascertained by another *Śāstric* procedure. This comes into experience only by devotion to the lotus feet of a genuine *guru* (spiritual director). So, nothing further has been described.

The same idea has been described by means of the first and the last verses in Spandakārikā :

"We bow to that *Śaṁkara* from whose expansion and contraction of *Śakti*, the world arises and dissolves and who is the source of all the glorious might of the multitude of *Śaktis*." (I, 1.).

"When one is rooted in the one place i.e., in the *spanda-tattva* consisting of the perfect I-consciousness, then controlling the rise and disappearance of it (i.e., the subtle body), one acquires the status of a real enjoyer, and then becomes the master of the group of *Śaktis*." (III, 19)

EXPOSITION

This *sūtra* describes a *Śāktopāya* (a discipline based on *Śakti*) as an aid to *Śāmbhavopāya*. In this, the entire manifestation of *Śakti* has to be realized by one-pointedness of mind as only a display of the *Svātantrya Śakti* of *Śiva*. Then the entire universe appears as a form of consciousness. It is no longer a mere material object, completely separate from consciousness, but only an expression of consciousness in a particular form. Then there is *viśvasaṁhāra* i.e. disappearance of the universe as something external to consciousness. *Viśvasaṁhāra* in this context does not mean *pralaya* or final dissolution of the universe but the disappearance of the universe as some thing separate from consciousness and its reduction to sameness with consciousness, its assimilation to consciousness itself. After this the mind of the aspirant is prepared for the reception of a sudden awareness of the full I-consciousness of Śiva (*Śāmbhava upāya*).

INTRODUCTION TO THE 7TH SŪTRA

TEXT

एवमुपसंहृतविश्वस्य न समाधिव्युत्थानभेदः कोऽपि इत्याह—

TRANSLATION

Thus to the individual in whom the universe has been assimilated to the inner *Śiva*-consciousness, there is no difference between *Samādhi* and *vyutthāna*. (*Samādhi* means collectedness of mind in meditation and *vyutthāna* means rising up from meditation. It is not only during *samādhi* that one has unity-consciousness, but also in the usual course of life).

Sūtra-7

जाग्रत्स्वप्नसुषुप्तभेदे तुर्याभोगसंभवः ॥ ७ ॥

Jāgratsvapnasuṣuptabhede turyābhogasambhavaḥ

NOTES

जाग्रत् = the waking state of consciousness.

स्वप्न = the dream state of consciousness.

सुषुप्ति = the state of consciousness in profound sleep in which there are no ideas. भेद = difference.

तुर्य = the fourth i.e. the fourth state of consciousness which is the witness of the other three states.

आभोग = rapturous experience: सम्भवः Lit. production, coming into existence; but abiding, remaining in this context. "Even during the three different states of consciousness in waking, dreaming and profound sleep, the rapturous experience of I-consciousness of the fourth state abides."

COMMENTARY

TEXT

समनन्तरनिरूपयिष्यमाणानां जाग्रत्स्वप्नसुषुप्तानां भेदे नानारूपे पृथक्त्वावभासे 'उद्यमो भैरवः' (१–५) इति लक्षितस्य स्फुरत्तात्मनः सर्वदशानुस्यूतस्य तुर्यस्य य आभोगश्चमत्कारः तस्य संभवो नित्यमेव तुर्यचमत्कारमयत्वं प्रोक्तमहायोगयुक्तस्य भवतीत्यर्थः । केचित् संभव इत्यत्र संविदिति स्पष्टार्थं पठन्ति ।

TRANSLATION

Even when there is *bheda* i.e. even when there is appearance of difference in the states of consciousness in waking, dreaming, and profound sleep which are to be expounded soon after, the rapturous experience of I-consciousness[1] of the fourth state[2] indicated in the *sūtra* 'udyamo bhairavaḥ', which is a glow of the inner light and which runs uninterruptedly in all the states abides permanently in the experient who is united with the Śiva-consciousness by the great *Yoga* already described (i.e. by *Śāmbhava Yoga* or *upāya*). Some adopt the reading *Saṁvid* in place of *sambhava*, the meaning of which is perfectly clear (i.e. in that case the meaning would be, there abides the *experience* (saṁvid) of the rapture of I-consciousness of the fourth state).

NOTES

1. *Ābhoga* is *camatkāra* i.e. the joyous, rapturous I-consciousness of Śiva which is present in every body in the fourth state.

2. *Turya* = the fourth state of consciousness. It holds together the consciousness of the other three states of waking, dreaming

and profound sleep. It is the everpresent consciousness without which even the other three cannot be known as states. It is integral awareness.

TEXT

एतच्च

'यथेन्दुः पुष्पसंकाशः समन्तादवभासते ।
आह्लादनसमूहेन जगदाह्लादयेत्क्षणात् ॥
तद्वद्देवि महायोगी यदा पर्यटते महीम् ।
ज्ञानेन्दुकिरणैः सर्वैर्जंगच्चित्रं समस्तकम् ॥
आह्लादयेत्समन्तात्तदवीच्यादिशिवान्तकम् ।'

इत्यादिना श्रीचन्द्रज्ञाने जागरादौ तुर्याभोगमयत्वं महायोगिनो दर्शितम् । स्पन्दे तु

'जागरादिविभेदेऽपि .... ।'

इति कारिकया संगृहीतम् ॥ ७ ॥

TRANSLATION

In *Candrajñāna* also it has been shown in the following verse that the rapturous experience of I-consciousness of the fourth state is present in the case of the great Yogi in waking state etc.

"As the moon pure like a flower shines all round and by the assemblage of its gladdening rays gladdens the world in a trice, even so, oh goddess, (addressed to Pārvatī), a great Yogī, when he moves about in the world, gladdens all round with the rays of his moon-like spiritual awareness the entire variegated world from *avīci* (a particular hell) upto *Śiva*.

In Spandakārikā also, the same idea has been expressed in the following verse.

"Even during the occurrence of different states of consciousness like waking etc. (i.e. waking, dreaming, profound sleep), that (i.e. the consciousness of the fourth state which is *Śiva*-consciousness) continuing to be the same (*tadabhinne*), one never departs from one's natural state of being the knower or the experient (in all the states)."

EXPOSITION

In the 5th *sūtra*, it has been shown that by *Śāmbhava Yoga*, there is sudden emergence of a deeper consciousness which is *Bhairava*-consciousness, which is the I-consciousness of *Śiva*.

In this *sūtra*, the attention of the aspirant has been drawn to five important points.

(1) The fourth state of consciousness is the everpresent witnessing consciousness of all the three. Even the three states of waking, dreaming, and profound sleep could not be experienced as three different states without a consciousness, a knower that knows all the three. That fourth state is, then, our real Self. It is the everpresent, immortal *ātman*, the deathless, ceaseless consciousness that witnesses all that we feel, think, and do. It is the changeless permanent I that witnesses all our changing I's.

(2) Our states of waking, dream, and profound sleep are interrupted. When we are in the waking state, there is no dream state; when we are in the dream state, there is no awareness in that state of our waking, and when we are in the state of profound sleep, there is no awareness in that state of our waking and dreaming state.

Further, each state is due to certain conditions which are not present in the other state. In the waking state, the body, *prāṇa*, senses, and *manas* are active. In the dream state, the eye, ear, touch etc. do not work. In one word, the function of the senses stops. Their function is taken up by the mind, by imagination. In dream, we see, hear, run, eat etc.—all mentally, In it only *prāṇa* and *manas* are active.

In profound sleep, even the function of *manas* stops; only *prāṇa* functions. So, that is also a separate state altogether.

Is there then nothing that remains the same in all these differing states ?

There is, declares the *Śaiva* philosophy. It is the fourth state (*turya* or *turīya*) of consciousness which is not involved in all the three states, which stands as witnessing consciousness to all the three. It should be borne in mind that it is called the fourth with reference to the other three. The word fourth is applied to it relatively owing to the limitation of language. In reality, any numerical term cannot be applied to it. It is ever present reality.

(3) *Turya* consciousness always remains as the background of all we feel, think, and do, but we are unaware of it in our normal consciousness. It is always there. It is *siddha* i.e. eternally present, not *sādhya* i.e. it is not reality that can be produced by our effort, by any *Yogic* discipline or technique. If it were to be produced, it would no longer be eternal. It cannot be ordered about. Then why all this pother about gaining the *turya* consciousness ? What is the value of the *upāyas* or *Yogic* disciplines mentioned in the *Śiva-Sūtras* ?

The answer is that though it remains as the background of all we are and do, we are unaware of it. It is not a feature of our normal consciousness. The *upāyas* are mentioned so that we may prepare ourselves for its reception.

The *Śāmbhavopāya* is for very advanced souls whose mind is already prepared for its reception. In them, there is *ut+yama* (*udyama*). In this context *udyama* does not mean exertion as some have unfortunately interpreted it, but as Kṣemarāja points out, it means *unmajjana, udyantṛtā—emergence.* When we are prepared by righteous living and by deconditioning our habitual consciousness, the *turya* emerges from its cryptic cell, so to speak, takes possession of our normal consciousness and becomes its active feature.

(4) In the words of Kaṭhopaniṣad, it is a *prabhava* or in the words of Śiva-Sūtra (7), it is a *sambhava*, the birth of a new awareness for ourselves. In that condition, even though states of waking, dream, and deep sleep differ, it abides as a constant active awareness in all of them. It brings about a transformation of our normal consciousness. In all the differing states, there is an integral awareness. We then live *sub specie aeternitatis.*

(5) Turya consciousness in *Śaiva* philosophy is not merely *prakāśa*, not merely *Sākṣi caitanya*, witnessing consciousness as in *Śāṁkara Vedānta*, but it is also *vimarśa*, full of *turyābhoga*, i.e. of rapturous experience of the perfect consciousness of Śiva.

INTRODUCTION TO THE 8th, 9th AND 10th SŪTRAS

एतज्जाग्रदादित्रयं सूत्रत्रयेण लक्षयति—

TRANSLATION

The *sūtrakāra* defines the waking state etc. by means of the next three sūtras.

ज्ञानं जाग्रत् ॥ ८ ॥
स्वप्नो विकल्पाः ॥ ९ ॥
अविवेको मायासौषुप्तम् ॥ १० ॥

8. *Jñānaṁ Jāgrat.*
9. *Svapno vikalpāḥ.*
10. *Aviveko māyāsauṣuptam.*

8. ज्ञानम् = knowledge; जाग्रत् = waking state of consciousness.

"All knowledge obtained by direct contact with the external world is included (in a wide sense) in the category of the waking state of consciousness (when the subject is in contact with the objective world around him on any plane)."

9. स्वप्नः = dream state of consciousness. विकल्प = all ideation; all knowledge obtained by the independent activity of the mind when one is not in direct contact with the external world.

"All knowledge obtained by independent activity of the mind when the Subject is not in direct contact with the external world (around him on any plane) is included in the category of *svapna* or dreaming state of consciousness (in a wide sense)."

10. अविवेकः = The word *aviveka* has been used here in the sense of non-discernment, lack of awareness. मायासौषुप्तम् The word *māyā* has been used here in the sense of *mohamayam* (of the form of delusion).

So the sūtra means "Lack of awareness on any plane is the profound sleep of delusion."

COMMENTARY

TEXT

सर्वसाधारणार्थविषयं बाह्येन्द्रियजं ज्ञानं लोकस्य जाग्रत् जागरावस्था । ये तु मनोमात्रजन्या असाधारणार्थविषया विकल्पाः स एव स्वप्नः स्वप्ना-

वस्था; तस्य एवंविधविकल्पप्रधानत्वात्। यस्तु अविवेको विवेचनाभावोऽख्या-तिः, एतदेव मायारूपं मोहमयं सौषुप्तम् । सौषुप्तं लक्षयता प्रसङ्गात् उच्छे-द्याया मायाया अपि स्वरूपमुक्तम् ।

TRANSLATION

(Kṣemarāja at first gives the usual, conventional sense of the three states of consciousness, viz., waking, dreaming, and dreamless sleep).

The waking state of consciousness is that in which knowledge of objects is produced in people by means of the external senses and the objects have a common connotation for all.

The dream state of consciousness is that in which knowledge is produced only by the mind (without contact with the external world), which is merely a thought-construct (*vikalpāḥ*) and which has an uncommon object (i.e. which is a particular kind of knowledge for each individual). It is called dream because it is characterized by such uncommon ideation.

That which is a state of *aviveka* i.e. complete lack of awareness is delusive deep sleep. While defining *suṣupta* state, the *sūtra* incidentally describes also the nature of Māyā which is to be eliminated.

TEXT

इत्थमपि च ईदृशेनाप्यनेन लक्षणेन तिसृष्वपि जागरादिदशासु त्रैरूप्य-मस्तीति दर्शितम् । तथा चात्र यद्यत् स्वप्नदशोचितं प्रथममविकल्पकं ज्ञानं सा जागरा । ये तु तत्र विकल्पाः स स्वप्नः । तत्त्वाविवेचनं सौषुप्तम् । सौषुप्ते यद्यपि विकल्पा न संचेत्यन्ते, तथापि तत्प्रविविक्षायां तथोचितजाग्र-ज्ज्ञानमिव तदनन्तरं संस्कारकल्पविकल्परूपस्तदुचितः स्वप्नोऽप्यस्त्येव ।

(Now Kṣemarāja interprets these states of consciousness in a wider, philosophical sense)

Thus by this kind of definition, the threefold character (of these states) has been indicated in all of the three states of waking etc. (i.e. waking, dreaming, and dreamless sleep).

(To take for illustration the dreaming state of consciousness), the initial undifferentiated state of knowledge characteristic of the dream state is the waking state; the reveries that follow constitute the dreaming state; the unawareness of any reality constitutes the state of dreamless sleep.

In deep sleep, though there is no mental activity as such, yet just when one is about to enter the state of deep sleep, there is a slightly vague awareness characteristic of the state of deep sleep which may be likened to the awareness of waking state. After that there is dreaming state also inasmuch as there are *vikalpas* (reveries) in the form of their residual traces.

(Kṣemarāja now describes the three states with reference to the *Yogī*).

TEXT

किं च योग्यभिप्रायेण प्रथमं तत्तद्धारणारूपं ज्ञानं जाग्रत्, ततः तत्प्रत्यय-प्रवाहरूपा विकल्पाः स्वप्नः, ग्राह्यग्राहकभेदासंचेतनरूपश्च समाधिः सौषुप्तम्, इत्यप्यनया वचोयुक्त्या दर्शितम्। अत एव श्रीपूर्वशास्त्रे जागरादीनां परस्परानुवेधकृतो योग्यभिप्रायेणापि

'........अबुद्धं बुद्धमेव च ।
प्रबुद्धं सुप्रबुद्धं च........॥'

इत्यादिना भेदो निरूपितः ॥ ८ ॥ ९ ॥ १० ॥

TRANSLATION

With reference to the *Yogī*, at first his knowledge in the form of *dhāraṇā* or fixing the mind on particular object is his waking state, then his *vikalpas* (reverie) in the form of a continuous flow of the idea of that object of his concentration is his dream state; (finally) *Samādhi* in the form of absence of difference between the thinker and the thought is his state of deep sleep. This has been shown by an appropriate application of words.

Therefore in Pūrvaśāsıra (i.e. Mālinīvijaya tantra) the varieties of waking state etc. (i.e. dreaming and deep sleep) have been expounded by means of the transmission of one state into the other with reference to *yogi* in the following verse:

चतुर्विधं तु पिण्डस्थमबुद्धं बुद्धमेव च ।
प्रबुद्धं सुप्रबुद्धं च पदस्थं तच्चतुर्विधम् ॥

(Mālinī Vijaya, II, 43).

The experience of one staying in the objective consciousness is of four kinds, viz; *abuddha* i e. unawakened, *buddha* i.e. awakened, *prabuddha* i.e. well awakened, and *suprabuddha* i.e. perfectly well-awakened. So also there are four kinds of experience of those who are staying in *pada*, (and also of those who are staying in *rūpa*).

EXPOSITION

The wider sense of dreaming, deep sleep as given in the text is quite clear, But Mālinīvijaya quoted by Kṣemarāja gives certain other details which require clarification.

According to Mālinīvijaya, the various states of waking, dream etc. are to be ascertained with reference to the *pramātā*, the knower or the subject. Whenever an object is known only as an external object, (*prameya*) i.e. when it is the objective side that is mostly prominent, we have the state of waking consciousness. It may be called *jāgrat-jāgrat* state, since it is a waking condition in an actual waking state. From the stand-point of the *Yogī*, it is an *abuddha* or unawakened state.

When in the waking state, it is not so much the external object but the knowledge (*pramāṇa*) of the object which is prominent in consciousness, it is the *jāgrat-svapna* state i.e. it is a kind of dream during the waking state. From the stand-point of the *Yogī*, it is the *buddha* or awakened state.

When in the waking state, it is the *pramātā*, the knower or the subject who is prominent in consciousness, then it is a state of *jāgrat-suṣupti* i.e. the knower is awake with regard to the subject, but asleep with regard to the object. From the yogic standpoint, it is *prabuddha* or well-awakened state.

When in the waking state, there is predominance only of consciousness as such (*pramiti*) it is known as the *jāgrat-turya* state. From the *yogic* standpoint, it is called *suprabuddha* state i.e. perfectly awakened state.

From the standpoint of the common man, all these pertain to *jāgrat-avasthā*. The *Yogīs* call all these states as *piṇḍastha*, i.e. states referring to the objective side. The *jñānīs* (those who have complete Śiva -consciousness) call this state *sarvatobhadra*, because according to them, the entire objective world is full of the glory of divine existence; the entire manifestation is an expression of Śiva, a play of *saṁvid* or consciousness.

Now let us take up the four states in *svapna* (dream). The common characteristics of the dream state are that (1) it is a plane of *vikalpas* i.e. ideas, fancies, reveries and that (2) it is *abāhya* i.e. independent of the external world, confined only to the dreamer.

When the dream world fabricated by the *vikalpas* (ideation) appears in dream as very clear, precise and stationary, it is the state of *svapna-jāgrat* (waking condition in dream). Mālinīvijaya calls it *gatāgata*, because in this state the movement of *prāṇa* and *apāna* is very prominent on account of which the dream-world appears to be very clear.

When in the dream state, the entire dream-phenomena appear to be hazy, vague, and disorderly, then it is known as *svapna-svapna* i.e. a dreamy condition within the dream state. Mālinī-vijaya calls this state *suvikṣipta*, because the dream-phenomena are in this state chaotic, disorderly.

When in the dream state, the dreamer is able to establish a clear connexion between one dream object and another, then it is called *svapna-suṣupti*, because the dreamer enjoys full, peaceful sleep without feeling any incongruity among his dream-objects. The *jñānins* call this state *saṁgata*, because the dreamer feels in this kind of dream a congruity or consistency among his dream-objects.

When during the entire phantasmagoria of his dream state, the dreamer does not lose hold of his self-consciousness, when he is fully aware of himself and knows that he is only dreaming, then this state is known as *svapna-turya*. This is also called *susamāhita* state, because in this state the dreamer is a fully integrated individual.

To the common man, the dream state is just a *svapna* or dream state in which he views the various *vikalpas* of his dream without any contact with the external world.

The *Yogī* includes all these four states in one blanket term, called *padastha*, because by means of *yoga*, he abides in the *pada* or state of his own Self in all these conditions. *Gatāgata*, *suvikṣipta*, *saṁgata* and *susamāhita* are only phases of the *padastha* state.

As already said, from the point of view of the *Yogīs*, this is a *padastha* state. From the point of view of the *jñānī*, this is a state of *vyāpti* or pervasion, for the *jñānī* experiences the pervasion of his own being in all these phases of the dream state.

Let us now take up the *suṣupti* state, the state of profound sleep. There are four phases of this also. First of all, there is the *suṣupti-jāgrat*, waking in deep sleep. This is also called *udita* (risen), because in this there is the residual impression of the entire objective world in a latent form.

The *Susupti-svapna* state is known as *vipula* in the *tantras*. The word *vipula* means thick, increased. This state is called *vipula*, because in this state the residual traces of the experience of the objective world are fostered so that they become stronger.

The *suṣupti-suṣupti* of this state is known as *śānta* in the *tantras*, because the residual traces of objective experience become subdued and tranquil.

The *suṣupti-turya* state is known as *suprasanna* in the *tantras*, because in this state the *yogī* enters the full I-consciousness of Śiva and is full of peace and joy.

So there are four phases of the *rūpastha* state of the *Yogī*, viz; *udita*, *vipula*, *śānta*, and *suprasanna*.

Briefly it may be said that the waking state is that in which the aspect of the known or the objective experience is prominent, the dream state is that in which knowledge or mentation is prominent, and *suṣupti* or dreamless state is that in which the knower or the subject aspect is prominent.

In the *turya* state, there are only three phases, viz. *turya-jāgrat*, *turya-svapna* and *turya-suṣupti*.

The *turya-jāgrat* is that state in which mind as we know it retires completely. Its function ceases and the *Super-mind* becomes active. This is called *manonmana*. In this state, the activity of the normal mind stops, and *unmanā* or *Super-mind* supervenes.

Turya-svapna is that state in which the *Yogī* crosses the boundary of limitation (of knowledge) and enters the region of unlimitedness (of knowledge). Hence in the *tantras*, it is called *ananta*, i.e. unlimited.

Turya-suṣupti is known as *sarvārtha* in the *tantras*, because in this state every thing appears as a form of divine *Śakti*.

There is no such phase as *turya-turya*.

In *turya* state, the aspirant is identified with *Śiva*-consciousness. The common man simply calls it the *turya* or fourth state, because it is beyond the three known states of waking, dream, and deep sleep. He has no experience of the *turya* state. The *yogī* calls it *rūpātīta*, because in this state, the common form of both the object and the subject is transcended. The *jñānī* calls it *pracaya* which means collectivity, because in this condition, the *jñānī* sees everything steeped in the sap of divine delight.

Turyātīta is that state which is full of uninterrupted divine rapture of I-consciousness. There is no question of phases of this state. It is the state of fullest realization. There is no need of any *Yogic* practice now. The *jñānī* calls this state *mahāpracaya*. In it even the distinction between the transcendent and the immanent disappears. To one who has entered this state, everything is *Śiva*.

INTRODUCTION TO THE 11th SŪTRA

TEXT

एवं लोकयोग्यनुसारेण व्याख्याते जागरादित्रये शक्तिचक्रसंधानाद्विश्वसंहारेण यस्य तुर्याभोगमयत्वमभेदव्याप्त्यात्मकं स्फुरति स तद्धाराधिरोहेण तुर्यातीतं पूर्वोक्तं चैतन्यमाविशन्——

TRANSLATION

Thus the *Yogī* in whom the rapturous experience of I-consciousness which is full of the consciousness of non-difference shines through the cancellation of the universe (as something separate from consciousness) by the process of uniting with the group of *Śaktis* through constant awareness in all the three states of waking, dream, and deep sleep which have been explained both from the point of view of the common folk and the *yogī*, enters the *turyātīta* state (i.e. the state beyond the *turya*) which has been previously described as *caitanya* by following up the stream (of that rapturous experience of I-consciousness) (He is then).

Sūtra—11

त्रितयभोक्ता वीरेशः ॥ ११ ॥

Tritayabhoktā vīreśaḥ

त्रितय = triad; भोक्ता = enjoyer; वीरेशः = master of the senses.

"Being an enjoyer of the rapture of I-consciousness in the triad (of waking, dreaming and deep sleep), he is verily the master of his senses.

COMMENTARY

एतज्जागरादित्रयं शक्तिचक्रानुसंधानयुक्त्या तुर्यानन्दाच्छुरितं यः तत्परामर्शानुप्रवेशप्रकर्षाद्विगलितभेदसंस्कारमानन्दरसप्रवाहमयमेव पश्यति स त्रितयस्यास्य भोक्ता चमत्कर्ता ।

तत एव

'त्रिषु धामसु यद्भोग्यं भोक्ता यश्च प्रकीर्तितः ।
वेदैतदुभयं यस्तु स भुञ्जानो न लिप्यते ॥'

इति नीत्या निःसपत्नस्वात्मसाम्राज्योऽयं परमानन्दपरिपूर्णो भवभेदग्रसनप्रवणानां वीराणामिन्द्रियाणामीश्वरः स्वामी; श्रीमन्थानभैरवसत्तानुप्रविष्टो महाम्नायेषूच्यते । यस्तु एवंविधो न भवति स जागराद्यवस्थाभिर्भुज्यमानो लौकिकः पशुरेव । योग्यपि इमां धारामनधिरूढो न वीरेश्वरः; अपि तु मूढ एवेत्युक्तं भवति ।

TRANSLATION

Whoever observes this triad of waking etc. as steeped in the delight of the fourth state by means of the awareness of his union with the multitude of *śaktis*, as full of the flow of the experience of delight, as that in which all the residual traces of difference have been dissolved by the intensity of the joyous experience of the fourth state, he becomes the enjoyer of the rapture of the divine I-consciousness in all the three states.

Therefore,

"He who (as witnessing consciousness) knows both what is said to be the object of experience and the subject of experience in all the three states is not tainted (with the condition of these) even while he is aware of both the subject and the object."

In this way, he enjoys unrivalled Self-sovereignty, is full of the highest bliss, and becomes the master of his senses[1] (vīrāṇām) that are (now) intent upon dissolving all worldly differences.

In the *mahāmnāyas*[2] (great scriptures), he is said to have entered the being of Manthāna Bhairava.[3]

One who is not of this sort becomes an object of enjoyment of the forces of the waking and other states, and remains simply the usual empirical subject. Even a *yogī* who has not risen up along this stream cannot be the master of his senses; he will remain only a confounded being. This is what is meant to be said.

NOTES

1. *Vīrāṇām* : of the senses. When the senses function ordinarily in common life, they are merely *vṛttis* i.e. modes of acquiring objective (in the case of the outer senses) and subjective (in the case of the *manas*) experience. When, however, the subject consciously acquires the experience of the fourth state, then his senses become *śaktis* i.e. divine powers intent on abolishing all sense of difference. They are not merely *indriyas*, but *vīras* now. The experient now becomes their master. He uses them for the higher purpose of life, and is no longer used by them.

2. *Mahāmnāyas* : *Śaiva* Philosophy has been expounded from three standpoints viz. (1) from the predominantly *abheda* or non-difference point of view. The *śāstras* of this stand-point are known as Bhairava *śāstras*. These are also called *mahāmnāyas* (great scriptures). These are 4 in number; (2) from the predominantly *bhedābheda* point of view (from the standpoint of identity in difference). The *śāstras* of this standpoint are known as *Rudra Śāstras*. They are 18 in number; (3) from the predominantly *bheda* (difference) point of view. The *śāstras* of this standpoint are known as *Śiva Śāstras*. They are 10 in number.

3. Manthāna Bhairava— one who churns the objective experience, withdraws it in himself and then again brings it forth, one who has *svātantrya*-absolute freedom of knowing and doing everything.

TEXT

एतच्च

'योगी स्वच्छन्दयोगेन स्वच्छन्दगतिचारिणा
स स्वच्छन्दपदे युक्तः स्वच्छन्दसमतां व्रजेत् ।'

इत्यादिना श्रीस्वच्छन्दादिशास्त्रेषु वितत्य दर्शितम् । स्पन्देऽपि
'तस्योपलब्धिः सततं त्रिपदाव्यभिचारिणी ।'
इति कारिकया संगृहीतमेतत् ॥ ११ ॥

TRANSLATION

This point has been explained in detail in *Svacchanda Śāstra*[1] etc.[2] in the following and other verses:

"The *Yogī*[3] functioning freely by means of *svacchanda yoga* is united with the status of *Svacchanda*[4] and acquires equality with *Svacchanda*." (VII, 260)

The same idea has been expressed in the following verse in *Spandakārikā* :

"The consciousness of the Highest Self abides in the *Suprabuddha* (perfectly well-awakened person) in all the three states of waking, dream, and deep sleep without any interruption." (I,17).

NOTES

1. *Svachanda śāstra* is known as *Svacchanda Tantra.*
2. Etc. includes *Vijñānabhairava, Spandakārikā.*
3. *Svacchanda Yoga.* This means union with *Svātantrya*, the Divine I-consciousness which is the quintessential nature of *Śiva.*
4. *Svacchanda*—the absolute Free Will of Bhairava.

EXPOSITION

Those who are united with the *turya* consciousness enjoy the rapturous I-consciousness of *Śiva* in all the states of waking, dreaming, and deep sleep, and acquire full control over their senses.

Even a *Yogī*, if he has not realized the *turya*-consciousness, will find himself identified with the three states of consciousnes, and will not be able to acquire full control over his senses.

Bhāskara in his *Vārttika* interprets *tritaya* as the three *guṇas*, but as *tritaya* comes immediately after *jāgrat*, *svapna* and *suṣupti*, it is better to interpret it as three states of consciousness as *Ksemarāja* has done.

INTRODUCTION TO THE 12th SŪTRA

TEXT

किमस्य महायोगिनः काश्चित् तत्त्वाधिरोहप्रत्यासन्ना भूमिकाः सन्ति ? याभिस्तत्त्वोर्ध्ववर्तिनी भूमिर्लक्ष्यते । सन्ति, इत्याह—

TRANSLATION

In the experience of that great *yogī*, are there certain stations closely connected with his ascent to Reality through which a high position in the *tattvas* (i.e. the 36 creative principles) may be marked. There are, says the present *sūtra*

Sūtra-12

विस्मयो योगभूमिकाः ॥ १२ ॥

Vismayo Yogabhūmikāḥ.

विस्मयः = fascinating wonder.
योगभूमिकाः = the stations and stages of *yoga*.
The stations and stages of *yoga* constitute a fascinating wonder.

COMMENTARY

TEXT

यथा सातिशयवस्तुदर्शने कस्यचित् विस्मयो भवति तथा अस्य महायोगिनो नित्यं तत्तद्वेद्यावभासामर्शाभोगेषु निःसामान्यातिशयनवनवचमत्कारचिद्घनस्वात्मावेशवशात् स्मेरस्मेरस्तिमितविकसितसमस्तकरणचक्रस्य यो विस्मयोऽनवच्छिन्नानन्दे स्वात्मनि अपरितृप्तत्वेन मुहुर्मुहुराश्चर्यायमाणता; ता एव योगस्य परतत्त्वैक्यस्य संबन्धिन्यो भूमिकाः; तदध्यारोहविश्रान्तिसूचिकाः परिमिता भूमयो, न तु कन्दबिन्द्वाद्यनुभववृत्तयः । तदुक्तं श्रीकुलयुक्तौ

'आत्मा चैवात्मना ज्ञातो यदा भवति साधकैः ।
तदा विस्मयमात्मा वै आत्मन्येव प्रपश्यति ॥'

इति । एतच्च

'तमधिष्ठातृभावेन स्वभावमवलोकयन् ।
स्मयमान इवास्ते यस्तस्येयं कुसृतिः कुतः ॥

इति कारिकया संगृहीतम् ॥ १२ ॥

TRANSLATION

As a person is struck with wonder by seeing something extraordinary, even so there is a pleasant surprise for the great *yogī* who notices in mute wonder an expansion (in the power) of his entire complex of senses, as they come fully under the influence of the inner Self which is a mass of consciousness and full of unique, pre-eminent and ever-new delight of I-consciousness which blossoms forth in the experience of the various objects of perception. The *yogī* has this experience in himself that is full of uninterrupted joy—a joy with which he never feels satiated. This facinating wonder betokens the various stations and stages of *yoga* which means communion with the Highest Reality. These are definite stations indicative of the repose of the *yogī* in the higher consciousness during the powers of his ascent to the Highest Reality, not experiences which one may notice in *mūlādhāra*[1] or the psychic centre[2] between the eyebrows.

The same idea has been expressed in *Kulayukti* (in the following verse):

"When aspirants realize the Self by themselves, then the Self experiences a pleasant surprise within itself."

The same idea has also been expressed in the following verse in Spandakārikā:

"How can there be the wretched transmigratory existence for him who observing his Self as the presiding power over every thing abides (in that consciousness) full of pleasant surprise." (I,11)

NOTES

1. *Mūlādhāra* : This is a psychic centre at the root of the spinal column below the genitals. This has been called *Kanda* in the text.

2. Psychic centre between the eye-brows refers to Ājñā Cakra. This has been called *vindu* in the text.

The author means to say that the experience in these centres is inferior to the experience of the full-blown I-consciousness of *Śiva.*

INTRODUCTION TO THE 13th SŪTRA

TEXT

ईदृग्योगभूमिकासमापन्नस्यास्य योगिनः—

TRANSLATION

Of the *yogī* who has reached the station of this kind.

Sūtra-13

इच्छा शक्तिरुमा कुमारी ॥ १३ ॥

Icchā śaktir umā kumārī.

इच्छाशक्ति := Will power उमा = Light or splendour of Śiva. (श्रोः शिवस्य मा लक्ष्मीरिव—mā, meaning *Lakṣmī* and 'u' meaning *Śiva* i.e. splendour of Śiva).
कुमारी—unwedded maiden; virgin.

The Will-power of the *yogī* who is in communion with Śiva is *Umā* (splendour of Śiva) who is Kumārī.

COMMENTARY

(Kṣemarāja interprets this sūtra from three standpoints—(1) *abheda* i.e. non-difference or identity (2) *bhedābheda* i.e. identity in difference (3) *bheda* i.e. difference or dualistic standpoint).

TEXT

योगिनः परभैरवतां समापन्नस्य या इच्छा सा शक्तिरुमा; परैव पारमेश्वरी स्वातन्त्र्यरूपा, सा च कुमारी विश्वसर्गसंहारक्रीडापरा 'कुमार क्रीडायाम्' इति पाठात् ।

TRANSLATION

(This interpretation is from the *abheda* or nondualistic standpoint. It is in accordance with *Śāmbhavopāya*).

The will-power of the *Yogī* who has reached the status of the Highest Bhairava is *Umā* i.e. the highest *svātantrya śakti*[1] of the Lord. This *Śakti* is *Kumārī* i.e. intent on the play of manifesting the universe and (finally) withdrawing it (within Herself). This interpretation is based on the root 'kumāra' (of the uṇādi class, Kumārayati), meaning to play.

NOTES

1. *Svātantrya Śakti* is ever present I-consciousness of Śiva which is absolutely free in knowing and doing every thing.

TEXT

अथ च कुं भेदोत्थापिकां मायाभूमिं मारयति अनुद्भिन्नप्रसरां करोति तच्छीला । कुमारी च परानुपभोग्या भोक्त्रैकात्म्येन स्फुरन्ती ।

TRANSLATION

(Now *Kṣemarāja* interprets the *sūtra* from the *bhedābheda* point of view. It is in accordance with *Śāktopāya*). Or *Ku* may mean the state of Māyā which brings about a sense of difference, and *mārī* may mean one who destroys i.e. one who does not allow the power of Māyā to spread. So *Kumārī* is one whose nature is of this sort. *Kumārī* (virgin) is one who remains always in the state of *bhoktrī* or enjoyer (bhoktraikātmyenasphurantī), never a *bhogyā* i.e. never to be enjoyed by others (parairanupabhogyā).

TEXT

अथवा यथा उमा कुमारी परिहृतसर्वासङ्गा महेश्वरैकात्म्यसाधनाराधनाय नित्योद्युक्ता तथैव अस्येच्छा, इत्यस्मद्गुरुभिरित्थमेव पाठो दृष्टो व्याख्यातश्च ।

TRANSLATION

(Now *Kṣemarāja* interprets the *sūtra* from the stand point of *bheda* or difference. This is in accordance with *āṇavopāya*).

Or as virgin *Umā* abandoning all attachment was always engaged in her devotion which may bring about her union with lord *Śiva*, even so is the will of this *yogī*. My revered teacher found this reading also and interpreted it in this way also. This reading would be (*Yoginaḥ*) *Icchā Kumārī Umāśaktiḥ*.

TEXT

अन्यैस्तु 'शक्तितमा' इति पठित्वा ज्ञानक्रियापेक्षोऽस्याः प्रकर्षो व्याख्यातः। एवं न लौकिकवत् अस्य योगिनः स्थूलेच्छा, अपि तु परा शक्तिरूपैव सर्वत्राप्रतिहता । तदुक्तं श्रीमत्स्वच्छन्दे

'सा देवी सर्वदेवीनां नामरूपैश्च तिष्ठति ।
योगमायाप्रतिच्छन्ना कुमारी लोकभाविनी ॥'

इति । श्रीमृत्युञ्जयभट्टारकेऽपि

'सा ममेच्छा परा शक्तिरवियुक्ता स्वभावजा ।
वह्नेरूष्मेव विज्ञेया रश्मिरूपा रवेरिव ॥
सर्वस्य जगतो वापि सा शक्तिः कारणात्मिका ॥

इति । तदेतत्

'नहीच्छानोदनस्यायं प्रेरकत्वेन वर्तते ।
अपि त्वात्मबलस्पर्शात्पुरुषस्तत्समो भवेत् ॥'

इति कारिकया भङ्ग्या प्रतिपादितम् ॥ १३ ॥

TRANSLATION

Others adopt the reading (*Icchā Śaktitamā Kumārī*)[1] and thus interpret the *sūtra* as pointing out the superiority of Wili over cognition and conation. Thus the desire of such a *yogī* is not coarse like that of the common folk, but it is like *parāśakti* itself, unimpeded everywhere. The same idea has been expressed in the following verse in *Svacchanda Tantra* also:

"That highest Divine *Śakti* abides in all the goddesses in different names and forms, remains concealed by the *yogamāyā*[2], is a virgin, and fulfils the desire of all people (X, Verse 727).

In *Mṛtyuñjaya*[3] also, it has been said, "That Highest Śakti is only my Will power, inseparable from me. She should be considered as natural to me. She is to be known (in the same relation to me), as heat to the fire and rays to the sun. That Śakti is the cause of the entire world." (I, 25-26)

The same idea has been expressed in another way in the following verse of Spandakārikā.

"A person cannot become the impeller of the goad of desire by himself. It is only by contact with the power residing in the Self that he can be like that Self." (I, 8)

NOTES

1. *Bhāskara* adopts this reading in his *Vārttika*.
2. *Yogamāyā* means māyā that has the power of veiling the

essential nature. This *māyā-śakti* arises by Yoga. i.e. by identification with the Highest Reality.

3. *Mṛtyuñjaya* is another name for *Netratantra*.

EXPOSITION

Kṣemarāja interprets this *Sūtra* from three standpoints. From the standpoint of (1) *abheda* (non-difference) he interprets *Icchā* (of the great *Yogī*) as identical (*abhinna*) with the *svātantrya śakti* of *Śiva*, and *Kumārī* as that *svātantrya śakti* engaged in the play of bringing about the manifestation and withdrawal of the universe. This explanation is in accordance with *Śāmbhavopāya*. From the standpoint of (2) *bhedābheda*, he shows that the Icchā is designated as Kumārī, because the consciousness of difference (*bheda*) brought about by Māyā (*ku*) is destroyed by her (*mārī*). So this shows the *abheda* of *Icchā* with *Śiva* in the midst of the difference brought about by *Māyā*. This explanation is in accordance with *Śāktopāya*. From the standpoint of *bheda*, he shows that just as *Kumārī Umā* was always intent on being united with *Śiva*, so the *Icchā* of the *Yogī* is always intent on being united with *Śiva*. This explanation is in accordance with *āṇavopāya*. In the concluding portion of his commentary on this *sūtra*, *Kṣemarāja* shows his preference for its interpretation from the *abheda* standpoint.

INTRODUCTION TO THE 14th SŪTRA

TEXT

ईदृशस्य महेच्छस्य—

TRANSLATION

Of such a kind of *Yogī* who has developed the great Will power.

Sūtra—14*th*

दृश्यं शरीरम् ॥ १४ ॥

Dṛśyaṁ Śarīram.

दृश्यम्—all phenomena outer or inner.

शरीरम्—(are like his own) body.

All objective phenomena outer or inner are like his own body.

COMMENTARY

TEXT

यद्यद् दृश्यं बाह्यमाभ्यन्तरं वा, तत्तत् सर्वम् 'अहमिदम्' इति-सदाशिववन्महासमापत्त्या स्वाङ्गकल्पमस्य स्फुरति; न भेदेन ।

शरीरं च देहधीप्राणशून्यरूपं नीलादिवद् दृश्यं; न तु पशुवद्द्रष्टृतया भाति । एवं देहे बाह्ये च सर्वत्रास्य मयूराण्डरसवदविभक्तैव प्रतिपत्तिर्भवति । यथोक्तं श्रीविज्ञानभैरवे

'जलस्येवोर्मयो वह्नेर्ज्वालाभङ्ग्यः प्रभा रवेः ।
ममैव भैरवस्यैता विश्वभङ्ग्यो विनिर्गताः ॥'

इति । एतच्च

'भोक्तैव भोग्यभावेन सदा सर्वत्र संस्थितः ।'

इत्यनेन संगृहीतम् ॥ १४ ॥

TRANSLATION

(*Kṣemarāja* interprets this *sūtra* in two ways. The first interpretation is based on *dṛśyaṁ śarīram*).

"Whatever is perceptible whether inwardly or outwardly, all that appears to this *Yogī* like his own body, i.e. identical with himself and not as something different from him. This is so because of his great accomplishment (of identity with the Universal consciousness). His feeling is 'I am this', just as the feeling of *Sadāśiva* with regard to the entire universe is 'I am this'.

(Now Kṣemarāja's interpretation of this sūtra is based on *Śarīraṁ dṛśyam*).

To the Yogī, the body appears as an objective perceptible phenomenon like blue etc, and not like a perceiver as in the case of the ignorant empirical beings, whether that body is in the form of *deha* or the physical body (as in waking consciousness), or in the form of *dhī* or the mind (as in dream) or *prāṇa* (as in deep sleep) or as *śūnya* or mere void (as in the case of the *śūnya-pramātā*).

So, in the body and in everything external, his awareness is one of undifferentiated consciousness as the plasma of the peacock's egg is undifferentiated plasma.

As has been said in *Vijñānabhairava* :

"Just as waves are modes of water, sparks of fire, light of the sun, even so the various modes of the universe have gone out of me, viz., Bhairava." (Verse 110)

The same idea has been expressed in the following line of Spandakārikā;

"The experient himself continues in the form of the object of experience always and everywhere." (II,4)

INTRODUCTION TO THE 15th SŪTRA

TEXT

यच्चेदं सर्वस्य दृश्यस्य शरीरतया, शून्यान्तस्य च दृश्यतया, एकरूपं प्रकाशनमुक्तं नैतत् दुर्घटम् ; अपि तु—

TRANSLATION

It has been said that all perceptible phenomena right up to the void appears to the *Yogī* uniformly like his own body. This is not impossible, Rather,

Sūtra—15

हृदये चित्तसंघट्टाद्दृश्यस्वापदर्शनम् ॥ १५ ॥

Hṛdaye cittasaṁghaṭṭād dṛśyasvāpadarśanam.

हृदये—on the core of consciousness; चित्तसंघट्टात् 'by meeting or union of the mind; दृश्यस्वापदर्शनम् there is the appearance of an observable phenomena and even a state of void as a form of consciousness.

"When the mind is united to the core of consciousness, every observable phenomenon and even the void appear as a form of consciousness".

COMMENTARY

TEXT

विश्वप्रतिष्ठास्थानत्वात् चित्प्रकाशो हृदयं; तत्रसंघट्टात् चलतश्चलतः तदेकाग्रभावनात् दृश्यस्य, नीलदेहप्राणबुद्ध्यात्मनः; स्वापस्य च, एतदभावरूपस्य शून्यस्य; दर्शनं, त्यक्तग्राह्यग्राहकविभेदेन यथावस्तु स्वाङ्गकल्पतया प्रकाशनं भवति । चित्प्रकाशतामभिनिविशमानं हि चित्तं तदाच्छुरितमेव विश्वं पश्यति । तदुक्तं श्रीविज्ञानभैरवे

'हृद्याकाशे निलीनाक्षः पद्मसंपुटमध्यगः ।
अनन्यचेताः सुभगे परं सौभाग्यमाप्नुयात्' ॥

इति । परं हि अत्र सौभाग्यं विश्वेश्वरतापत्तिः । तत्त्ववृत्तिसमापन्नं महायोगिनमुद्दिश्य श्रीमत्स्वच्छन्देऽपि

'स च भूतेषु सर्वेषु भावतत्त्वेन्द्रियेषु च ।
स्थावरं जङ्गमं चैव चेतनाचेतनं स्थितम् ॥
अध्वानं व्याप्य सर्वं तु सामरस्येन संस्थितः ।'

इति । स्पन्दे तु

'तथा स्वात्मन्यधिष्ठानात्सर्वत्रैवं भविष्यति ॥ ३६ (कारिका)

इत्यनेनैव एतत्संगृहीतम् ॥ १५ ॥

TRANSLATION

Hṛdaya (in this context) means the light of consciousness inasmuch as it is the foundation of the entire universe.

Cittasaṁghaṭṭāt means the concentration of the fickle mind on that (foundational consciousness), *Dṛśyasya* means 'of all objective phenomena like blue, body, *prāṇa* and mind.'

Svāpasya[1] means of the void i.e. of the absence of every objective phenomenon.

Darśanam means the appearance of everything as it is in its essential reality devoid of the distinction between subject and object like a component of oneself.[2] (The sum and substance of the whole *sūtra* is):—

The individual mind intently entering into the universal light of foundational consciousness sees the entire universe as saturated with that consciousness.

The same thing has been said in *Vijñānabhairava* :

"He whose mind together with the other senses is merged in the ether of the heart, who has entered mentally into the centre of the two bowls of the heart-lotus[3], who has excluded everything else from consciousness acquires the highest fortune, O beautiful one." (Verse 49)

Here the highest fortune refers to the acquisition of the lordship of the universe.

Svacchanda Tantra also referring to the great *Yogī* who has attained to the state of highest Reality says:

"He who has realized his identity with the Highest Reality pervading the two aspects (*adhvā*) (of *Varṇa*, *pada*, and *mantra*, and *kalā*, *tattva* and *bhuvana*) manifest in the unconscious entities like the unmoving ones and conscious beings like the moving ones abides as identical with Bhairava in all beings, objects, *tattvas* like earth etc. and the senses." (IV, verse 310).

The same idea has been expressed in the following verse in *Spandakārikā*:

"As when the *Spanda* principle pervades the body then all knowledge and action appropriate to that condition are possible, even so if he abides in his Real Self, his omniscience and omnipotence can function everywhere." (III, 7).

NOTES

1. *Kṣemarāja* has taken the word *svāpa* in the sense of the void. *Svāpa*, according to him, is complete absence of objectivity.

2. *Kṣemarāja* has interpreted the word *darśanam* in the sense of *abhedadarśanam* i.e. by concentrating on Central Reality one sees all phenomena as non-different from the Universal consciousness.

3. *Padmasampuṭamadhyagaḥ* : In his commentary on Vijñānabhairava, Sivopādhyāya says that one bowl of the heart lotus is *pramāṇa* (knowledge), the other bowl is *prameya* (objects), *madhya* or centre of this heart lotus is *pramātā* (the knower i.e. the Self). It is in this centre i.e. the Self into which one has to plunge mentally. 'This is Śāktopāya.'

EXPOSITION

The 14th *Sūtra* says that to the *Yogī* in whom Icchāśakti (Will Power) has been developed, the entire objective world including the body appears as a form of consciousness.

The 15th *Sūtra* says that the above is not merely a metaphysical chimera. If the individual mind is united with the Central, foundational consciousness, if the *citta* (the individual mind) is brought into communion with *Cit* (the Universal consciousness) which is the core of Reality, one can find for oneself that the objective world is only an expression of that Consciousness. Then the consciousness of the individual is steeped in the universal consciousness and the sense of difference disappears. This describes a *Śāktopāya* for being established in the Universal Consciousness.

Just as in the plasma of the peacock's egg, there is one uniform liquid without any differentiation, even so for the realization of universal Consciousness, the differentiation between subject and object, object and object disappears.

INTRODUCTION TO THE 16th SŪTRA

TEXT

अत्रैव उपायान्तरमाह—

TRANSLATION

Another means for acquiring Śiva-Consciousness is described below :—

Sūtra—16

शुद्धतत्त्वसंधानाद्वाऽपशुशक्तिः ॥ १६ ॥

Śuddha-tattva-sandhānād vā apaśuśaktiḥ.

वा = or.

शुद्धतत्त्व = the Pure Principle i.e. the Highest *Śiva.*

संधानात् = by constant awareness.

अपशुशक्तिः = he becomes like one in whom the binding power existing in the limited self is absent.

Or by constant awarenes of the Pure Principle, he becomes like one in whom the binding power existing in the limited self is absent.

COMMENTARY

TEXT

शुद्धं तत्त्वं परमशिवाख्यं, तत्र यदा विश्वमनुसंधत्ते 'तन्मयमेव एतत्' इति, तदा अविद्यमाना पश्वाख्या बन्धशक्तिर्यस्य तादृगयं तदाशिववत् विश्वस्य जगतः पतिर्भवति । तदुक्तं श्रीमल्लक्ष्मीकौलार्णवे

'दीक्षासिद्धौ तु ये प्रोक्ताः प्रत्ययाः स्तोभपूर्वकाः ।
संधानस्यैव ते देवि कलां नार्हन्ति षोडशीम् ॥'

इति । श्रीविज्ञानभैरवे तु

सर्वं देहं चिन्मयं हि जगद्वा परिभावयेत् ।
युगपन्निर्विकल्पेन मनसा, परमोद्भवः ॥'

इति । तदेतत्

'इति वा यस्य संवित्तिः क्रीडात्वेनाखिलं जगत् ।
स पश्यन्सततं युक्तो जीवन्मुक्तो न संशयः ॥'

इति कारिकया संगृहीतम् ॥ १६ ॥

TRANSLATION

Śuddha tattva means *Parama Śiva* or the Highest *Śiva,* the Absolute Principle, when in that (i.e. Pure Principle of Śiva or Absolute Consciousness), he (i.e. the aspirant) becomes aware of the universe as that itself i.e. as Śiva, then he becomes the lord of the world like Sadāśiva, and like him becomes *a-paśuśakti* i.e. one in whom the binding power designated by *paśu* (*paśvākhyā bandhaśakti*) is absent (*avidyamānā*).

The same idea has been expressed in *Lakṣmīkaulārṇava* in the following verse :

"O goddess, all the religious disciplines together with joyful exclamations of praise which are prescribed for the success of initiation are not worth even the sixteenth part of that awareness which is centred on you."

In *Vijñāna-bhairava* also, it is said :

"One should consider the entire body or the entire world simultaneously without thought-construct as a form of consciousness, then he will experience the emergence of the highest consciousness." (Verse 63). (This is *Śāktopāya*).

The same idea has also been expressed in the following verse in Spandakārikā :

"He who knows thus (i.e. it is the experient himself who appears in the form of the object of experience), and regards the whole world as play (of the Divine), being ever united (with the universal consciousness) is, without doubt, liberated even while alive." (II, 5). (This again is Śāktopāya).

NOTES

The *Vārttika* of *Bhāskara* splits this *sūtra* into two different ones, viz., *Śuddha-tattva-sandhānāt vā* (16) and *svapada-śaktiḥ* (17). The first means "By intensive awareness of the pure principle i.e. Śiva, one acquires Śiva-consciousness." The second means "*Svapada*=*Śiva*; his *Śakti* is *jñāna* and *kriyā*". The first refers to *Śiva-caitanya*; the second refers to *Śakti-caitanya.* There is no special point in splitting the 16th *sūtra* into two different ones.

INTRODUCTION TO THE 17th SŪTRA

TEXT

ईदृग्ज्ञानरूपस्य अस्य योगिनः—

TRANSLATION

Of the yogi who has realized that the universe is only a form of Śiva.

Sūtra—17

वितर्क आत्मज्ञानम् ॥ १७ ॥

Vitarka ātmajñānam.

वितर्क=unwavering awareness.

आत्मज्ञानम्=knowledge of Self.

Note : Vitarka in this context does not mean deliberation which is merely thought-construct, but unwavering awareness, an awareness with full conviction "unwavering awareness (that I am Śiva) constitutes the knowledge of Self."

COMMENTARY

TEXT

'विश्वात्मा शिव एवास्मि' इति यो वितर्को विचारः, एतदेव अस्य आत्मज्ञानम् । तदुक्तं श्रीविज्ञानभैरवे

'सर्वज्ञः सर्वकर्ता च व्यापकः परमेश्वर : ।
स एवाहं शैवधर्मा इति दाढर्याच्छिवो भवेत् ॥'

इति । स्पन्देऽपि

'............अयमेवात्मनो ग्रहः ।'

इत्यनेन एतदुक्तम् । तत्र हि आत्मनो ग्रहणं ग्रहो ज्ञानम् एतदेव, यद्विश्वात्मकशिवाभिन्नत्वम् ; एषोऽपि अर्थो विवक्षितः ॥ १७ ॥

TRANSLATION

Of this Yogi, the unwavering awareness that I am *Śiva*, the Self of the universe constitutes the knowledge of Self. (This is *Śāktopāya*). The same idea has been expressed in *Vijñānabhairava* in the following Verse :

"The Highest Lord is omniscient, omnipotent and omnipresent. As I have the characteristic of *Śiva*, I am that very Śiva. With this strong conviction, one becomes Śiva Himself." (Verse, 102) (This is also *Śāktopāya*).

The same thing has also been said in the following verse in *Spandakārikā*;

The realization of oneself as *Śiva* is the acquisition of ambrosia. This is verily the veritable seizure of the Self. This constitutes the *dīkṣā*[2] for *Nirvāṇa* and this confers on one self the realization of one's identity with *Śiva*." (II, 7).

In this verse 'the seizure of Self' means 'the knowledge of Self' By this phrase it is also intended to express the idea that oneself is non-different from *Śiva*, the Self of the universe.

NOTES

1. Dīkṣā : *svarūpasambodhadānātmako bhedamayabandha-kṣapaṇalakṣaṇaśca saṁskāraviśeṣaḥ* (Rāmakaṇṭha) i.e. *dīkṣā* is a particular consecration ceremony for initiation into the higher life, conferring on the initiate the gift of knowing oneself, and casting away the impurity due to the sense of difference that binds oneself.

2. *Nirvāṇa* : *nirvāṇaṁ nirvṛtir-dvaitapratyayalakṣaṇakṣobha-parikṣayād ātyantikī praśāntiḥ saṁvidaḥ svasvabhāvavyavasthitiḥ* (Rāmakaṇṭha) i.e. *Nirvāṇa* is beatitude which means absolute peace resulting from the destruciton of the mental disturbance caused by harbouring belief in dualism; it is the establishment of consciousness in its natural state.

EXPOSITION

The 16th *sūtra* exhorts the aspirant to trace back the universe to its ultimate source, viz., *Śiva* and regard it as His epiphany, nay, as *Śiva* Himself.

The present *sūtra* now calls upon the aspirant to regard his Self as that very *Śiva*. The 16th *Sūtra* teaches that the objective world is in essence *Śiva*; the 17th teaches that the Subject is also *Śiva*.

This is to be realized not by *tarka* or logical reasoning, not by *vikalpa* or thought-construct, but by *vitarka* or an awareness in which all *tarka* has disappeared by an indomitable, irresistible conviction of the Self being *Śiva*.

INTRODUCTION TO THE 18th SŪTRA

TEXT

किं च अस्य—

TRANSLATION

However of this *Yogī*.

Sūtra—18

लोकानन्दः समाधिसुखम् ॥ १८ ॥

Lokānandaḥ samādhisukham.

लोक means both whatever is observed and the observer, both the subject and the object.

आनन्दः = the delight that the *Yogī* feels in abiding in his nature of a knower in respect of both.

समाधिसुखम् = (his) delight of continuously maintaining the awareness of knowership.

"The delight that the *yogī* feels in abiding in his nature as the knower in respect of both the subject and object in the world, is his delight of *samādhi*".

Note:—The word *samādhi* in this context does not mean absorption or trance. It means maintaining continuous awareness of knowership.

COMMENTARY

TEXT

लोक्यते इति लोको, वस्तुग्रामः ; लोकयति इति च लोको ग्राहकवर्गः ; तस्मिन्स्फुरति सति

'ग्राह्यग्राहकसंवित्तिः सामान्या सर्वदेहिनाम् ।
योगिनां तु विशेषोऽयं संबन्धे सावधानता ॥'

इति श्रीविज्ञानभट्टारकनिरूपितनीत्या प्रमातृपदविश्रान्त्यवधानतश्चमत्कारमयो य आनन्द एतदेव अस्य समाधिसुखम् । तदुक्तं तत्रैव

'सर्वं जगत्स्वदेहं वा स्वानन्दभरितं स्मरेत् ।
युगपत्स्वामृतेनैव परानन्दमयो भवेत् ॥'

इति । एतच्च

'इयमेवामृतप्राप्तिः . . . .।' ३२ (कारिका)

इत्यनेन संगृहीतम् ।

अथ च यत् अस्य स्वात्मारामस्य समाधिसुखं, तदेव तत्तादृशम् अवलोकयतां लोकानाम् आनन्दसंक्रमणयुक्त्या स्वानन्दाभिव्यक्तिपर्यवसायि भवति । एतदपि श्रीचन्द्रज्ञानग्रन्थेन प्रागुक्तेन (२३ पृ० सू० ७) सुसंवादम् ॥ १८ ॥

TRANSLATION

"The word *loka* has to be construed in two senses: (1) that which is perceived i.e. the multitude of objects, (2) he who perceives i.e. the class of subjects. Though this distinction of subject and object is evident in the world, the *yogī* experiences a unique delight of I-consciousness which results from his mindfulness of his repose in the state of a knower in every case. This is his *samādhi-sukha*[1] i.e. this is his delight of continuous awareness of knowership. This has been referred to in the following verse in *Vijñānabhaṭṭāraka* :[2]

"The consciousness of object and subject is common to all the embodied ones. The *Yogīs* have, however, this distinction that they are mindful of this relation."[3] (verse 106).

In the same book, it has also been said

"One should regard the whole world or his own body as full of the delight inherent in his Self. Simultaneously (with this world-view), he will find himself full of the highest delight which is simply due to the ambrosia (i.e. the spiritual delight) welling up in his Self." (Verse 65)[4]

The same idea has been brought out in the following verse in Spandakārikā.

"This is the acquisition of ambrosia (i.e. immortality). This is the veritable seizure of the Self. This constitutes the *dīkṣā* for *Nirvāṇa,* and this confers on oneself the realization of one's identity with *Śiva.*" (ii, 7)

(Now *Kṣemarāja* gives a further interpretation of the *sūtra* by arranging it as *Samādhisukhaṁ lokānandaḥ* i.e. the continuous delight of knowership of the *yogī* infuses delight into the people also).

"Moreover, the delight of knowership which the *yogī* experiences by continuous repose and delight within himself ends in making his delight manifest among those people also who carefully observe him in that state (*tat tādṛśam*). This happens by the process of transmission of delight. This is quite in agreement with the quotation given before from *Candrajñāna.*[5]

NOTES

1. *Samādhisukham* = The delight resulting from continuous mindfulness of knowership. The word *samādhi* in this context does not mean absorption or trance, but mindfulness of the Self as being the subject of every knowledge.

2. *Vijñānabhaṭṭāraka* is the same as *Vijñānabhairava.* The word *bhaṭṭāraka* is a term of respect.

3. The verse means to say that for all embodied beings, there is always subject-object relationship in every bit of knowledge, but the common man is only mindful of the object, not of the subject. The *yogī*, however, is always mindful of the relation of the object to the *subject* without which relation the object could not be known at all.

4. The Self is not only *cit* (consciousness), but *cidānanda* (consciousness-bliss). The surface-view of things denotes distress, disharmony, but there is wonderful harmony at the heart of the universe. That harmony, delight, bliss is the characteristic of consciousness which forms the warp and woof of the universe. The *yogī* who can penetrate beneath the surface and realize the underlying bliss will always be full of the highest delight, for his own Self is nothing but that blissful consciousness.

5. The quotation referred to is given in *Sūtra.* 7.

EXPOSITION

The present *sūtra* says that it is not necessary for the aspirant to lock himself up in a room and plunge into trance in order to realize the delight of Self. He can find this delight in the ordinary, normal course of life if he is mindful of the subject-object relation which is involved in every bit of knowledge. When a person knows a thing, he is extroverted, wholly involved in the external environment but if on the occasion of every bit of knowledge, he looks within, he will have a *feel* of the Self which alone makes that knowledge possible. In that *feel* of the Self, he will experience the perennial joy of I-consciousness. This is the ever-present joy of *samādhi.*

Further, this delight is not confined to the *Yogī.* He radiates it all round among the people who care to observe him in that state. His delight is infectious.

INTRODUCTION TO THE 19th SŪTRA

TEXT

अथ ईदृशस्य अस्य योगिनो विभूतियोगं दर्शयति—

TRANSLATION

Now the next *sūtra* shows the supernormal powers of this *Yogī*.

Sūtra—19

शक्तिसन्धाने शरीरोत्पत्तिः ॥ १९ ॥

Śaktisandhāne Śarīrotpattiḥ

शक्तिसन्धाने = On being united with (*Icchā*) *Śakti* with one-pointedness.

शरीरो पत्तिः = (there can be) creation of body. (According to the *Yogī's* desire).

When with one-pointedness the *yogī* is fully united with *Icchā Śakti*, then he can acquire the power of creating any kind of body according to his desire."

COMMENTARY

TEXT

'इच्छा शक्तिरुमा कुमारी' (१—१३) इति सूत्रेण या अस्य शक्तिरुक्ता, तामेव यदा अनुसंधत्ते, दार्ढ्येन तन्मयीभवति, तदा तद्वशेन अस्य यथाभिमतं शरीरमुत्पद्यते । तदुक्तं श्रीमृत्युञ्जयभट्टारके

'ततः प्रवर्तते शक्तिर्लक्ष्यहीना निरामया ॥
इच्छा सा तु विनिर्दिष्टा ज्ञानरूपा क्रियात्मिका ॥'

इत्युपक्रम्य

'सा योनिः सर्वदेवानां शक्तीनां चाप्यनेकधा ।
अग्नीषोमात्मिका योनिस्तस्यां सर्वं प्रवर्तते ॥'

इति । शक्तिसंधानमाहात्म्यं लक्ष्मीकौलार्णवे

'न संधानं विना दीक्षा न सिद्धीनां च साधनम् ।
न मन्त्रो मन्त्रयुक्तिश्च न योगाकर्षणं तथा ॥'

इत्यादिना प्रतिपादितम् । एतच्च

'यथेच्छाभ्यर्थितो धाता जाग्रतोऽर्थान्हृदि स्थितान् ।
सोमसूर्योदयं कृत्वा संपादयति देहिनः ॥'

इत्यनेन संगृहीतम् । देहिनः अत्यक्तदेहवासनस्य योगिनो हृदि स्थितान् अर्थान् तत्तदपूर्वनिर्माणादिरूपान् धाता महेश्वरः प्रकाशानन्दात्मतया सोमसूर्यरूप-

वाहोन्मीलनेन सोमसूर्यसामरस्यात्मनश्च शक्तेरुदयं कृत्वा बहिर्मुखवाहित्वेन तामासाद्य संपादयति; इति हि अस्यार्थः

'तथा स्वप्नेऽप्यभीष्टार्थान् .... ।'

इत्येतच्छ्लोकप्रतिपादितस्वप्नस्वातन्त्र्यं प्रति दृष्टान्ते योजितः, इति स्पन्द-निर्णये मयैव दर्शितम् ॥ १६ ॥

TRANSLATION

When the *Yogī* is united with the Will Power indicated in the 13th *Sūtra* i.e. when he is firmly and completely at-one-ment with that (*dārḍhyena tanmayībhavati*), then through it, he can bring into being (any kind of) body according to his desire.

The same fact has been indicated in *Mṛtyuñjaya bhaṭṭāraka* (i.e. Netra Tantra) in the verse, beginning with

"Thence proceeds that Power which has been indicated, as Icchā which is beyond purview and beyond the province of Māyā (lit. beyond any disease, or distemper) and which expresses itself in the form of knowledge and activity" and ending with.

"She (i.e. *Parā śakti*) is the source (*yoni*) of all the gods, and of all the *Śaktis*. She is of the nature of *agni* and *soma*[1]. Every thing proceeds from her." (VII, Verse 36-40)*

The greatness and power of the intensity and fixedness of awareness of Śakti (Śakti-sandhāna) has been described in Lakṣmīkaulārṇava in the following and other verses.

"Without *sandhāna* (union with intensity and fixedness of awareness), no initiation ceremony is effective, nor can there be successful completion of supernormal powers, nor can *mantra*, nor any stratagem of *mantra* succeed nor application of *yoga*."*

The same point has also been made out in the following verse in *Spandakārikā*:

"As the supporter of the universe (i.e. *Śiva*) when eagerly entreated with desire accomplishes all the desires existing in the heart of the embodied *yogī* who is awake after causing the rise of the moon and the sun.[2] (III.1)

*The above translation is according to the interpretation of Kṣemarāja. Svāmī Lakṣmaṇa joo interprets *Yoni* in the sense of indispensable means. Through her the *devas* (gods) realize their non-difference from *Śiva* (*Śāmbhavopāya*). Through her the *Śaktis* acquire spiritual realization by means of *Śāktopāya*, and it is through her that empirical beings realize their spiritual goal by *āṇavopāya*.

The meaning of this verse is that the supporter of the universe or the great lord (*Śiva*) accomplishes (i.e. brings into existence) outwardly the desires (e.g. the desires of various kinds of unique creation etc.) existing in the heart of the *yogī* who has not yet abandoned the desire of remaining in the body. He does this by inducing in him (the *yogī*) the feeling of *prakāśa* and *ānanda*, by opening out the flow of the *apāna* (*soma* i.e. moon) and *prāṇa* (*sūrya* i.e. sun) currents and by arousing the *śakti* (i.e. *samāna śakti*) which brings about equilibrium between *apāna* (*soma*) and *prāṇa* (sūrya).

As has been shown by me in *spandanirṇaya*, the matter explained in the above verse has been used as an example to show the *yogi's* freedom in dream also, (as will be clear from the following verse of Spandakārikā). "So also in dream, Śiva, by appearing in the central *nāḍī* (madhya) always clearly reveals the desired objects to the *yogī* in accordance with his entreaty." (III.2)

NOTES

1. *Agni* and *Soma*—literally fire and moon do not mean the obvious fire and moon that we see every day. *Agni* and *soma* are symbolic terms. *Agni* symbolizes the *prāṇa śakti* and *soma* symbolizes the *apāna śakti*. The *prāṇa* and *apāna śaktis* are associated with the *prāṇa* and *apāna* breaths. *Prāṇa* is the breath of expiration and *apāna* is the breath of inspiration.

2. *Soma-sūrya* (moon and sun) : Here again these are symbolic words. Moon or soma symbolizes the *apāna śakti* and sun or *sūrya* symbolizes the *prāṇa śakti*. This is so in connexion with *āṇavopāya*. In connexion with *Śāktopāya*, *soma* or moon symbolizes *jñāna śakti* (knowledge) and *sūrya* or sun symbolizes Kriyāśakti (activity). In connexion with Śāmbhavopāya, *soma* symbolizes *Vimarśa* and *sūrya* symbolizes *prakāśa*.

3. *Madhya* or Central *nāḍī* (channel, nerve) is the *susumnā* in the spinal column.

EXPOSITION

This sūtra says that the *yogī* who is united with *Icchā Śakti* can develop certain *vibhūtis* or supernormal powers. He can, for instance, create any kind of body that he desires. It should be borne in mind that he can do so only by being in contact with the Divine Will Power (Icchā or Parā Śakti).

Quoting a verse from Spandakārikā, *Kṣemarāja* describes how he can do so. In his waking condition, he has to pray to the Divine for the accomplishment of a certain desired object. Afterwards when he goes into *samādhi* (complete mental absorption), his *prāṇa* and *apāna* functions stop, but when he rises from the *Samādhi* and is in the waking condition again, the functions of his *prāṇa* and *apāna* are re-established, and he finds that his desired object has been fulfilled by the Divine Power to which he prayed and with which he was united. If the *Yogī* wants to experience certain supernormal objects in dream, that again is fulfilled by the Divine Power with which he is in contact.

INTRODUCTION TO THE 20th SŪTRA

TEXT

अन्या अपि अस्य यथाभिलषिताः सिद्धय एतन्माहात्म्येनैव घटन्ते इत्याह—

TRANSLATION

Through the pre-eminence of the union with this Icchāśakti other supernormal powers as desired (by him) accrue to the *Yogī*. This is what the next *sūtra* says.

Sūtra—20

भूतसंधानभूतपृथक्त्वविश्वसंघट्टाः ॥ २० ॥

Bhūtasandhāna-bhūtapṛthaktva-viśvasaṁghaṭṭāḥ.

भूत = existent entities; संधान = putting together or joining; भूतसंधान = putting together or joining the components of existents; भूतपृथक्त्व = disjoining or separating the components of existents; संघट्ट = assembling, collecting, joining, uniting; विश्व = everything; all; विश्वसंघट्टः = the power of uniting, bringing together every thing (removed by space and time).

The other supernormal powers of the *yogī* are: (1) The power of joining or putting together elements or parts in all existents i.e. synthetical power; (2) the power of separating elements of existents i.e. analytical power and (3) the power of bringing together everything (removed by space and time).

COMMENTARY

TEXT

भूतानि शरीरप्राणभावाद्यात्मकानि; तेषां क्वचित् आप्यायनादौ संधानं, परिपोषणं; व्याध्याद्युपशमादौ पृथक्त्वं, शरीरादेर्विश्लेषणं; देशकालादिविप्रकृष्टस्य च विश्वस्य संघट्टो, ज्ञानविषयीकार्यत्वादिकः; अस्य पूर्वोक्तशक्तिसंधाने सति जायते । एतच्च सर्वागमेषु साधनाधिकारेषु अस्ति । तदेव स्पन्दे ।

'दुर्बलोऽपि तदाक्रम्य यतः कार्ये प्रवर्तते ।
आच्छादयेद्बुभुक्षां च तथा योऽतिबुभुक्षितः ॥'

इति ।

'ग्लानिर्विलुण्ठिका देहे तस्याश्चाज्ञानतः सृतिः ।
तदुन्मेषविलुप्तं चेत्कुतः सा स्यादहेतुका ॥'

इति ।

'यथा ह्यर्थोऽस्फुटो दृष्टः सावधानेऽपि चेतसि ।
भूयः स्फुटतरो भाति स्वबलोद्योगभावितः ॥
तथा यत्परमार्थेन येन यत्र यथा स्थितम् ।
तत्तथा बलमाक्रम्य न चिरात्संप्रवर्तते ॥'

इत्यादिना विभूतिस्पन्दे सोपपत्तिकं दर्शितम् ॥ २० ॥

TRANSLATION

Bhūta means all existents like body, *prāṇa*, objects etc. *Sandhāna* means their addition or putting together for promoting growth etc. So *bhūtasaṁdhāna* means the power of joining elements of existence for augmentation or promotion of growth in some cases. *Bhūtapṛthaktva* means the power of separating of elements from body etc. for curing physical ailments, etc. *Viśvasaṅghaṭṭāḥ* means the power of bringing together all (*viśva*) things removed by space and time, etc. by making them objects of his own knowledge. All these powers accrue to him when he is able to unite his consciousness with Icchā Śakti as said before. This has been given in all the *āgamas* in the chapter on *Sādhana* (the means of accomplishing, mastering, overpowering).

In the *Spandakārikā* such powers have been described in a well-reasoned manner in the chapter dealing with supernormal powers (*vibhūti*), e.g.,

"Just as even a weak person proceeds to do his work by taking hold of that power (of *spanda*)[1], so even he who is exceedingly hungry can subdue his hunger..,[2] (III, 6).

"Just as a thief carries away the valuables of the house, even so depression saps away the vitality of the body. This depression proceeds from ignorance. If that ignorance disappears by *unmeṣa*[3], how can that depression last in the absence of its cause.'[4] (III, 8)

"As a thing which was dimly perceived at first in spite of the attentiveness of mind becomes clearer when observed again with all the exertion of the Will, even so that thing which existed in reality (*yat paramārthena*) in whichever form (*yena*), in whichever place or time (*yatra*), in whichever way (*yathā*) becomes manifest immediately again (in the same form, place or time and way) to one who takes resort to the power of *spanda*."[5] (III, 4 and 5).

NOTES

1. 1. *Spanda* = the Divine creative pulsation; the creative power inherent in I-consciousness.

2. The *yogī* acquires control over hunger, thirst etc. by *spandaśakti*. This describes the power of controlling physical instincts.

3. *Unmeṣa*—In *Śaiva Yoga*, *unmeṣa* means the unfoldment of spiritual consciousness by concentrating on the inner consciousness which is the background of all thought-process.

4. This verse describes the power of controlling all emotions.

5. This describes the power of bringing back to consciousness all past objects and events which are unknown.

EXPOSITION

The 19th *Sūtra* says that the *Yogī* who can unite his consciousness with the Divine *Icchāśakti* can acquire the power of creating any kind of body according to his desire. The present *sūtra* describes further supernormal powers of the *yogī*, e.g. power of joining together certain elements in a body for growth and nourishment (synthetical power), the power of separating elements from a body or object (analytical power), and the power of bringing back to consciousness all objects and events far removed in space and time (the occult power of reading past events and knowing objects far away in space).

INTRODUCTION TO THE 21st SŪTRA

TEXT

यदा तु मितसिद्धीरनभिलष्यन् विश्वात्मप्रथामिच्छति तदा अस्य--

TRANSLATION

When, however, he does not desire simply limited powers, but wants to acquire the form of universal Consciousness, there accrues to him.

Sūtra—21

शुद्धविद्योदयाच्चक्रेशत्वसिद्धिः ॥ २१ ॥

Śuddhavidyodayāccakreśatva-siddhiḥ.

शुद्धविद्योदयात् = through the appearance of *Śuddhavidyā*;
चक्रेशत्वसिद्धिः = full acquisition of mastery over the collective whole of the Śaktis.

"Full acquisition of mastery over the collective whole of the Śaktis through the appearance of Śuddhavidyā."

COMMENTARY

TEXT

वैश्वात्म्यप्रथावाञ्छया यदा शक्तिं संधत्ते तदा 'अहमेव सर्वम्' इति शुद्धविद्याया उदयात् विश्वात्मकस्वशक्तिचक्रेशत्वरूपं माहेश्वर्यमस्य सिद्ध्यति । तदुक्तं स्वच्छन्दे

'तस्मात्सा तु परा विद्या यस्मादन्या न विद्यते ।
विन्दते ह्यत्र युगपत्सार्वज्ञ्यादिगुणान्परान् ॥

वेदनानादिधर्मस्य परमात्मत्वबोधना ।
वर्जनापरमात्मत्वे तस्माद्विद्येति सोच्यते ॥
तत्रस्थो व्यञ्जयेत्तेजः परं परमकारणम् ।
परस्मिंस्तेजसि व्यक्ते तत्रस्थः शिवतां व्रजेत् ॥'

इति । तदेतत्

'दिदृक्षयेव सर्वार्थान्यदा व्याप्यावतिष्ठते ।
तदा किं बहुनोक्तेन स्वयमेवावभोत्स्यते ॥'

इत्यनेनैव संगृहीतम् ॥ २१ ॥

TRANSLATION

When he (the *yogī*) unites his consciousness with *Śakti* through intensive awareness with a desire to gain universal consciousness, then through the appearance of *Śuddhavidyā*, he succeeds in acquiring the supreme power of *Śiva* in the form of complete mastery over His universal collective whole of *śaktis*.

The same has been said in *Svacchanda Tantra* in the following verses:

"Therefore, as there is no other *Vidyā* (power of supreme knowledge) like her, she is the highest *vidyā*. In this (i.e. on the appearance of this *vidyā*) the *yogī* acquires the greatest qualities like omniscience, etc. all at once.

She is designated *Vidyā*, because she brings about investigation of the beginningless characteristic of *Śiva*, viz; *Svātantrya Śakti*, because she brings about the knowledge of the Highest Self and because she dispels all that is not that Highest Self. Established in that (i.e. the *Unmanā* state), one can manifest the highest light[3], the highest cause. If one is established in that manifest highest Light, he can attain to the state of *Śiva*." (IV, verses 396, 397).

The same idea has been expressed in the following verse in Spandakārikā:

"When the *Yogī* desirous of seeing stands fixed (in concentration) covering all objects with the light of his consciousness, (then he will experience the entire objective world in one sweep in himself), then what is the use of talking much, he will have the experience (of universal knowership) for himself." (III,11)

NOTES

1. *Śuddhavidyā*—This *Śuddha vidyā* is not the *Śuddha Vidyā tattva* which is above the *Māyā tattva*. *Śuddha vidyā* in this context means that supreme consciousness in which every thing appears as Self. It is the *unmanā avasthā*.

2. *Vidyā*—This word is derived from the root *vid*—which means both 'to deliberate' and 'to know'. The meaning of deliberation is brought out in वेदनानादिधर्मस्य and the meaning of knowledge is brought out in परमात्मत्वबोधना।

3. This light is the light of the primal *cit*.

4. The highest light is also the highest cause, i.e. Śiva.

EXPOSITION

14th to 20th *sūtras* describe limited supernormal powers acquired by the *yogī* who is united with *Ichhā Śakti*. The 21st *sūtra* describes the power of universal consciousness or cosmic consciousness acquired by the *Yogī*. After acquiring this power, the *Yogī* realizes the entire universe as his Self in one sweep, not in bits. In *sūtra* 14, it has been shown that the *Yogī* feels his identity with every object. His consciousness is of the form 'Ahmidam' or 'I am this' with regard to every object separately. The 21st *Sūtra* says that when the *Yogī* acquires universal consciousness, his consciousness is of the form *Ahameva Sarvam* i.e. 'I myself am all.'

INTRODUCTION TO THE 22nd SŪTRA

TEXT

यदा तु स्वात्मारामतामेव इच्छति तदा अस्य—

TRANSLATION

When, however, he desires only the delight of repose within himself (and not any supernormal power), then he has :

Sūtra—22

महाह्रदानुसंधानान्मन्त्रवीर्यानुभवः ॥ २२ ॥

Mahāhradānusandhānānmantravīryānubhavaḥ.

महाह्लद = the great lake, the infinite reservoir of Divine Power. अनुसंधानात् = by mental union मन्त्रवीर्यानुभवः = experience of the Supreme I-consciousness which is the generative source (*vīrya*) of all *mantras.*

"By uniting with the great lake (the infinite reservoir of Divine Power), (he has) the experience of the Supreme I-consciousness which is the generative source (*vīrya*) of all *mantras.*"

COMMENTARY

TEXT

परा भट्टारिका संवित् इच्छाशक्तिप्रमुखं स्थूलमेयपर्यन्तं विश्वं वमन्ती, खेचरीचक्राद्यशेषवाहप्रवर्तकत्व-स्वच्छत्वानावृतत्व-गभीरत्वादि-धर्मयोगान्महा-ह्लदः तस्यानुसंधानात्, अन्तर्मुखतया अनारतं तत्तादात्म्यविमर्शनात्; वक्ष्यमाणस्य शब्दराशिस्फारात्मकपराहन्ताविमर्शमयस्य मन्त्रवीर्यस्यानुभवः, स्वात्मरूपतया स्फुरणं भवति । अत एव श्रीमालिनीविजये

'या सा शक्तिर्जगद्धातुः .... ।'

इत्युपक्रम्य इच्छादिप्रमुखपञ्चाशद्भेदरूपतया मातृका-मालिनीरूपताम् अशेष-विश्वमयीं शक्तेः प्रदर्श्य, तत एव मन्त्रोद्धारो दर्शितः ; इति परैव शक्ति-र्महाह्लदः; ततः तदनुसंधानात् मातृका-मालिनीसतत्त्वमन्त्रवीर्यानुभव इति युक्तमुक्तम् ।

एतदेव

'तदाक्रम्य बलं मन्त्राः .... ।'

इत्याद्युक्त्या भङ्ग्या प्रतिपादितम् ।

TRANSLATION

The most venerable supreme Consciousness (parā-*saṁvit*)[1] positing *Ichhā Śakti* as the primary *Śakti*, projecting the universe (from the most subtle) upto gross objects, is a great lake. It is so-called, because it sets in motion the entire group of khecarī[2] and other currents, because it is limpid (inasmuch as it reflects the entire universe in it), because it is not shrouded (i.e. though it reflects the universe, the universe is unable to cast a pall over it), because it is deep (inasmuch as it is not easily understandable).

It is because of its association with such and other characteristics that it is rightly called the great lake.

By being mentally united with it (*anusandhānāt*) i.e. by being inwardly aware of ceaseless identity with it, there is the experience of the *mantra* of the supreme I-consciousness which is the generative source of all other *mantras* and which expands in the form of a multitude of words to be described in the sequel. This experience gleams forth as a form of one's own Self.

Therefore *Mālinīvijaya* beginning with :

"She is the *Śakti* of the creator of the world and is said to be in constant and intimate union with Him, and becomes, O goddess, *Icchā* (desire) of that lord desirous to create" (III, 5)

And after showing that this *Śakti* appears as the entire universe in the form of *Mātṛkā* and *Mālinī* with a variety of fifty letters with Ichhā Śakti (Divine Will Power) taking the leading part, it has described the emergence of the *mantra* of I-consciousness through that Śakti (*tata eva*).

Thus the highest Śakti herself is the great lake. Therefore, it has been rightly said that by uniting the mind with her, the *Yogī* has the experience of the potency of the *mantra* of the nature of *Mātṛkā* and *Mālinī*.

This very point has been explained in another way in the following verse in Spandakārikā;

"The *mantras* resorting to that power of *Spanda* (by identifying themselves with that power) proceed to perform their respective functions even as the senses of the embodied ones do."[3] (II, 1)

NOTES

1. *Parā saṁvit*, *parāśakti*, *parāhantā*, *parāvāk*, and *svātantrya* are synonymous terms denoting the Supreme I-consciousness of *Śiva*.

2. *Khecarī cakra* and other currents—The group of power-currents referred to here are—*Khecarī*, *gocarī*, *dikcarī* and *bhūcarī*. *Khecarī* is connected with the *pramātā*, the experient; *gocarī* is connected with his *antaḥkaraṇa* or the inner psychic apparatus; *dikcarī* is connected with the *bahiṣkaraṇa* i.e. the outer senses; *bhūcarī* is connected with the *bhāvas*, existents or the outer objects.

The *śakti cakras* indicate the processes of the objectification of the universal consciousness. By *Khecarī Cakra*, one is reduced from the position of an all-knowing consciousness to that of a limited experient; by *gocarī cakra*, he becomes endowed with an inner psychic apparatus; by *dikcarī cakra*, he is endowed with outer senses; by *bhūcarī cakra*, be becomes confined to *bhāvas* or external objects.

Khecarī is one that moves in *kha* or *ākāśa*. *Kha* or *ākāśa* is here a symbol of consciousness. This *Śakti* is called Khecarī, because her sphere is *kha* or consciousness. *Gocarī* is so-called, because her sphere is the inner psychic apparatus. The *Saṁskṛta* word 'go' indicates movement. The *antaḥkaraṇa* is the seat of the senses, and sets them in motion; it is the dynamic apparatus of the spirit par excellence. Hence it is said to be the sphere of *gocarī*. *Dikcarī* is the *Śakti* that moves in *dik* or space. The outer senses are concerned with space; hence they are said to be the sphere of *Dikcarī*. The word *bhū* in *Bhūcarī* means existence. Hence existent objects are the sphere of *bhūcarī Śakti*.

3. *Mātṛkā-Mālinī* : *Mātṛkā* connotes the fifty letters of the *Saṁskṛta* alphabet in the regular order. *Mātṛkā* means the unknown mother i.e. the mother whose mystery is not realized. The etymology of Mālinī is "malate, viśvam antaḥ dhatte" i.e. *Mālinī* is one who holds the universe within herself. *Mālinī* connotes the fifty letters of the *Saṃskṛta* alphabet in an irregular order as given below:

न ॠ ऋ ॡ ऌ थ च ध ई ण उ ऊ ब क ख ग घ ङ इ अ व
भ य उ ढ ठ झ ञ ज र ट प छ ल आ स अः ह ष क्ष म श अं त
ए ऐ ओ औ द फ

Conclusion of the First Section

COMMENTARY

TEXT

तदेवं 'चैतन्यमात्मा' (१-१) इत्युपक्रम्य तत्स्वातन्त्र्यावभासिततदख्यातिमयं सर्वमेव बन्धं यथोक्तोद्यमात्मकभैरवसमापत्तिः प्रशमयन्ती, विश्वं स्वानन्दामृतमयं करोति, सर्वाश्च सिद्धीः मन्त्रवीर्यानुप्रवेशान्ता ददाति ।

इति शाम्भवोपायप्रथनात्मा अयं प्रथम उन्मेष उक्तः । अत्र तु मध्ये शक्तिस्वरूपमुक्तं, तत् शाम्भवरूपस्य शक्तिमत्ताप्रदर्शनाभिप्रायेण इति शिवम् ॥२२॥

इति श्रीमन्महामाहेश्वराचार्याभिनवगुप्तपादपद्मोपजीवि-श्रीक्षेमराजविरचितायां शिवसूत्रविमर्शिन्यां शाम्भवोपायप्रकाशनं नाम प्रथम उन्मेषः ॥

TRANSLATION

This first section has been designated as the display of Śāmbhavopāya[1], for the acquisition of Bhairava-consciousness which, as has been already described (in Sūtra 5), is sudden emergence of the Supreme I-consciousness, which sets at naught all bondage (*āṇava*, *māyīya* and *kārma*) which is of the nature of ignorance brought about by the absolute freedom of consciousness (the characteristic of *ātmā* expounded in *Sūtra* 1) which makes the universe full of ambrosia through its own bliss, and which secures all the supernormal powers right up to one's establishment into that *mantra*[2] of Supreme I-consciousness which is the generative source of all other *mantras*.

In between, the nature of *Śakti* has also been described. That is with purpose of showing the power of Śāmbhava consciousness. May there be prosperity for all.

Here ends the first Section of the *Vimarśinī* Commentary on the *Śiva Sūtras* pertaining to *Śāmbhavopāya* by *Kṣemarāja* dependent on the lotus feet of the glorious *Abhinavagupta*, the best among the venerable great *Śaiva* teachers.

NOTES

1. *Śāmbhavopāya* : *upāya* = means of spiritual realization. *Śāmbhavopāya* connotes the means of spiritual realization of which the source is *Śambhu* (Śiva) Himself and which has been handed down by Him. For further details, see the Introduction.

2. *Mantra*—See Note No. 4 under the first *Sūtra* of the Second Section.

EXPOSITION

This sūtra says that by uniting his mind with *parāśakti*, the aspirant realizes the Supreme I-consciousness of *Śiva*. This is not power so much as the highest Spiritual experience. This I-consciousness is the source of all the *mantras*.

SECOND SECTION

INTRODUCTION TO THE 1st SŪTRA

TEXT

इदानीं शाक्तोपायः प्रदर्श्यते । तत्र शक्तिः मन्त्रवीर्यस्फाररूपा इति प्रथमोन्मेषान्तसूत्रिततत्स्वरूपविवेचनपुरःसरमुन्मेषान्तरमारभमाणो मन्त्रस्वरूपं तावत् निरूपयति--

TRANSLATION

Now *Śāktopāya* is being described. In the last *sūtra* of the first section, it was pointed out that *Śakti* signifies the expansion of the potency of *mantra*. The second section starting with an examination of *mantra* first ascertains its essential characteristic.

SŪTRA—1

चित्तं मन्त्रः॥ १ ॥

Cittam mantraḥ.

चित्तम्—in this context means that by which the Highest Reality is cognised.

मन्त्रः—a formula consisting of a word or a set of words addressed to a deity. In this context, *mantra* means that mental awareness by which one feels one's identity with the Highest Reality enshrined in a *mantra* and thus saves oneself from a sense of separateness and difference.

"By intensive awareness of one's identity with the Highest Reality enshrined in a *mantra* and thus becoming identical with that Reality the mind itself becomes *mantra*."

COMMENTARY

TEXT

चेत्यते विमृश्यते अनेन परं तत्त्वम् इति चित्तं, पूर्णस्फुरत्तासतत्त्वप्रासादप्रणवादिविमर्शरूपं संवेदनम्: तदेव मन्त्र्यते गुप्तम्, अन्तर् अभेदेन विमृश्यते

परमेश्वररूपम् अनेन, इति कृत्वा मन्त्रः। अत एव च परस्फुरत्तात्मकमनन-धर्मात्मता, भेदमयसंसारप्रशमनात्मक-त्राणधर्मता च अस्य निरुच्यते।

अथ च मन्त्रदेवताविमर्शपरत्वेन प्राप्ततत्सामरस्यम् आराधकचित्तमेव मन्त्रः, न तु विचित्रवर्णसंघट्टनामात्रकम्। यदुक्तं श्रीमत्सर्वज्ञानोत्तरे

'उच्चार्यमाणा ये मन्त्रा न मन्त्रांश्चापि तान्विदुः।
मोहिता देवगन्धर्वा मिथ्याज्ञानेन गर्विताः॥'

इति। श्रीतन्त्रसद्भावेऽपि

'मन्त्राणां जीवभूता तु या स्मृता शक्तिरव्यया।
तया हीना वरारोहे निष्फलाः शरदभ्रवत्॥'

इति। श्रीश्रीकण्ठीयसंहितायां तु

'पृथङ्मन्त्रः पृथङ्मन्त्री न सिद्ध्यति कदाचन।
ज्ञानमूलमिदं सर्वमन्यथा नैव सिद्ध्यति॥'

इत्युक्तम्। एतच्च स्पन्दे

'सहाराधकचित्तेन तेनैते शिवधर्मिणः॥'

इति भङ्ग्या प्रतिपादितम्॥ १॥

TRANSLATION

Citta is that which ponders over the Highest Reality. In other words, it is consciousness that ponders over *prāsāda*,[2] *praṇava*[3] and other *mantras* which constitute the essential characteristic of the perfect I-consciousness.

That by which one deliberates secretly i.e. ponders inwardly as being non-different from the Highest Lord is *Mantra*.[4] Thus that *citta* itself (*tadeva*) is *mantra*. The etymological interpretation of *mantra* points to its characteristic of *manana* i.e. pondering over the highest light of I-consciousness and the other characteristic of *trāṇa* i.e. protection by terminating the transmigratory existence full of difference.

The mind of the devotee intent on intensive awareness of the deity inherent in the *mantra* acquires identity with that deity and thus becomes that *mantra* itself. It is this mind itself which is *mantra*, not a mere conglomeration of various letters.

It has been rightly said in *Sarvajñānottara*—

"Those are not really *mantras* which are only a matter of enunciation. Elated with the pride of false knowledge, even *devas* and *Gandharvas* are deluded in this matter." (Verse 16-17).

In *Tantrasadbhāva* also, it has been said,

"She who is considered to be the imperishable *Śakti* (*Śaktiravyayā*)[5] is the soul of all *mantras.* O fair one, without her, (i.e. the *śakti*), they (*mantras*) are useless like autumnal clouds."

In *Śrīkaṇṭhī-Saṁhitā*, it has been said:

"If the practiser of the *mantra* is different from the *mantra*, then his *mantra* will never be successful. Knowledge (of the divine I-consciousness) alone is the root of all this. Without it, a *mantra* will never be successful".[6]

In *Spandakārikā* also the same idea has been explained in the following verse in another way :

"Not knowable as objective existents (*nirañjanāḥ*)[7] and full of peace (*śāntarūpāḥ*)[8] they (i.e. the *mantras*) together with the mind of their devoted practisers get absorbed in that very *Spanda.*[9] Therefore, *mantras* have the characteristic of *Śiva*[10] (*Śivadharmiṇaḥ*)" (II. 2).

NOTES

1. *Citta* in this context is not used in the usual sense of mind, but in the sense of aspiring mind, mind aspiring for communion with the Supreme I-consciousness of Śiva.

2. Prāsāda is a technical word of this system which will not be found in any dictionary. It is the name of the *mantra sauḥ* (सौः). It contains within itself the entire panorama of manifestation. The *mantra* is formed by (स्+औ +:. The first letter स् represents सत् or existence from the earth upto *māyā* (the 31 *tattvas* of *Śaiva* philosophy). सत् is formed from the root अस् + the suffix अत्. According to the rule of Sanskrit Grammar, the अ of अस् is dropped and स्+अत् i.e. सत् is formed which means 'existence.'

In order to form the mantra सौः the त् of this सत् is dropped. As said before, this स् represents the 31 *tattvas* from earth upto *māyā.* Now to the letter स् is added औ. 'औ' represents *Śuddha vidyā*, *Īśvara* and *Sadāśiva* who are full of *jñāna* and *kriyā*. Now remains *visarga* i.e. : The upper dot of the *visarga* represents

Śiva and the lower dot represents *Śakti*. Thus सौः represents all the 36 *tattvas*. It refers to *Parama Śiva* who is the *fons et origo* of the entire world-process. This *mantra* is known as *hṛdaya-bīja* the heart-seed of *Śiva*. He who can enter into the spirit of this *mantra* will be identified with the Supreme I-consciousness and will be liberated.

3. *Praṇava* is the mystic sacred syllable. According to *Śaivāgama*, there are four kinds of *praṇava*, (1) the *Śaiva Praṇava* which is हुं, (2) the *Śākta praṇava* which is क्लीं, (3) the *māyā praṇava* which is ह्रीं and (4) the Vedic *praṇava* which is ओऽम्. The *praṇava* referred to in this *sūtra* is the *Śaiva-praṇava*.

4. *Mantra*—This word is formed from the roots √*man*+*trai*— *man* means to ponder over, to ruminate mentally, and *trai* means to protect. *Mananāt trāyate iti mantraḥ* i.e. *mantra* is that which by pondering over the Supreme I-consciousness protects or saves one from transmigratory existence.

5. This *śaktiravyayā* or imperishable *Śakti* is the *Śakti* of Supreme I-consciousness.

6. The meaning is that the performer of the *mantra* should identify himself with the deity invoked in the *mantra*, if it is to succeed.

7. Nirañjanāḥ—According to Abhinavagupta, this means *na añjyante prakaṭīkriyante* (*prameya-rūpeṇa*) *iti nirañjanāḥ*—those which can never be known as objects are *nirañjanāḥ*. The *mantras* are full of I-consciousness; therefore they are always subjects and can never be reduced to the category of objects.

8. *Śāntarūpāḥ* here means 'which remain only as pure consciousness, which have negated all difference.'

9. The *Spanda* referred to is the power of the Supreme I-consciousness.

10. *Śiva-dharmiṇaḥ* or have the characteristic of Śiva means that the *mantras* are endowed with the qualities of Śiva like omniscience, etc.

EXPOSITION

The main technique of Śāktopāya is mantra, but *mantra* in this context does not mean incantation or muttering of some sacred formula. The word, *Mantra* is used here in its etymological signification. That which saves one by pondering over the light of Supreme I-consciousness is *mantra.* The divine Supreme I-consciousness is the dynamo of all the *mantras.* What is that which ponders over the central significance of every *mantra* ? It is *Citta.* But it is not any and every *Chitta.* It is the *Citta* (the individual mind) that is oriented towards the Divine, that is intent on seeking its own source. This *citta* itself is *mantra.* The key of *Śāktopāya* is *jñāna.* Therefore it is also called *jñānopāya.*

INTRODUCTION TO THE SŪTRA 2.

TEXT

अस्य च—

TRANSLATION

Of this mantra.

SŪTRA—2

प्रयत्नः साधकः ॥ २ ॥

Prayatnaḥ Sādhakaḥ.

प्रयत्नः—zealous and spontaneous close application.
साधकः—effective in fulfilment.

"Zealous and spontaneous close application is effective in fulfilment.

COMMENTARY

यथोक्तरूपस्य मन्त्रस्य अनुसंधित्साप्रथमोन्मेषावष्टम्भप्रयतनात्मा अकृतको यः प्रयत्नः स एव साधको, मन्त्रयितुर्मन्त्रदेवतातादात्म्यप्रदः । तदुक्तं श्रीतन्त्रसद्भावे

'आमिषं तु यथा खस्थः संपश्यञ्शकुनिःप्रिये ।
क्षिप्रमाकर्षयेद्यद्वद्वेगेन सहजेन तु ॥
तद्वदेव हि योगीन्द्रो मनो बिन्दुं विकर्षयेत् ।
यथा शरो धनुःसंस्थो यत्नेनाताड्य धावति ॥
तथा बिन्दुर्वरारोहे उच्चारेणैव धावति ॥'

इति । अन्यत्रापि

'तद्ग्रहो मन्त्रसद्भावः .... ।'

इति । अत्र हि तद्वत् इति, अकृतकनिजोद्योगबलेन योगीन्द्रो मनः (कर्म), बिन्दुं विकर्षयेत् परप्रकाशात्मतां प्रापयेत् इति । तथा बिन्दुः परप्रकाशः अकृतकोद्यन्तृतात्मना उच्चारेण धावति, प्रसरति इत्यर्थः । एतच्च स्पन्दे

'अयमेवोदयस्तस्य ध्येयस्य ध्यायिचेतसि ।
तदात्मतासमापत्तिरिच्छतः साधकस्य या ॥'

इत्यनेनोक्तम् ॥ २ ॥

TRANSLATION

Prayatna means the natural or spontaneous close application in firmly taking hold of the initial emergence of the desire for quest of the spirit of the *mantra*. It is this close application which becomes effective in fulfilment i.e. in bringing about identity of the contemplator of the *mantra* with the deity inherent in it. The same point has been made out in the following verses in *Tantrasadbhāva*:

"As a kite in the sky seeing a piece of meat, flying back with a spring draws it immediately towards itself with natural onset, O dear one, even so the great *yogī* should draw forth his mind to the light of the Self.

As an arrow placed on a bow runs after its target, if the bow is stretched with intensive effort, even so, O fair one, the knowledge of the Self expands through intensive awareness."

Elsewhere also it has been said.

"Apprehension of the Self constitutes the real being of the *mantra*."

In the above verse, the word *manaḥ* should be treated as an objective case, and the expression *tadvat* (even so) means to say that the great *yogī*, by means of spontaneous effort, draws the mind to *bindu*. i.e. should make the mind attain to the highest light (the light of Supreme I-consciousness). The meaning of the last line of the verse is, "Even so, *bindu* i.e. the highest light (of Self) runs i.e. expands by *uccāra* (maintenance of full awareness) resulting from spontaneous emergence of quest. The same idea has been expressed in the following verse in *Spandakārikā*:

"The appearance, in the mind of the contemplator of the deity contemplated on (really) means this—that the aspirant realizes his identity with the nature of the deity contemplated on in the *mantra* with intence desire (*icchataḥ*)[2] (i.e. with a mind free of thought-construct)" (II,6).

NOTES

1. *Uccāra* in this context does not mean utterance or pronunciation. *Uccāra* literally means *ut+cāra,* moving up, rising. It is in this etymological sense that the word has been used here. It means the movement of the mind upwards i.e. towards the light of the supreme I-consciousness.

2. *Icchataḥ* is an adjective of *sādhakasya*—of an aspirant who is full of intense desire for union with the deity.

INTRODUCTION TO THE 3rd SŪTRA

TEXT

ईदृशसाधकसाध्यस्य मन्त्रस्य पूर्वोपक्षिप्तं वीर्यं लक्षयति—

TRANSLATION

The next sūtra points to the previously referred to potency of the *mantra* which is to be accomplished with the above kind of spontaneous effort by the aspirant.

SŪTRA—3

विद्याशरीरसत्ता मन्त्ररहस्यम् ॥ ३ ॥

Vidyāśarīra-sattā mantrarahasyam.

विद्या = the knowledge of the highest non-dualism.

शरीर = *svarūpa* or essence.

सत्ता = being i.e. the luminous being of the perfect I-consciousness which is non-different from the world. मन्त्र-रहस्यम् the secret of *mantra.*

"The luminous being of the perfect I-consciousness inherent in the multitude of words whose essence consists in the knowledge of the highest non-dualism is the secret of *mantra.*"

COMMENTARY

TEXT

विद्या पराद्वयप्रथा, शरीरं स्वरूपं, यस्य स विद्याशरीरी भगवान् शब्दराशिः; तस्य या सत्ता, अशेषविश्वाभेदमयपूर्णाहंविमर्शनात्मा स्फुरत्ता, सा मन्त्राणां रहस्यम्, उपनिषत् । यदुक्तं श्रीतन्त्रसद्भावे

'सर्वे वर्णात्मका मन्त्रास्ते च शक्त्यात्मकाः प्रिये ।
शक्तिस्तु मातृका ज्ञेया सा च ज्ञेया शिवात्मिका ॥'

इति ।

TRANSLATION

Vidyā means knowledge of the highest non-dualism, 'Śarīra' means *svarūpa* i.e. own form, essence. *Vidyā-śarīra* means that multitude of words whose essence consists in *vidyā* i.e. the knowledge of highest non-dualism: Sattā means being i.e. the luminous being of the perfect I-consciousness which is non-different from the entire cosmos. Vidya-śarīra-sattā therefore, means the luminous being of the perfect I-consciousness which is non-different from the entire cosmos and which is inherent in the multitude of words whose essence consists in the knowledge of the highest non-dualism. *Mantrarahasyam* means the secret of *mantra*.

The whole *sūtra*, therefore, means—

"The luminous being of the perfect I-consciousness which is non-different from the entire cosmos and which is inherent in the multitude of words whose essence consists in the knowledge of the highest nondualism is the secret of *mantra*."

As has been said in *Tantrasadbhāva* :

"O dear one, all *mantras* consist of letters. The letters are a form of *śakti*. That *śakti* should be known as *mātṛkā*. *Mātṛkā* should be known as the very form of *Śiva*."

COMMENTARY

TEXT

तत्रैव च अयमर्थः अतिरहस्योऽपि वितत्य स्फुटीकृतः । तथा च

'न जानन्ति गुरुं देवं शास्त्रोक्तान्समयांस्तथा ।
दम्भकौटिल्यनिरता लौल्यार्थाः क्रिययोज्झिताः ॥

अस्मात्तु कारणाद्देवि मया वीर्यं प्रगोपितम् ।
तेन गुप्तेन ते गुप्ताः शेषा वर्णास्तु केवलाः ॥'

इति-पीठिकाबन्धं कृत्वा

'या सा तु मातृका देवि परतेजःसमन्विता ।
तया व्याप्तमिदं विश्वं सब्रह्मभुवनान्तकम् ॥
तत्रस्थं च सदा देवि व्यापितं च सुरार्चिते ।
अवर्णस्थो यथा वर्णः स्थितः सर्वगतः प्रिये ॥
तथाहं कथयिष्यामि निर्णयार्थं स्फुटं तव ।'

इत्युपक्रम्य

'या सा शक्तिः परा सूक्ष्मा निराचारेति कीर्तिता ॥
हृद्बिन्दुं वेष्टयित्वान्तः सुषुप्तभुजगाकृतिः ।
तत्र सुप्ता महाभागे न किञ्चिन्मन्यते उमे ॥
चन्द्राग्निरविनक्षत्रैर्भुवनानि चतुर्दश ।
क्षिप्त्वोदरे तु या देवी विषमूढेव सा गता ॥
प्रबुद्धा सा निनादेन परेण ज्ञानरूपिणा ।
मथिता चोदरस्थेन बिन्दुना वरवर्णिनि ॥
तावद्वै भ्रमवेगेन मथनं शक्तिविग्रहे ।
वेधात्तु प्रथमोत्पन्ना बिन्दवस्तेऽतिवर्चसः ॥
उत्थिता तु यदा तेन कला सूक्ष्मा तु कुण्डली ।
चतुष्कलमयो बिन्दुः शक्तेरुदरगः प्रभुः ॥
मथ्यमन्थनयोगेन ऋजुत्वं जायते प्रिये ।
ज्येष्ठाशक्तिः स्मृता सा तु बिन्दुद्वयसुमध्यगा ॥
बिन्दुना क्षोभमायाता रेखैवामृतकुण्डली ।
रेखिणी नाम सा ज्ञेया उभौ बिन्दू यदन्तगौ ॥
त्रिपथा सा समाख्याता रौद्री नाम्ना तु गीयते ।
रोधिनी सा समुद्दिष्टा मोक्षमार्गनिरोधनात् ॥
शशाङ्कशकलाकारा अम्बिका चार्धचन्द्रिका ।
एकैवेत्थं परा शक्तिस्त्रिधा सा तु प्रजायते ॥
आभ्यो युक्तवियुक्ताभ्यः संजातो नववर्गकः ।
नवधा च स्मृता सा तु नववर्गोपलक्षिता ॥
पञ्चमन्त्रगता देवि सद्य आदिरनुक्रमात् ।
तेन पञ्चविधा प्रोक्ता ज्ञातव्या सुरनायिके ॥
स्वरद्वादशगा देवि द्वादशस्था उदाहृता ।

अकारादिक्षकारान्ता स्थिता पञ्चशता भिदा ॥
हृत्स्था एकाणवा प्रोक्ता कण्ठे प्रोक्ता द्वितीयका ।
त्रिराणवा तु ज्ञातव्या जिह्वामूले सदा स्थिता ॥
जिह्वाग्रे वर्णनिष्पत्तिर्भवत्यत्र न संशयः ।
एवं शब्दस्य निष्पत्तिः शब्दव्याप्तं चराचरम् ॥'

इत्यादिना ग्रन्थेन परभैरवीयपरावाक्शक्त्यात्मकमातृका, अत एव ज्येष्ठा-रौद्री-अम्बाख्यशक्तिप्रसरसंभेदवैचित्र्येण सर्ववर्णोदयस्य उक्तत्वात्, वर्णसंघट्टनाशरीराणां मन्त्राणां सैव भगवती व्याख्यातरूपा विद्याशरीरसत्ता रहस्यम्—इति प्रदर्शितम् । प्रत्यागमं च मातृकामालिनीप्रस्तारपूर्वकं मन्त्रोद्धारकथनस्य अयमेव आशयः । रहस्यागमसारसंग्रहरूपत्वात् शिवसूत्राणाम् आगमसंवादे भरः अस्माभिः कृत इति नास्मभ्यम् असूयितव्यम् । एवमपि संवादिते आगमे यदि रहस्यार्थो न बुद्ध्यते, तस्मात् सद्गुरुसपर्या कार्या । एष च सूत्रार्थः

'तदाक्रम्य बलं मन्त्राः .... ।'

इत्यनेन कारिकाद्वयेन स्पन्दे दर्शितः ॥ ३ ॥

TRANSLATION

In that very book (i.e. *Tantrasadbhāva*), the following matter though very occult, has been elucidated in detail.

With the following introductory remarks—

"People do not know their spiritual director as full of divine power nor the established practices described in the scriptures. They are intent upon hypocrisy and crookedness, indulge in sense-pleasure and are devoid of practical performance.

On account of this, O goddess, the potency (of the *mantras*) has been concealed by me. On account of this concealment, they are concealed. What remain consist only of letters", the book starts (the exposition of the mystery) in the following way:

"O goddess, the universe from Brahmā upto the last *bhuvana* (gross physical world) is pervaded by *Mātṛkā* who is full of the highest lustre (of the Supreme I-consciousness); O goddess, venerated by all the gods that lustre always resides in *Mātṛkā* who is filled with it, I shall tell you clearly for your complete ascertainment how the letter 'a' (अ) pervades the entire alphabet.[1]

That *Śakti* who is described as supreme and subtle, and beyond the pale of religious practices (like worship, meditation etc.);

enclosing within herself the central *vindu*[2] sleeps coiled up in the form of a snake. O illustrious Umā; sleeping there, she is thoroughly incognizant.[3] Having cast within her womb the moon, fire, the sun, the stars and the fourteen worlds[4] she appears as if senseless owing to poison.

Then, O fair one, she gets awakened with the throb (ninādena)[5] of the highest knowledge, being churned by the *vindu* (Śiva's virile drop of light) present in her womb.

The churning goes on with whirling force in the body of the Śakti till with the penetration of Śiva's *Vindu* there appear at first many light-drops of great splendour.

When the subtle circular Śakti (kalā) is aroused by that creative throb of knowledge, then O dear one, the powerful four-phased[6] *vindu* existing in the womb of *Śakti* assumes a straight position by the union of the churner (Śiva) and that which is churned (Śakti). The Śakti that passes into the middle of the two *vindus* (viz. of Śiva and Śakti) is known as *Jyeṣṭhā*. Being agitated by that *vindu*, the straight line is known as *amṛta kuṇḍalī*. She is known as *rekhiṇī*[7] (one of straight line) at the ends of which are the two *vindus*. She is known as *Tripathā*[8] (having three tracks) and is named Raudrī. She is also known as *Rodhinī*,[9] because she stands as a bar to the path to liberation. *Ambikā* who is of the shape of a part of moon is like half moon.

Thus *Parā-śakti*[10] which is only one appears in three ways. Through these *Śaktis*[11] by various sorts of conjunction and disjunction, all the nine classes of letters are produced. She (*Parā śakti or Parāvāk*) characterized by nine classes[12] of letters is known in nine ways. O goddess, she pervades the five *mantras*[13] like *Sadyojāta* etc. successively. Therefore, O leadress of all the gods, she is described in five ways. She appears in the twelve vowels[14], therefore is she said to be existing in twelve. From 'a' to 'kṣa', she exists in fifty varieties.[15]

In the heart, she is said to be of one atom. In throat, she is of two atoms; always, situated in the root of the tongue, she is to be known as having three atoms.[16]

In the front of the tongue, there is successful production of letters. There is no doubt about this. In this way is the production of words. All existents moving and unmoving, are pervaded by words."

By all these statements the particular chapter in *Tantrasadbhāva* intends to show that Mātṛkā is a manifestation of Parāvāk who is only a *śakti* of the highest *Bhairava*. Therefore as it has been said that all letters come into being because of the varieties brought about by the conjunction of the extension of *Jyeṣṭhā, Raudrī* and *Ambā śaktis*, it is the Supreme I-consciousness (*vidyāśarīra-sattā*), as already explained, which is the secret of all the *mantras* which are embodied in the conjunction of letters. In every *Āgama*, this is the intention of the statement that *mantras* arise by means of the extension of *Mātṛkā* and *Mālinī*.

As the *Śiva-sūtras* are a sort of compendium of the essentials of the occult Āgamas, therefore have I undertaken all this labour to show their agreement with the *Āgamas*. So none need criticise me (for being prolix). If even in spite of all the agreement with the *Āgamas* that I have shown, the occult meaning is not understood, one should betake oneself to the reverential service of a good spiritual director.

This purport of the *Sūtra* has been shown in the following two verses of *Spandakārikā*.

"Resorting to the power of *Spanda*, *mantras* become endued with the power of omniscience and perform their functions just as the senses of the embodied ones do.

Not knowable as objective existents (*nirañjanāḥ*) and full of peace, they together with the mind of their devoted performers get absorbed in that very *spanda*. Therefore, they have the characteristic of *Śiva*. (II, 1 and 2).

NOTES

1. The letter 'a' (अ) representing *anuttara*, the highest *Śakti*. That is the origin of all letters.

2. *Vindu*—This is the integral virile creative drop of light of consciousness.

3. This sleep refers to the cosmic sleep (before a new creation) in which all the objective phenomena are withdrawn.

4. 'The moon......fourteen worlds': besides indicating the entire objective phenomena of the universe also symbolize the following :

Chandra or moon symbolizes *prameya* i.e. objects.
agni or fire symbolizes *pramātā* i.e. Knower or subject.
ravi or sun „ *pramāṇa* i.e. knowledge.
nakṣatra or stars „ *saṁkalpa-vikalpa*. i.e. thought constructs.

Caturdaśa bhuvanāni symbolizes the fourteen vowels from अ to औ (a to au).

5. *Nināda* is not sound in this context, but the throb of consciousness, the germinal emergence of the universe to be manifested.

6. The four-phased or *Catuṣkala vindu* consists of (1) *icchā* (2) *jñāna* (3) *kriyā* pertaining to Śakti and (4) *svātantrya*, pertaining to Śiva.

7. The *vindus* or points of *icchā*, *jñāna* and *kriyā* now form a straight line. This is known as *Rekhiṇī* (one having a *rekhā* or straight line). There are two *vindus* or points, one below and one at the top of this straight line. The lower *vindu* is that of *Śakti*, the higher one is that of *Śiva*.

8. *Raudrī* is a line of *icchā*, *jñāna*, and *kriyā* and is, therefore, known as *tripathā*.

9. *Rodhinī* is the dividing line between phenomena and noumena. On the lower side of this dividing line is *aśuddhādhvā*, the empirical manifestation; on the other or higher side of that line is the *Śuddhādhvā*, the metempirical manifestation. *Rodhinī* acts as a bar between the two. Only those who are completely purified are allowed to cross the bar.

10. *Parāśakti* appears in three ways i.e. (1) Anuttara or the letter अ (a) (2) *icchā* or the letter इ (i) and (3) *unmeṣa* (*jñāna*) or the letter उ (u).

11. Through these *Śaktis* i.e. through *Jyeṣṭhā*, *Raudrī* and *Ambikā śaktis*.

12. Nine classes of letters are the following.

(1) अ वर्ग which includes all the vowels of the Sanskrit alphabet.

(2) क वर्ग which includes क, ख, ग, घ, ङ

(3) च वर्ग ,, ,, च, छ, ज, झ, ञ
(4) ट वर्ग ,, ,, ट, ठ, ड, ढ, ण,
(5) त वर्ग ,, ,, त, थ, द, ध, न,
(6) प वर्ग ,, ,, प, फ, ब, भ, म
(7) य वर्ग ,, ,, य, र, ल, व,
(8) श वर्ग ,, ,, श ष स ह
(9) क्ष वर्ग ,, ,, only the letter क्ष

Some include क्ष in श वर्ग According to them, there are only eight classes of letters.

13. The five *mantras* are (1) *Sadyojāta* (2) *Tatpuruṣa* (3) *Īśāna* (4) *Vāmadeva* (5) *Aghora.*

14. The twelve vowels are all the vowels of Sanskrit alphabet with the exception of ऋ ॠ लृ and ॡ

15. The Sanskrit alphabet from अ to क्ष consists of fifty letters.

16. *Parāśakti* or *Parāvāk* is Kuṇḍalinī *Śakti.* She is the central creative power of the entire Mātṛkā of all the subjective and objective phenomena. Broadly, she expresses herself in three ways, Paśyantī, Madhyamā and Vaikharī. *Paśyanti* is that where the word and the object are identical. The division between word and object has not yet arisen. In this, there is only the light of consciousness. Therefore, this is the stage of vision, and that is why this *śakti* is known as *paśyantī.* She consists of one *aṇu.* She is said to be existing in the heart.

In the *Madhyamā* stage, though the division between the word and object has started, it is not fully pronounced yet. *Madhyamā* occupies an intermediate stage between *Paśyantī* and *Vaikharī.* That is why she is called *Madhyamā.* She is of two *aṇus* and resides in the throat. In the *Vaikharī* stage, the object is completely separated from the word. The word *Vikhara* means body. The body is the seat of gross speech. Therefore, gross speech is known as *Vaikharī.* She is said to exist in the root of the tongue and consists of three *aṇus.*

EXPOSITION

Śāktopāya is described in the second Section. In a general way, it has been said that *mantra* is the chief *Sāktopāya* for self-realization.

The first *Sūtra* tells us what *mantra* really means. "That by which one recognises one's identity with *Śiva*" is what is meant by *mantra*. It is not the letters which constitute *mantra*, but the realization of oneself as identical with the deity invoked in the *mantra* and finally with the supreme I-consciousness which is the core of all *mantras*. The purpose of *mantra* is to make the mind God-oriented. Indeed such a mind itself is *mantra*.

The third *sūtra* corroborates the main idea of the first *sūtra* with an amazing wealth of details.

It begins by saying that Vidyāśarīrasattā constitutes the secret of *mantra*. This *vidyāśarīra-sattā* is the awareness of that supreme I-consciousness of *Śiva* which is identical with the universe. The origin of all *mantras* is this divine I-consciousness and it is to this divine I-consciousness that all *mantras* have to be directed. The *mantras* consist of letters.

Reproducing a long quotation from *Tantrasadbhāva*, the commentary on this *sūtra* goes on to say that the supreme I-consciousness in its creative aspect is known as *Parāśakti* or *Parāvāk*. This *Parā-śakti* is the *śakti-kuṇḍalinī* which goes into cosmic sleep after the dissolution of the manifested world. Then there is churning process between *Śiva* and *Śakti*; in consequence the first letter 'a' (अ) comes into being. This' a' (अ) is the origin of all the lettters. So the letters of the *mantra* are not merely dead symbols, they point to the I-consciousness of *Śiva* which is their origin. It is, therefore to this I-consciousness that the mind should be directed in each *mantra*.

INTRODUCTION TO THE 4th SŪTRA

TEXT

येषां तु एवंविधमेतन्मन्त्रवीर्यं प्रोक्तमहाह्लदानुसंधानौपयिकमपि परमेश्वरेच्छात एव न हृदयङ्गमी भवति; अपि तु आनुषङ्गिकमात्रविन्दुनादादिकलाजनितासु मितसिद्धिषु चित्तं रोहति, तेषाम्—

TRANSLATION

Those to whom the potency of this kind of *mantra* which is a means to the mental union with the afore-said great lake does not appeal through God's will, but rather whose heart is set on unimportant secondary limited powers like *vindu* or light *nāda* or sound etc. which are produced by *śakti*, to them then accrues.

SŪTRA—4

गभ चित्तविकासोऽविशिष्टविद्यास्वप्नः ॥ ४ ॥

Garbhe Cittavikāso 'viśiṣṭavidyāsvapnaḥ

गर्भे = in the *māyic* powers; चित्त-विकास: satisfaction of mind; अविशिष्टविद्यास्वप्न: common, inferior knowledge confusing like a dream "(To them accrues) Mental satisfaction in *māyic*, limited powers which are only a form of common inferior knowledge confusing like a dream."

COMMENTARY

TEXT

गर्भः अख्यातिर्महामाया; तत्र तदात्मके मितमन्त्रसिद्धिप्रपञ्चे यश्चित्तस्य विकासः, तावन्मात्रे प्रपञ्चे संतोषः; असावेव अविशिष्टा, सर्वजनसाधारण-रूपा; विद्या, किञ्चिज्ज्ञत्वरूपा अशुद्धविद्या; सैव स्वप्नो, भेदनिष्ठो विचित्रो विकल्पात्मा भ्रमः । तदुक्तं पातञ्जले

'ते समाधावुपसर्गा व्युत्थाने सिद्धयः ॥' (३-३७)

इति । तदेतत्

'अतो विन्दुरतो नादो रूपमस्मादतो रसः ।
प्रवर्तन्तेऽचिरेणैव क्षोभकत्वेन देहिनः ॥'

इत्यनेन दर्शितम् ॥ ४ ॥

TRANSLATION

Garbhaḥ means primal ignorance, *mahāmāyā*. In that i.e. in *māyic* limited powers. *Cittasya vikāsaḥ* means satisfaction in the limited phenomenal powers.

This is merely common kind of knowledge i.e. limited inferior, impure knowledge. This is mere dream i.e. confusion full of strange fancies based on a sense of difference.

In *Patañjali's Yogasūtra* also, it has been said,

"They (i.e. the supernormal powers) are obstacles in *Samādhi* (contemplative absorption); on coming back to the normal consciousness, they are powers." (III,37).

This point has also been made out in the following verse in Spandakārikā:

"From this (i.e. *unmeṣa*) there appears in a short time *vindu* i.e. light (between the eye-brows), *nāda* i.e. unstruck sound of various kinds, *rūpa*, i.e. different kinds of forms even in darkness, *rasa*, i.e. pleasant taste in the mouth even in the absence of any thing edible. To the *Yogī* whose sense of identification with the body has not yet disappeared, these (supernormal experiences) act at once only as disturbance (in his progress of *Yoga*)," (III,10).

EXPOSITION

Bhāskara has given this *sūtra* differently in his *Vārttika*. He reads it thus—गर्भे चित्तविकासो विशिष्टोऽविद्यास्वप्नः। He interprets it thus—*Garbhe* i.e. in the bliss of the light of Supreme consciousness. When the mind is turned towards this light, then there is the highest development of the mind i.e. the mind is full of bliss. This being so, there is disappearance (*svapnaḥ* i.e. disappearance like a dream) of *avidyā* or primal ignorance.

INTRODUCTION TO THE 5th SŪTRA

TEXT

यदा तु आगतामपि मितसिद्धिं खिलीकृत्य परामेव स्थितिमवष्टभ्नाति योगी तदाः—

TRANSLATION

When, however, the *yogī*, rejecting even the accrued limited powers as useless, sticks firmly to the highest state, then.

SŪTRA—5.

विद्यासमुत्थाने स्वाभाविके खेचरी शिवावस्था ।। ५ ।।

Vidyāsamutthāne Śvābhāvike Khecarī Śivāvasthā.

विद्यासमुत्थाने—on the emergence of Supreme knowledge; स्वाभाविक natural, spontaneous; खेचरी moving in the vast expanse of consciousness; शिवावस्था—Śiva's state.

"On the emergence of spontaneous supreme knowledge, occurs that state of movement in the vast unlimited expanse of consciousness which is *Śiva*'s state i.e. the Supreme State of Reality."

COMMENTARY

TEXT

प्राङ्‌निर्दिष्टसतत्त्वाया विद्यायाः स्वाभाविके समुत्थाने, परमेशेच्छामात्र-घटिते मितसिद्धिन्यग्भाविनि सहजे समुन्मज्जने; खे बोधगगने चरति इति खेचरी मुद्रा अभिव्यज्यते । कीदृशी खेचरी, शिवस्य चिन्नाथस्य अवस्थातुः संबन्धिनी अवस्था, स्वानन्दोच्छलत्तारूपा । न तु

'बद्ध्वा पद्मासनं योगी नाभावक्षेश्वरं न्यसेत् ।
दण्डाकारं तु तावत्तन्नयेद्यावत्कखत्रयम् ।।
निगृह्य तत्र तत्तूर्णं प्रेरयेत् खत्रयेण तु ।
एतां बद्ध्वा महायोगी खे गतिं प्रतिपद्यते ।।'

इत्येवं संस्थानविशेषानुसरणरूपा; अपि तु

"............... पराम् ।
गतिमेत्यर्थभावेन कुलमार्गेण नित्यशः ।।
चरते सर्वजन्तूनां खेचरी नाम सा स्मृता ।'

इति—श्रीतन्त्रसद्भावनिरूपितपरसंवित्तिस्वरूपा । एवमिह भेदात्मकमायीय-समस्तक्षोभप्रशान्त्या चिदात्मकस्वरूपोन्मज्जनैकरूपं मन्त्रवीर्यं मुद्रावीर्यं च आदिष्टम् । तदुक्तं कुलचूडामणौ

'एकं सृष्टिमयं बीजमेका मुद्रा च खेचरी ।
द्वावेतौ यस्य जायेते सोऽतिशान्तपदे स्थितः ।।'

इति । स्पन्दे तु मन्त्रवीर्यस्वरूपनिरूपणेनैव मुद्रावीर्यं संगृहीतम् ।

'यदा क्षोभः प्रलीयेत तदा स्यात्परमं पदम् ।'

इत्यर्धेन अन्यपरेणापि चूडामण्युक्तं खेचरीस्वरूपं भङ्ग्या सूचितम् ॥ ५ ॥

TRANSLATION

On the appearance of the previously defined *Vidyā* (Supreme knowledge of non-dualism) i.e. on the spontaneous emergence of *Vidyā* which occurs merely by the wish of God and which rejects all limited power as worthless, *Khecarī mudrā*, meaning movement in the vast, unlimited expanse of consciousness, is manifested.

What kind of *Khecarī* ? It is a state of *Śiva* who as the possessor of that state is the lord of consciousness. It is Self's delight welling up from within. This *Khecarī* is not of the usual sort which is merely a disposition of certain parts of the body in a particular form as described in the following verse:

"A *Yogī* should be seated in a *Padmāsana* posture erect like a stick and should then fix his mind (lit. the chief of the senses) on the navel and should lead the mind upto *khatraya* or the three *śaktis* situated in the space in the head. Holding the mind in that state, he should move it forward immediately with the above. Disposed in this psycho-physical posture the great *Yogī* acquires the supernormal power of moving (flying) in the sky.

Khecarī is rather as described in the following verse:

"......he (the *yogī*) reaches the highest state in actuality always by the *Śākta* process (by following the occult process of Mātṛkā from 'a' to 'kṣa'). Only when his consciousness moves in all beings, only then is it genuine *Khecarī*."

Thus *Khecarī* as defined in *Tantrasadbhāva* is the highest form of consciousness. Accordingly in this *Yoga*, it is only the emergence of the essential nature of the divine consciousness by setting at naught all disturbances caused by *māyā* that has the nature of creating difference. It is this alone which constitutes the potency of *mantras* and the potency of *mudrā*.

The same thing has been said in *Kulacūḍāmaṇi* in the following verse :

"There is only one seed-*mantra* (of Supreme I-consciousness) which pervades the entire manifestation; there is only one *mudrā*, viz, *Khecarī* which pertains to highest Bhairava. He in whom these two appear is established in that state which transcends the merely immobile condition (i.e. he is established in Spanda which is the creative pulsation").

In Spandakārikā the potency of *mudrā* has been hinted at only in the exposition of the nature of the potency of *mantra.* In the following half verse, however, *Spandakārikā* indirectly indicates the nature of *Khecarī mudrā* described in *Cuḍāmaṇi*, though there it has been described from another point of view.

"When his agitation ceases then will accrue to him the highest state." (I,9)

NOTES

1. *Khecarī* : This literally means that which moves in the sky or empty space. *Kha* or empty space is a symbol of consciousness. One of the meanings of *Khecara* is *Śiva. Khecarī mudrā*, therefore, means a *mudrā* pertaining to *Śiva* or *Śivāvasthā* as the above *sūtra* puts it.

Mudrā : Lit, means a seal, a token of divine attribute impressed on the body; intertwining of the fingers in a particular way; a disposition of certain parts of the body in a particular shape. *Khecarī Mudrā* is that particular disposition of the psychophysical posture which enables the experient to move freely in the expanse of consciousness.

Khecarī mudrā is of various sorts. *Śaiva āgama* does not set any store by *mudrā* in the sense of disposition of certain parts of the physical body. It interprets *mudrā* in a higher sense in three ways, viz. (1) *mudam* (*harṣam*) *rāti* (*dadāti*)—that which gives *muda* or joy, (2) *muṁ drāvayati*—that which dissolves *mu* or bondage (3) *mudrayati iti*—that which seals up (the universe into *turīya*).

The ideal of mudrā is expressed in the following verse by *Abhinavagupta:*

मुदं स्वरूपलाभाख्यं देहद्वारेण चात्मना ।
रात्यर्पयति यत्तेन मुद्रा शास्त्रेषु वर्णिता ॥

(Tantrāloka-32nd āhnika)

That which enables living beings to acquire Self-realization in all the states of the embodied ones is *Mudrā.* By *dehadvāreṇa* is meant all the bodily states—waking (physical body) dreaming (subtle body) deep sleep (*paradeha* or the causal body).

So *Khecarī mudrā* in *Śaiva āgama* means a state of universal consciousness which is the state of *Śiva*.

2. *Khatrayam*—Lit. it means the triad of space or void. The triad referred to is *Śakti*, *Vyāpinī*, and *Samanā*, extending from the middle of the eyebrows up to *Brahmarandhra*.

EXPOSITION

This sūtra says that the potency of *mantra* or of *mudrā* consists in enabling the aspirant to aquire *Khecarī* which is *Śiva*—consciousness.

This is possible only when one realizes the secret of *mantra* which is the Supreme I-consciousness of Śiva, the I-consciousness that is also the world-consciousness.

INTRODUCTION TO THE 6th SŪTRA

TEXT

तदत्र मुद्रामन्त्रवीर्यासादनेऽपि—

TRANSLATION

Now in acquiring the potency of *mudrā* and *mantra*.

SŪTRA—6

गुरुरुपायः ॥ ६ ॥

Gururupāyaḥ.

गुरुः = the spiritual director

उपायः = means.

"The Guru who has attained Self-realization can alone help the aspirant in acquiring it."

COMMENTARY

TEXT

गृणाति उपदिशति तात्त्विकमर्थमिति गुरुः; सोऽत्र व्याप्तिप्रदर्शकत्वेन उपायः । तदुक्तं श्रीमालिनीविजये

'स गुरुर्मत्समः प्रोक्तो मन्त्रवीर्यप्रकाशकः ।'

इति । स्पन्दे तु एवमादिप्रसिद्धत्वात् न संगृहीतम् ।

'अगाधसंशयाम्भोधिसमुत्तरणतारिणीम् ।
वन्दे विचित्रार्थपदां चित्रां तां गुरुभारतीम् ॥

इति-पार्यन्तिकोक्त्या च एतदपि संगृहीतमेव ।

गुरुर्वा पारमेश्वरी अनुग्राहिका शक्तिः । यथोक्तं श्रीमालिनीविजये

'शक्तिचक्रं तदेवोक्तं गुरुवक्त्रं तदुच्यते ।'

इति । श्रीमन्त्रिशिरोभैरवेऽपि

'गुरोर्गुरुतरा शक्तिर्गुरुवक्त्रगता भवेत् ।'

इति । सैव अवकाशं ददती उपायः ॥ ६ ॥

TRANSLATION

Guru is one who teaches the essential Truth. So he is the means for leading one to the attainment of the potency of *mantra* and *mudrā*.

In Mālinivijaya, it has been said (Śiva addressing Pārvatī says)

"One, who knows all the principles in their essentials, being able to throw light on the virility or efficiency of *mantras*, is a *guru* like myself." (II,10).

In Spandakārikā, such matters being well known have not been treated. But in a way this matter has also been treated there in the last verse which is as follows:

"I offer my homage to that wonderful teaching of my *guru*, serving as a boat in crossing the fathomless ocean of doubts and full of such words as express wonderful, uncommon ideas." (IV 1).

Or *guru* may be said to be the power of divine grace. As has been said in Mālinīvijaya "That (the power of grace) has been said to be the collective whole of *śaktis*, that has been said to be the mouth of the *guru*, i.e. the *guru's* power of grace."

In Mantriśirobhairava also, the same idea has been expressed in the following way.

"*Guru's* power of grace inherent in the mouth of the *guru* is greater than the *guru* himself." That power of grace affording a favourable opportunity to the aspirant is the means (to the unravelling of the secret of the *mantra*).

INTRODUCTION TO THE 7th SŪTRA

TEXT

तस्माद्गुरोः प्रसन्नात्—

TRANSLATION

Therefore, from a pleased guru.

SŪTRA—7

मातृकाचक्रसम्बोधः ॥ ७ ॥

Mātṛkācakrasambodhaḥ.

मातृकाचक्र = the group of letters; सम्बोधः enlightenment."

"(From a pleased guru) accrues enlightenment regarding the group of letters."

COMMENTARY

TEXT

शिष्यस्य भवतीति शेषः । श्रीपरात्रिंशकादिनिर्दिष्टनीत्या अहंविमर्शप्रथमकला अनुत्तराकुलस्वरूपा, प्रसरन्ती आनन्दस्वरूपा सती, इच्छेशनभूमिकाभासनपुरःसरं, ज्ञानात्मिकामुन्मेषदशां ज्ञेयाभासासूत्रेणाधिक्येन च ऊनतां प्रदर्श्य, इच्छामेव द्विरूपां विद्युद्विद्योतनकल्पतेजोमात्ररूपेण, स्थैर्यात्मना च एषणीयेन रञ्जितत्वात् र-लश्रुत्या आरूषितेन, अत एव स्वप्रकाशात्मीकृतमेयाभासत्वतः अमृतरूपेण, मेयाभासारूषणमात्रतश्च बीजान्तरप्रसवासमर्थतया, षण्ढाख्यबीजचतुष्टयात्मना रूपेण प्रपञ्च्य, प्रोक्तानुत्तरानन्देच्छासंघट्टेन त्रिकोणबीजम्, अनुत्तरानन्दोन्मेषयोजनया च क्रियाशक्त्युपगमरूपमोकारं, प्रोक्तैतद्बीजद्वयसंघट्टेन षट्कोणं शूलबीजं च, इच्छाज्ञानशक्तिव्याप्तपूर्णक्रियाशक्तिप्रधानत्वात् शक्तित्रयसंघट्टनमयं प्रदर्श्य, इयत्पर्यन्तविश्वैकवेदनरूपं बिन्दुमुन्मील्य, युगपदन्तर्बहिर्विसर्जनमयबिन्दुद्वयात्मानं विसर्गभूमिमुद्दर्शितवती, अत एव अन्तर्विमर्शनेन अनुत्तरे एव एतद्विश्वं विश्रान्तं दर्शयति, बहिर्विमर्शेन तु कादि-मान्तं पञ्चक-पञ्चकम् अ-इ-उ-ऋ-लृशक्तिभ्यः पुरुषान्तं समस्तं प्रपञ्चयति । एकैकस्याश्च शक्तेः पञ्च शक्तित्वमस्ति, इत्येकैकतः पञ्चकोदयः । आभ्य एव शक्तिभ्यः शिक्षोक्तसंज्ञानुसारेण अन्तः-पुंभूमौ नियत्यादिकञ्चुकत्वेन अवस्थानात् अन्तःस्थाख्यान्प्रमातृभूमिधारणेन विश्वधारणात् धारणाशब्देन

आम्नायेषु उक्तान्, तदुपरि भेदविगलनेन अभेदापत्त्या उन्मिषितत्वात् ऊष्माभिधानान् चतुरो वर्गानाभासितवती। अत्र च अन्ते सर्वसृष्टिपर्यन्तवर्ति परिपूर्णममृतवर्णं प्रदर्श्य, तदन्ते प्राणबीजप्रदर्शनं कृतम् ; तत् अनुत्तरशक्त्याप्यायितानाहतमयम्, इयद्वाच्यवाचकरूपं षडध्वस्फारमयं विश्वम्; इति प्रत्यभिज्ञापयितुम् । अतएव प्रत्याहारयुक्त्या अनुत्तरानाहताभ्यामेव शिवशक्तिभ्यां गर्भीकृतम् एतदात्मकमेव विश्वम्; इति महामन्त्रवीर्यात्मनोऽहंविमर्शस्य तत्त्वम् । यथोक्तमस्मत्परमेष्ठिश्रीमदुत्पलदेवपादैः

'प्रकाशस्यात्मविश्रान्तिरहंभावो हि कीर्तितः ।
उक्ता सैव च विश्रान्तिः सर्वापेक्षानिरोधतः ॥
स्वातन्त्र्यमथ कर्तृत्वं मुख्यमीश्वरतापि च ।'

इति । तदियत्पर्यन्तं यन्मातृकायास्तत्त्वं तदेव ककार-सकारप्रत्याहारेण अनुत्तरविसर्गसंघट्टसारेण कूटबीजेन प्रदर्शितमन्ते; इत्यलं रहस्यप्रकटनेन । एवंविधायाः

'............न विद्या मातृकापरा ।'

इत्याम्नायसूचितप्रभावाया मातृकायाः संबन्धिनश्च कस्य प्रोक्तानुत्तरानन्देच्छादिशक्तिसमूहस्य चिदानन्दघनस्वस्वरूपसमावेशमयः सम्यक् बोधो भवति । एतच्चेह दिङ्मात्रेणोट्टङ्कितम् । विततं तु अस्मत्प्रभुपादैः श्रीपरात्रिंशकाविवरण-तन्त्रालोकादौ प्रकाशितम् । उक्तं च श्रीसिद्धामृते

'सात्र कुण्डलिनी बीजजीवभूता चिदात्मिका ।
तज्जं ध्रुवेच्छोन्मेषाख्यं त्रिकं वर्णास्ततः पुनः ॥
आ इत्यवर्णादित्यादि यावद्वैसर्गिकी कला ।
ककारादिसकारान्ता विसर्गात्पञ्चधा स च ॥
बहिश्चान्तश्च हृदये नादेऽथ परमे पदे ।
बिन्दुरात्मनि मूर्धान्ते हृदयाद्व्यापको हि सः ।
आदिमान्त्यविहीनास्तु मन्त्राः स्युः शरदभ्रवत् ।
गुरोर्लक्षणमेतावदादिमान्त्यं च वेदयेत् ॥
पूज्यः सोऽहमिव ज्ञानी भैरवो देवतात्मकः ।
श्लोकगाथादि यत्किञ्चिदादिमान्त्ययुतं यतः ॥
तस्माद्विदंस्तथा सर्वं मन्त्रत्वेनैव पश्यति ।'

इति । एतच्च स्पन्दे

'सेयं क्रियात्मिका शक्तिः शिवस्य पशुवर्तिनी ।
बन्धयित्री स्वमार्गस्था ज्ञाता सिद्ध्युपपादिका ॥'

इत्यनेनैव भङ्ग्या सूचितम् ॥ ७ ॥

TRANSLATION

'Accrues to the disciple'—this is the remaining part of the *sūtra*. According to the process described in *Parātriṁsakā* etc. the first aspect (*spanda*) of *anuttaraśakti* is the Supreme I-Consciousness which assumes the form of *akula*[1] i.e. that of which the body (*kula*) is 'a' (the letter अ). (This 'a' is the expression of *Cit-śakti* of *Śiva*). As there is further expansion of the world-manifesting power of *aham* or I-consciousness, *ānanda śakti* (bliss) comes into play which assumes the form of the letter 'ā' (आ), then bringing forward *icchā śakti* (will power), that I-consciousness displays 'i' (इ) in the *akṣubdha*[2] state of *icchā* and ī (ई) in its *kṣubdha* state which is an expression of *īśāna* or *īśitrī* (the power of mastery); then with *jñāna śakti* in its *akṣubdha* state, she displays *unmeṣa* (knowledge) which is represented by the letter 'u' (उ) and in the *kṣubdha* state of *jñāna śakti* displays *ūnatā* (deficiency in *jñāna* as mere *jñāna*) which becomes the cause of objective appearance. This is represented by the letter 'ū' (ऊ).

(After this there is a slight reverse movement in the progressive manifestation of the universe).

Just as in the flash of lightning there is at first merely a faint glimmer, and then there is more bright light, so 'i' of *akṣubdha icchāśakti* combining with 'r' becomes ऋ (ṛ) ; and 'i' of Kṣubdha *icchā* combining more firmly with 'r' becomes ॠ; 'r' is the seed letter of 'fire'. So also 'i' of *akṣubdha icchā śakti* combining with 'l' (ल) becomes 'ḷ' (ऌ) and 'i' of *kṣubdha icchā śakti* combining more firmly with 'l'(ल)becomes ॡ (ḹ);'r' is the seed letter of 'earth' (fixity, steadiness). The letters 'ṛ' and 'l' are only implicitly heard sounds (they are not actually produced letters). Inasmuch as they i.e. 'ṛ' and 'ḷ', the seed letters of fire and earth are mere subtle objects of *icchā śakti* and are imposed on it merely by the sound[3] of 'ṛ' and 'ḷ' and inasmuch as these four letters (ऋॠऌॡ) are assimilated to their own light (i.e. they rest only in themselves), they are said to be *amṛta* (imperishable) letters (i.e. they are not subject to any change; they do not give rise to other letters). As they are coloured merely by semblance of objectivity, so they are unable to produce any other letter. These four are, therefore, designated eunuch vowels[4].

The previously mentioned *anuttara* i.e. the letter 'a' (अ) and *ānanda* i.e. the letter 'ā' (आ) combining with 'i' of *icchā* form the triangular[5] e (ए) vowel.

With the combination of *anuttara* (i.e. the letter अ) *ānanda* (i.e. the letter आ) and *unmeṣa* (i.e. the letter उ) there is the formation of the letter 'o' (ओ) which denotes the inclusion of *kriyā śakti*.

With the combination of the previously mentioned two letters (i.e. with अ or आ + ए) there is the formation of the hexagonal letter[6]—(ऐ) and with the combination of 'a' or 'ā' and 'o' there is the formation of the trident[7] 'au' (औ). In the formation of the letter औ, there is the union of all the three *śaktis* viz, *icchā*, *jñāna* and *kriyā* with the predominance of *kriyā* in its clearest form.

Then the Supreme I-consciousness expresses the undivided knowledge of the universe in the form of a dot (*vindu*) in the letter 'am' (अं)[8]. It shows further the *visarga* stage in the form of two (perpendicular) dots indicating simultaneously inner and outer manifestation.[9]

Thus the creative I in its inner awareness shows the entire panorama of manifestation only as resting within the *anuttara* state and from the standpoint of outer awareness exhibits the expansion of a group of five *tattvas* in each group of five letters. through a, i, u, ṛ, ḷ, (अ,इ,उ,ऋ,लृ) *Śaktis*. Each group of five letters from *ka* to *ma* expresses *tattvas* from *pṛthivī* upto puruṣa.[10]

Each of these (a, i, etc.) has five *Śaktis*.[11] Therefore from each of these there arises a group of five (letters). With these very *śaktis* together with the *niyati* and other coverings of *māyā* which are located within the *Puruṣa* or the limited experient, the I-consciousness displays those letters which are known as *antaḥstha*.[12] (i.e. ya, ra, la, va) in Śikṣā.[13] Their names as *antaḥstha* (i.e. located within) are justified because they are the products of the *māyic* forces located within man (*pumbhūmau*)

They are known as *dhāraṇā* in the *āgama* scriptures (*āmnāyeṣu*), because they hold the universe by seizing the consciousness of the subjects (knowers).

Above Māyā (*tadupari*) with the disappearance of difference and the appearance of non-difference with her essential nature, the I-consciousness (with the zealous heat of this identity-consciousness) displays the four *ūṣmā* letters (viz., *Śa*, *Ṣa*, *Sa*, and *ha*)[14] [The word ūṣmā means heat, passion, eagerness]. In these *ūṣmā* letters she (I-consciousness) shows perfect *amṛta* letter[15] (*sa*) occurring as the penultimate one of the entire manifestation of letters and after that at the end she displays the *prāṇa bīja* (*ha* letter) in order to make one realize the fact that this universe consisting of words (*vācaka*) and their objects (*vācya*) and of the form of expansion of *ṣaḍadhvā*[16] is brought to its completion in the letter *ha* (*anāhata-maya*[17]) by the *anuttara śakti*.

Therefore the essence of the supreme virility of the great *mantra* in the form of the Supreme I-consciousness consists in showing by means of *pratyāhāra*[18] that the universe lies in the womb of 'a' and 'ha' (*aham* or I) which are symbolic of *anuttara* (a) and *anāhata* (ha) or in other words of *Śiva* and *Śakti*[19]. As has been said by *Utpaladeva*, our great grand teacher.

"The I-concept connotes resting of the light of consciousness within itself. Inasmuch as it excludes all (external) expectancy, it is known as Repose (within itself) or Composure. It is also absolute freedom, main doership and sovereign power." (Ajadapramātṛ-siddhi, 22-23).

Thus so far what has been described as the essence of Mātṛkā that very thing has been shown at the end by the *Kūṭabīja*[20] (*kṣa* letter) which is a combination of ka and sa and which results by the combination of the essence of *anuttara* (i.e. 'ka'[21]) and the essence of *visarga* (i.e. *sa*). So enough of expressing the mysterious.

Thus sambodha means full enlightenment consisting of communion with one's Self which is of the nature of consciousness-bliss. *Mātṛkā-cakra* means the collective whole (*cakra*) of the previously described *anuttara*, *ānanda*, *icchā* and other *śaktis* connected with the *Mātṛkā* the efficacy of which has been described in the scriptures in the following words "There is no knowledge higher than that of *Mātṛkā*."

This matter has been dealt with here merely by way of brief indication. It has been expressed in detail by my teacher (Abhinavagupta) in his commentary on *Parātriṁśakā*, *Tantrāloka* etc. It has been said in *Siddhāmṛta* also :

"That divine consciousness in its form as creative energy is known as *Kuṇḍalinī*. She is the seed and life of[22] all (बीजजीवभूता). From her is produced the group of three letters, viz; *dhruva* i.e. *anuttara* indicating 'a' *icchā* (indicating 'i') and *unmeṣa*, (indicating 'u').

From this triad are produced the various letters, e.g. ā' (आ) from 'a' (अ), 'ī' from 'i', ū from 'u' etc. right up-to the *visarga* aspect (i.e. अ:).

The letters from *Ka* (क) to *sa* (स) are produced by the creative energy (*visarga*)[23] of *Śiva*. That *visarga* is manifested in *five* ways, *one* outside (in the form of the expansion of the universe), and *four* inside (1) in the heart (2) in *nāda* i.e. in the throat (3) in the great stage (*parame pade*) i.e. between the two eyebrows and (4) in Brahmarandhra Thus it pervades from the heart up to the top of the skull.

Mantras devoid of the initial letter 'a' and the final letter 'ma' (i.e. अहं (*aham*) or I) are like autumnal clouds (i.e. just as autumnal clouds do not rain and so are useless, even so such *mantras* are useless).

The essential characteristic of a real spiritual director is that he should explain (to his disciples) the *mantra* beginning with 'a' and ending with 'ma' (aham). That sage, Bhairava-like, god-like guru deserves worship like myself (this is addressed to *Pārvatī* by *Śiva*). As he (the *guru*) feels even a hymn of praise (*śloka*) or a laudatory song (*gāthā*) or any thing else as connected with the Supreme I-consciousness, therefore, knowing everything in that way (i.e. as connected with I-consciousness), he perceives everything as a *mantra*.

The same idea has been expressed in another way in *Spanda kārikā* :

"That operative energy of *Śiva* (i.e. the divine *spanda*) existing in the limited experient (i.e. the empirical individual) binds the individual (when unrealized). When, however, it is realized as forming a path to *Śiva* who is one's own Self, it secures supreme power." (III,16).

NOTES

1. *Akula* : *Kula* is the state in which Śiva and Śakti remain in indistinguishable unity. *Akula* is a state different from it i.e. it is a state of Śiva. This is one meaning of *akula*, Secondly, *kula* means body. . Akula means that of which the body is the letter 'a' (which is the expression of *Cit-Śakti*). So there is a double entendre in the word *akula*. It is impossible to bring this out in the translation.

2. *Akṣubdha* and *Kṣubdha* : *Akṣubdha* (lit, unagitated) is the state in which *Icchā Śakti* has simply decided to manifest externally, but is still unaffected by objectivity. *Kṣubdha* (i.e. agitated) is the state when *Icchā Śakti* is coloured by objectivity.

The same holds true of the *akṣubdha* and *kṣubdha* states of *unmeṣa*.

3. ऋ-लृ-श्रुत्या: merely by the sound of 'ṛ', 'ḷ'. These letters are only heard as sound, they are not actually produced.

4. They are said to be *Ṣaṇḍha* or eunuch, because they are neither purely vowels nor purely consonants; they have a semblance of both, just as a eunuch has the semlance of both male and female. Secondly they are called eunuch because they are unable to produce any other letter.

5. This is called triangular vowel (त्रिकोणबीजम्) because firstly the letter 'e' (ए) is written in Śāradā Script as Ñ (indicating three angles) and secondly because all the three *Śaktis cit*, *ānanda* and *icchā* operate in its formation.

6. 'ai' (ऐ) is called षट्कोण or hexagonal, because as written in *Śāradā* script, it forms six angles.

7. औ is called शूलबीजं or त्रिशूलबीजं i.e. trident, because all the three *Śaktis*, *icchā*, *jñāna* and *kriyā* are present in this in the clearest form.

8. The idea is that the dot or *vindu* indicates that in spite of all these projections or emanations in the form of a, ā, i, ī, etc. the *anuttaraśakti* remains the highest knower or subject. The Sanskrit word *vindu* means both 'dot' and knower. *Vetti iti vinduḥ* i.e. *Vindu* means one who knows. In spite of all

objectivity issuing from *anuttara śakti* or the Supreme I-consciousness, this (i.e. I-consciousness) remains the changeless eternal Subject. In spite of all objectivity, there is no deviation from its position of a changeless subject.

9. The two dots of *visarga* (:) indicate the truth that from the point of view of *Śakti* symbolized by the lower dot there is an expansion of an outer world, but at the same time from the point of view of *Śiva* symbolized by the upper dot, the entire universe rests in the I-Consciousness of *Śiva*.

10. Each group of five letters as *vācaka* (i.e. names) has a corresponding group of *tattvas* as *vācya* (i.e. objects of those names). This will be clear from the following table :

Sl. No.	Name of the Śakti from which each class of letters is produced.	Names of the letters.	Name of the corresponding *tattvas*.
1.	अ	क, ख, ग, घ, ङ	पृथिवी, जल, अग्नि, वायु, आकाश —5 gross elements.
2.	इ	च, छ, ज, झ, ञ.	शब्द, रस, रूप, स्पर्श, गंध —5 Tanmātrās.
3.	ॠ	ट, ठ, ड, ढ, ण	उपस्थ, पायु, पाद, पाणि, वाक् —5 organs of action
4.	ॡ	त, थ, द, ध, न	घ्राण, रसना, चक्षुष्, त्वक्, श्रोतृ —5 organs of sense.
5.	उ	प, फ, ब, भ, म,	मन, अहंकार, बुद्धि, प्रकृति, पुरुष —the psychic apparatus the primal matter, and the limited experient.

11. A doubt may arise as to how from each *Śakti*, say from only one '*a*' of *anuttara*, there arises a group of five letters, viz, *ka, kha, ga, gha, ṅa,* similarly how from '*i*' of *icchā*, there arises a group of five letters, viz, *ca, cha, ja, jha, ña* and so on. To remove this doubt, *Kṣemarāja* says that each of these i.e. 'a' of

anuttara, 'i' of *icchā* etc. has all the five *Śaktis*, e.g., the 'a' of *anuttara* has all the five *śaktis* of *cit*, *ānanda*, *icchā*, *jñāna*, and *kriyā*; similarly 'i' of *icchā* has *icchā*, *cit*, *ānanda*, *jñāna* and *kriyā* and so on. Inasmuch as each of these has the power of five *śaktis*, therefore from each of these, there arises a group of five letters as *vācaka* (indicator) and a corresponding group of five *tattvas* as*vācya* (indicated or objects).

12. *Antaḥstha varṇas* are *ya*, *ra*, *la*, *va*. *Kṣemarāja* thinks that they are known as *antaḥstha* because they are determined by *māyā* and her *Kañcukas* (coverings) which operate from within the mind of man. Thus '*ya*' is determined by *niyati*; '*ra*' is determined by *kāla*, 'la' by *rāga* and *vidyā*, and 'va' by *Māyā* and *Kalā*.

Abhinavagupta, however, says in Tantrāloka 3rd Āhnika, (verses 154 to 156) that when *kṣubdha* and *akṣubdha Icchā śakti* is oriented towards *anuttara* (which is *cit*), then it produces '*ya*'. When ऋ which is identified with *Icchā śakti* is oriented towards *anuttara*, then *ra* appears, and when ऌ which is identified with *Icchā Sakti* is oriented towards *anuttara* then *la* appears. Similarly when *unmeṣa* is oriented towards *anuttara*, *va* appears.

In the same *Āhnika* in verse 158 *Abhinavagupta* says that since the formation of these *antaḥstha* letters (*ya*, *ra*, *la*, *va*) is due to *icchā* and *unmeṣa śaktis*, and since these are inner (*antaḥ*) forces and are identified with the *pramātā* (the subject), the letters *ya*, *ra*, *la*, *va* are rightly called *antaḥstha*. The *Sikṣā* works, however, call them *antaḥstha*, because they lie in between vowel and consonant i.e. they are neither purely vowel nor purely consonant.

13. *Sikṣā*—the science of phonetics.

14. Abhinavagupta says that *Icchā Śakti* appears in three forms, viz., 'i', 'ṛ' and 'ḷ' and these inspired by the inner light of Self appear outwardly as *śa*, *ṣa*, and *sa*. '*Ha*' is only a gross form of *visarga*. *Ś*a, *ṣa*, *sa*, represent *Śuddha vidyā*, *Īśvara*, and *Sadā-śiva* respectively.

15. Sa (स) is called परिपूर्ण अमृत वर्ण or perfect *amṛta* letter, because it includes within itself the manifestation of the universe. According to Śaiva Philosophy, the manifestation of the universe by *Śiva* is not a derognation from His essential

nature, but a fulfilment of it. The four letters ऌ ॡ ऋ ॠ are called simply *amṛta* without any adjective, because they only rest within themselves and do not produce anything. Besides 'sa' represents the state of *Sadāśiva*. Hence its importance.

16. *Ṣaḍadhvā* : The universe may be said summarily to consist of *varṇa, mantra* and *pada* on the *vācaka* or the subjective side and (1) *kalā* (2) *tattva* (3) and *bhuvana* on the *vācya* or objective side. *Ṣaṭ* means six and *adhvā* means course or path.

17. 'Ha' is a form of *Śiva's visarga śakti*. So 'ha' (ह्) in its subtle form is constantly being sounded inside each creature without any effort on its part.

It is called *avyakta hakalātmaḥ* by Abhinavagupta (T. III, verse 146). Jayaratha comments on this as follows :

अव्यक्ता नादमात्ररूपत्वादनुद्भिन्नवर्णप्रविभागा येयं हकलाहकारार्धार्धभाग: तदात्मकोयं विसर्ग:

(pp. 142-148)

This visarga pertaining to ह् is only a vibration inside, not uttered in the form of a distinct letter.

Again on p. 149, Jayaratha quotes the following verse :

नास्योच्चारयिता कश्चित् प्रतिहन्ता न विद्यते ।
स्वयमुच्चरते देव: प्राणिनामुरसि स्थित: ।।

No one (deliberately) pronounces it, nor can any body prevent its being sounded (as an inner vibration). This is self-sounded in the breast of beings.

It is spontaneous, ceaseless sound going on inside without utterance, without effort on the part of any one. Hence it is called *anāhatamaya* i.e. not struck or uttered by the vocal organs. 'Ha' indicates *śakti*. As such, it is the source of all prāṇa (प्राणबीज).

18. *Pratyāhāra* : This word has been used here in the technical sense of Sanskrit Grammar. It means the 'comprehension of several letters or affixes into one syllable, effected by combining the first letter of a *sūtra* with the final indicatory letter'. The *pratyāhāra* of 'a' the first letter and 'ha' the final letter is 'aha' which suggests 'aham', meaning 'I' or Self. 'Aha' includes all

the letters of the Sanskrit alphabet, and since each letter is indicative of an object, 'aha' suggests the sum total of all objects i.e. the universe. The Philosophical truth that is pointed out is that the entire universe lies in Śiva or Highest Reality in an undifferentiated state.

The full word for I in Sanskrit is 'aham' written as अहं with a *vindu* or dot on the letter 'ha'. This *vindu* or dot is full of high philosophical significance.

In the definite calm of *anuttara* or Highest Reality, there arises a metaphysical Point of Stress. This is known as *vindu.* In this, the universe to be is gathered up into a Point. This *vindu* is *ghanībhūtā śakti*, the creative force compacted into a Point. It is as yet undifferentiated into subjects and objects. It is the *cidghana* or massive consciousness in which lie potentially in an undifferentiated mass all the worlds and beings to be manifested. The dot or *vindu* on 'ha' joins 'a' and 'ha' into oneness and shows that all manifestation though appearing emanated and different is actually resting in *śiva* and is not different from Him. 'A' represents *Śiva* and 'ha' represents *Śakti*, the *vindu* on 'ha' represents the fact that though Śiva is manifested right up to the earth through *Śakti* he is not divided thereby, he remains undivided whole. *Vindu* means that which knows. It is derived from the root 'vid' which means 'to know'. *Vetti iti vinduḥ. Vindu* is that which knows. That is why Abhinavagupta calls it *avibhāgaḥ prakāśo yaḥ. Avibhāgah prakāśo yaḥ sa vinduḥ paramo hi naḥ* (I. III A, verse III). "That which is undivided light, that which in spite of all differentiation does not change, remains unaffected and does not deviate from its inherent oneness is for us *Vindu.*"

19. अ of अह represents *Śiva* and 'ha' of this word represents *Sakti.*

20. *Kūṭabīja*—The word *kūṭa* means highest, most excellent, mysterious. *Kūṭabīja* is a mystical name of the letter *kṣa* (क्ष). Kūṭa is a technical name for a letter which results from the combination of two *halanta* letters. Here the two *halanta* letters are 'k' (क्) and 's' (स्). Their combination results in *kṣa* (क्ष) Therefore 'kṣa' is called a Kūṭa letter.

21. *Anuttara* is said to be the essence of *ka* class of tetters,

because as described before, '*ka*' is formed by the vowel 'a' (अ) which is the symbol of *anuttara*.

22. In the unmanifest state, *Kuṇḍalinī* is *bīja* i.e. the seed of all manifestation; in the manifest state she is *jīva* i.e. the life of all.

The word *Kuṇḍalinī* means the divine creative Energy—*Visarga-Śakti* of *Śiva's* I-consciousness. It is coiled in three and a half folds. One fold represents the objective aspect (*prameya*) of the Supreme I-Consciousness, another fold represents the *pramāṇa* or knowledge aspect, the third fold represents the *pramātā* or the subjective aspect; the remaining half represents *pramā* aspect which contains within itself both the subjective and the objective aspect in indistinguishable unity.

When the *parā-śakti* (the Highest creative *Śakti* of *Śiva*) though creative, is not yet functioning but lies like a sleeping serpent coiled in three and a half folds, she is known as *Śakti Kuṇḍalinī*. When she is oriented externally to manifest life, she is known as *Prāṇa Kuṇḍalinī*. At this stage, *Saṁvit* or consciousness is transferred into *prāṇa* or life. This Prāṇa Kuṇḍalinī is present in every living being. In the reverse movement back from life to consciousness when she assumes her original form of consciousness, she is known as *Parā Kuṇḍalinī*. At this stage, there is the delightful unity-consciousness of I and the world, of Self and not-Self. Everything appears as a form of 'I'.

In the long verse quoted from *Siddhāmṛta*, the author shows how the creative *Śakti-Kuṇḍalinī* passes into the stage of *Prāṇa-Kuṇḍalinī* by manifesting both *vācaka* (words) and *Vācya* (their objects) and how her *Visarga Śakti* (creative energy) manifests itself in human life, and finally exhorts all aspirants to recapture their original divine I-consciousness from which alone the *visarga śakti* in the form of *Kuṇḍalinī* started the play of life.

Thus it gives all the three aspects of Kuṇḍalinī—(1) Śakti, (2) Prāṇa and (3) Parā Kuṇḍalinī.

23. *Visarga* : It literally means emanation, manifestation, projection. The verse says :

ककारादि सकारान्ता विसर्ग इति (जाता)

In this context *visarga* means *visarga śakti*, the projecting manifesting, creative energy of the Divine, the supreme Creative energy of *anuttara* (the Highest Reality).

There are three aspects of this *visarga.* (1) परविसर्ग (*para-visarga*) is आ (ā) (आनन्द). It is known as *ānandavisarga*, It is *śāmbhava visarga* showing *abheda* or non-difference. (2) परापरविसर्ग (*parāpara-visarga*) is अ : It is *śākta visarga* showing *bhedābheda* i.e. identity in the midst of difference. The lower dot of अ: denotes the expansion of the creative energy into the universe, indicating a difference from *Śiva*; the upper dot points to the identity of the universe with Śiva. Hence it is *parāpara.* The pharse बहिश्चान्तश्च signifies this *parāpara* aspect of *visarga.* (3) अपर विसर्ग (apara visarga) is ह (ha). This is also known as *bheda visarga*, showing *bheda* or difference. It is also known as *āṇava visarga.* It only refers to the manifestation of the universe without making any reference to its source.

EXPOSITION

Manifestation consists of *vācaka* and *vācya* or *nāma* and *rūpa*, words and objects. At the highest level of Reality they are one. In manifestation, they bifurcate into *vācaka* and *vācya.* In manifestation, the *vācaka* is the subjective side and the *vācya* is the objective side.

All human activities are carried on through *vācaka* or words. *Vācaka* consists of *Mātṛkā. Mātṛkā* means letters or lettered sound. It is through *mātṛkā*, therefore, that all human activities are carried on. So long as the mystery of the *mātṛkā* is not understood, we are only involved in the 'fret and fever' of life. "We nod and hurry and pass by, and do not for once possess our soul." If a man wants to understand the mystery of life, if he wants to turn to the source of his being, he will have to understand the mystery of *Mātṛkā.* Mātṛkā not properly understood only confines us to the feverish activities of life, and thus becomes a source of bondage. If properly understood, she becomes our saviour.

The realization of the mysteries of *Matṛkā* is most important for the aspirant who is in quest of the source of his being. The *Śāktopāya* deals primarily with *mantra. Mantra* consists of words or letters, in other words, *Mātṛkā.* It is, therefore, of utmost importance for the aspirant to understand *Mātṛkā* and her host of *śaktis.*

This *sūtra*, therefore, exhorts the aspirant to have *sambodha*—full realization, perfect enlightenment of *Mātṛkā Cakra*, of the occult meaning of lettered sound which is the warp and woof of *mantra*.

The *Sūtra* tells us that all letters are only an expression of *Parāvāk* or *Parāśakti* or *Parāhantā* or *Anuttara śakti*—the Cosmic Creative Stress, the *Spanda* or pulsation of Supreme Creative Consciousness known as *Śiva*, This Creative Power of Śiva in its cosmic aspect is also known as *Śakti Kuṇḍalinī*.

There are five main *Śaktis* of *Śiva*, viz., *Cit* or *ANUTTARA Śakti*, *Ānanda*, *Icchā*, *Jñāna* and *Kriyā*. The *anuttara śakti* expresses itself in the vowel 'a' (अ); the *ānanda śakti* expresses itself in the vowel 'ā' (आ). *Icchā Śakti* expresses itself in two ways, viz. 'i' and 'ī' (इ, ई) and ऋ, ॠ, ऌ, and ॡ, the *jñāna Śakti* expresses itself in '*u*' and '*ū*' (उ, ऊ) and with the permutation and combination of 'a', 'i', 'u' in various ways, the *Kriyā* Śakti expresses itself in 'e', 'ai', 'o', 'au' (ए, ऐ, ओ, औ). The dot (बिन्दु) expresses the unification of all manifestation into one consciousness of Śiva and the *visarga* (two dots one above the other) points to Śiva's inner rest and the external expansion of His Śakti in the form of the universe. These vowels represent the inner life of *Śiva*. Of all the vowels, a (अ) the representative of *anuttara śakti* is the most important. As Jayaratha puts it in his commentary on Tantrāloka (Āhnika III, p. 120)

'अकारः सर्ववर्णानामन्तर्यामितया स्थितः

"A (अ) resides in all the letters as their inner controller."

The vowels अ, इ, उ, ऋ, ऌ give rise to the various consonants which symbolize the various *tattvas* from earth to *Sadāśiva*. It is Śiva, therefore, who dwells in the heart of all the letters and all the creatures and expresses all manifestation as identical with Himself.

Niṣkala or *Parama Śiva* is the transcendent *Śiva*, above all manifestation: *Śiva* is His first creative pulsation in whom arises I-Consciousness-(*aham*). This *aham* or I-consciousness known as *vimarśa* is like a mirror of rays of light which contains all the *varṇas* or letters (*vācakas*) and *vācya* (objects) in a latent, incipient form just as the plasma of a peacock's egg contains the variegated plumage of the peacock in a latent form.

The 'a' (अ) of *aham* symbolizes *anuttara* (the Highest Reality) and the 'ha' of this 'aham' symbolizes *Visarga Śakti*. Thus 'aham' is the matrix of fifty letters from 'a' to 'h'. This 'aham' is the *parā mātṛkā śakti* which contains within itself *icchā, jñāna* and *kriyā*. From this arise *icchātmaka paśyantī mātṛkā*, jñānātmaka *madhyamā mātṛkā* and *kriyātmaka vaikharī mātṛkā*. This '*aham*' contains the entire *vācaka* and *vācya* universe in a latent form.

A knowledge of the *Mātṛkā cakra* shows how all letters and all *tattvas* from earth upto *Sadāśiva* have evolved simultaneously from *aham*. The collective whole of *śaktis* (*cakra*) of Mātṛkā pertains to *icchā, jñāna* and *kriyā śaktis* of Śiva which evolve the world of words and objects.

The *sambodha* or clear realization of the significance of *Mātṛkā cakra* leads the aspirant to realize that his real I is the blissful I-consciousness of Śiva. This real I-consciousness is the secret of *mantra*. It liberates the aspirant from his pseudo I-consciousness, from his psycho-somatic self, and he now knows himself as identical both with *Śiva* and His manifestation in the form of the universe.

INTRODUCTION TO THE 8th SŪTRA

TEXT

ईदृशस्य अस्य मातृकाचक्रसंबोधवतः—

TRANSLATION

Of such a person who has fully realized the significance of the collective whole of Mātṛkā.

SŪTRA—8

शरीरं हविः ॥ ८ ॥

Śarīraṁ haviḥ

शरीरं—body; हविः—oblation.

"(Of such a person) the body becomes an oblation (to be poured into the fire of the highest consciousness).

COMMENTARY

सर्वैर्यत्प्रमातृत्वेन अभिषिक्तं स्थूलसूक्ष्मादिस्वरूपं शरीरं तत् महायोगिनः परस्मिन् चिदग्नौ हूयमानं हविः; शरीरप्रमातृताप्रशमनेन सदैव चिन्मातृताभिनिविष्टत्वात् । यदुक्तं श्रीविज्ञानभैरवे

'महाशून्यालये वह्नौ भूताक्षविषयादिकम् ।
हूयते मनसा साकं स होमः स्रुक्च चेतना ॥'

इति । श्रीतिमिरोद्घाटेऽपि

'यः प्रियो यः सुहृद्बन्धुर्यो दाता योऽतिवल्लभः ।
तदङ्गभक्षणाद्देवि ह्यु त्पतेद्गगनाङ्गना ॥'

इति । अत्र हि देहप्रमातृताप्रशमनमेव पिण्डार्थः । श्रीमद्भगवद्गीतास्वपि

'सर्वाणीन्द्रियकर्माणि प्राणकर्माणि चापरे ।
आत्मसंयमयोगाग्नौ जुह्वति ज्ञानदीपिते ॥'

इति । स्पन्दे तु ।

'यदा क्षोभः प्रलीयेत तदा स्यात्परमं पदम् ।'

इत्यनेनैव संगृहीतम् । क्षोभो देहाद्यहंप्रत्ययरूपः, इति हि तद्वृत्तौ भट्टश्रीकल्लटः ॥८॥

TRANSLATION

Of that great *Yogī*, all this gross, subtle and causal body which is affected with the idea of knower or I becomes an oblation to be offered to the highest consciousness-fire. Because of the annulment of the idea of the body being the Self, he is constantly steeped in the idea of pure consciousness only being his Self.

As has been said in *Vijñāna-bhairava*,

"One should pour into the fire of the Highest Consciousness all the elements, senses, and the objects of sense together with mind (that creates all these divisions). This is real *homa* (oblation). The (Self-inquiring) consciousness is the ladle (with which this oblation is to be performed)." (Verse 149).

In *Timirodghāta* also it is said,

"By the extinction of attachment in one who is dear, who is a friend, who is a relation, a donor, or who is greatly beloved, the *Śakti* of *cidākāśa* rises higher." Here the main purport is the extinction of the sense of the body as the Self. In the *Bhagavadgītā* also, it has been said,

"In the deep fire of *yoga* pertaining to self-control lighted with clear perception of reality do the *yogis* offer as oblation all the activities of the senses, and *prāṇa*." (IV, 27). (*Apara* in this verse has been explained as *agādha* (deep) by Abhinavagupta).

In the Spandakārikā also the same idea has been expressed in the following verse:

"When the disturbed condition of his mind in considering the Self as not-self and the not-Self as Self disappears, then will accrue to him the highest state (i.e. the realization of the Spanda principle". (I, 9)

Here *Kṣobha* means the idea of the body etc as the Self.

This is how *Bhaṭṭa Kallaṭa* has explained it in his commentary.

INTRODUCTION TO THE 9th SŪTRA

TEXT

अस्य च—

TRANSLATION

And of such a *yogī,*

SŪTRA—9

ज्ञानमन्नम् ॥ ९ ॥

Jñānam annam.

ज्ञानम्—limited knowledge which is the cause of bondage; अन्नम्—food to be devoured.

"The limited, vitiated knowledge which is the cause of bondage is the food to be devoured."

COMMENTARY

TEXT

यत्पूर्वं 'ज्ञानं बन्धः' (१–२) इत्युक्तं तत् अद्यमानत्वात्, ग्रस्यमानत्वात योगिनामन्नम् । यत्संवादितं प्राक्

'मृत्युं च कालं च कलाकलापं
विकारजातं प्रतिपत्तिसात्म्यम् ।
ऐकात्म्य-नानात्म्यवितर्कजातं
तदा स सर्वं कवलीकरोति ॥'

इति ।

अथ च यत्स्वरूपविमर्शात्मकं ज्ञानं तत् अस्य अन्नं, पूर्णपरितृप्तिकारितया स्वात्मविश्रान्तिहेतुः । तदुक्तं श्रीविज्ञानभैरवे

'अत्रैकतमयुक्तिस्थे योत्पद्येत दिनाद्दिनम् ।
भरिताकारिता सात्र तृप्तिरत्यन्तपूर्णता ॥'

इति । युक्तिर्हि तत्र द्वादशोत्तरशतभूमिकाज्ञान-रूपैव । एतच्च स्पन्दे

'प्रबुद्धः सर्वदा तिष्ठेत् . . . . ।'

इत्यनया कारिकया संगृहीतम् ॥ ६ ॥

TRANSLATION

"Limited knowledge is the cause of bondage" which has been mentioned previously (under I,2) becomes his food, because such limited knowledge is devoured by the *Yogī*.

This is in full conformity with what has been adduced earlier as testimony in the following verse of *Bhargaśikhā*.

"When he (the *yogī*) realizes his real Self, then he devours death, (death of the gross body), *kāla*—the presiding Spirit of death, the multitude of activities, all changes for the worse, identification with the knowledge of objects, all thought-constructs of non-difference, and difference."

(The *Sūtra* may be explained in another way) or his knowledge of the realization of Self is food inasmuch as by affording full satisfaction it becomes the means of rest in one's own Self. It has been said in *Vijñānabhairava*:

"By adopting any one of the means for Self-realization, the sense of fulfilment that occurs from day to day is, in this matter, a satisfaction denoting highest perfection." (Verse 148). The word *yukti* or means indicates here the knowledge of hundred and twelve kinds of *yoga*.

The same idea has been expressed in the following verse of Spandakārikā :

"One should always remain awake .e. should not lose sight of the fact that everything is *Śiva*) by observing the whole universe of objectivity with the knowledge (that everything is *Śiva*). He should consider everything as non-different from *Śiva*. Then he will not be afflicted with anything." (III, 12).

EXPOSITION

Kṣemarāja interprets this *sūtra* in two ways. In the first interpretation, he takes *jñāna* in the sense of 'limited knowledge', and *annam* in the sense of 'being devoured' and says that all limited knowledge should be devoured by the *yogī* i.e. all limited knowledge should be reduced to sameness with the Self.

In the second interpretation, he takes *jñānam* in the sense of *svarūpa-jñāna* (knowledge of Self), and *annam* in the sense of 'food that gives satisfaction' and interprets the *sūtra* as saying that Self-knowledge is the food that gives highest satisfaction. *Bhāskara* in his *Vārttika* interprets *jñāna* as *svarūpa-jñāna* (knowledge of Self), and so his interpretation of this *sūtra* agrees with the second interpretation given above.

INTRODUCTION TO THE 10th SŪTRA

TEXT

यदा तु एवं सततावहितो न भवति, तदा ज्ञानवतोऽपि अस्य अवधानावलेपात्—

TRANSLATION

When the *yogī* is not always on the alert, then even in the case of one who has acquired knowledge of the Self, there is, on the flagging of attention.

SŪTRA—10.

TEXT

विद्यासंहारे तदुत्थस्वप्नदर्शनम् ॥ १० ॥

Vidyāsaṁhāre taduttha-svapna-darśanam.

विद्यासंहारे—on the submergence of *Śuddha vidyā* तदुत्थस्वप्नदर्शनम्—there is appearance of thought-construct arising from it.

On the submergence of *Śuddha Vidyā* (pure overmental knowledge), (there is) appearance of all kinds of thought-constructs arising from it, (i.e. from the submergence of *Śuddha Vidyā*).

Bhāskara, in his *Vārttika*, interprets this *sūtra* differently. According to *Kṣemarāja*, *Vidyā* here means *śuddha vidyā*, but according to *Bhāskara, vidyā* here means knowledge, common to the ordinary folk of the world. So Bhāskara interprets the *sūtra* thus :

"When the knowledge common to the ordinary folk of the world dissolves (on the realization of one's true Self) then the previously apprehended delusive knowledge of the objects of the world is remembered only like a dream."

COMMENTARY

TEXT

प्रोक्तज्ञानस्फाररूपायाः शुद्धविद्यायाः संहारे, निमज्जने, तदुत्थस्य क्रमात्क्रमत्यक्तकृतविद्यासंस्कारस्य स्वप्नस्य, भेदमयस्य विकल्पप्रपञ्चरूपस्य दर्शनं स्फुटम् उन्मज्जनं भवति । तदुक्तं श्रीमालिनीविजये

'न चैतदप्रसन्नेन शङ्करेणोपदिश्यते ।
कथञ्चिदुपदिष्टेऽपि वासना नैव जायते ॥'

इत्युपक्रम्य

'वासनामात्रलाभेऽपि योऽप्रमत्तो न जायते ।
तमनित्येषु भोगेषु योजयन्ति विनायकाः ॥'

इति । तदेतत्

'अन्यथा तु स्वतन्त्रा स्यात्सृष्टिस्तद्धर्मकत्वतः ।
सततं लौकिकस्येव जाग्रत्स्वप्नपदद्वये ॥'

इत्यनेन स्पन्दे संगृहीतम् । अतश्च नित्यं शुद्धविद्याविमर्शनपरेणैव योगिना भाव्यम् इत्युपदिष्टं भवति । यथोक्तम्

'तस्मान्न तेषु संसक्तिं कुर्वीतोत्तमवाञ्छया ।'

इति—श्रीपूर्वे । श्रीस्पन्देऽपि

'अतः सततमुद्युक्तः स्पन्दतत्त्वविविक्तये ।
जाग्रदेव निजं भावमचिरेणाधिगच्छति ॥' इति

TRANSLATION

On the *saṁhāra* i.e. on the submergence of the previously mentioned *Śuddha Vidyā* which cannotes expansion of spiritual wisdom there is appearance of all kinds of pluralistic thought-constructs which arise from the gradual disappearance of the impressions of *Śuddha-Vidyā*. *Darśanam* means 'there occurs clear emergence (of such thought-constructs).

It has been said in Mālinī-vijaya :

"This is instructed by *Śaṅkara* (in the form of a *guru*) when he is fully pleased. But even when somehow the instruction is imparted, the impression of such knowledge does not remain."

Beginning with the above, *Mālinīvijaya* says further, "Even when one has obtained merely limited powers (vāsanāmātra lābhe-pi) but is not mindful, tempters who put obstacles in the progress of *yoga* egg him on to transient pleasures."

The same idea has been well set forth in *Spandakārikā* in the following verse;

"Otherwise (i.e. if he is not established in his real nature), Nature as is characteristic of her is quite free in presenting objects to him both in waking and dreaming states in the same way as she does in the case of ordinary worldly persons (i.e. like ordinary worldly people, he will be the plaything of the ordinary course of Nature)" (III, 3).

Therefore it is taught that the *yogī* should always be intent on the awareness of Śuddha Vidyā.

In *Mālinī-vijaya*, it has been said,

"Therefore, one who desires to realize the higher Self should not be attached to objects of pleasure."

In *Spandakārikā* also, it has been said

"Hence one who is always intent on having a clear vision of the *spanda* principle realizes very soon his real nature even in the waking state." (I, 21)

CONCLUSION OF THE SECOND SECTION

TEXT

एवं 'चित्तं मन्त्रः' (२–१) इत्यतः प्रभृति मन्त्रवीर्य-मुद्रावीर्यानु-संधिप्रधानम्

'उच्चाररहितं वस्तु चेतसैव विचिन्तयन् ।
यं समावेशमाप्नोति शाक्तः सोऽत्राभिधीयते ॥'

इत्याम्नातं शाक्तोपायं विविच्य, अवधानावलिप्तं प्रति 'विद्यासंहारे तदुत्थ-स्वप्नदर्शनम्' (२–१०) इति सूत्रेण एतदनुषङ्गेण आणवोपायप्रतिपादनस्य अवकाशो दत्तः । इति शिवम् ॥ १० ॥

TRANSLATION

Thus the second section beginning with the *sūtra* : *Cittam mantraḥ*, and showing that in *Śāktopāya*, the main emphasis is on the intensive awareness of the transforming power of *mantra* and *mudrā*, gives a clear conception of *śāktopāya*, according to the *āgama* scriptures in the following verse of Mālinīvijaya.

"That communion (with *Śiva*) which is obtained only by mental reflection on the reality which is beyond the process of enunciation is designated in this tradition as *Śākta*." (II, 22).

Further by the Sūtra *Vidyāsaṁhāre tadutthasvapnadarśanam* directed towards the aspirant who is unable to maintain continuous attention, this section provides in this connexion an occasion for expounding *āṇavopāya* (in the next section). May there be prosperity for all!

THIRD SECTION

INTRODUCTION TO THE 1st SŪTRA

TEXT

इदानीमाणवोपायं प्रतिपिपादयिषुः, अणोः तावत्स्वरूपं दर्शयति—

TRANSLATION

Now desirous of expounding *āṇavopāya*, the *Sūtrakāra* first of all describes the nature of *aṇu*.

SŪTRA—1.

आत्मा चित्तम् ॥ १ ॥

Atmā Cittam.

आत्मा—the individual Self.

चित्तम् = mind

"The individual Self is mind (constituted by *buddhi*, *aham*, and *manas*)."

COMMENTARY

TEXT

यदेतत् विषयवासनाच्छुरितत्वात् नित्यं, तदध्यवसायादिव्यापारबुद्ध्यहङ्कृन्मनोरूपं चित्तं, तदेव अतति, चिदात्मकस्वस्वरूपाख्यात्या सत्त्वादिवृत्त्यवलम्बनेन योनीः संचरति, इति आत्मा अणुरित्यर्थः । न तु चिदेकरूपस्य अस्य अतनमस्ति । अत एव 'चैतन्यमात्मा' (१–१) इति स्वभावभूततात्त्विकैतत्स्वरूपप्रतिपादनाशयेन पूर्वमात्मा लक्षितः । इदानीं तु एतदीयसंकोचावभासप्रधानाणवदशौचित्येन, इति न पूर्वापरवैषम्यम् ॥ १ ॥

TRANSLATION

Citta or mind is that which coloured with the desire for sense-objects is always engaged in the activity of their ascertainment, appropriation to self and thought-construct. These activities are carried on respectively by *buddhi*, *ahaṁkāra* and *manas*. It is these that constitute *citta* It is this *citta* which is the individual *ātmā* or *aṇu*. It is called *ātmā*, because the word *ātman* is derived from the root *at* which means to move constantly'. *Atati iti ātmā*—that which moves on constantly is *ātmā*. Owing to primal ignorance of its real nature which is pure foundational consciousness, it moves on to various forms of existence by clinging to *sattva*, *rajas* and *tamas*.[1] That is why it is known as *ātmā* or *aṇu*.[2]

Really speaking, there is no wandering of *ātmā* which is purely consciousness. Therefore in the first Sūtra of the first section, viz., 'Caitanyam Ātmā' i.e. ātma is consciousness', *ātmā* has been, at first, so defined with the intention of expounding its inherent, essential nature. Now, however, the definition is being given mainly from the standpoint of its appearance in limitation. This definition is suitable to its condition of limitation (āṇava daśā). Therefore, there is no inconsistency between the previous and the later definition.

NOTES

1. *Sattva* : is prakāśa, visibility or manifestation. This is predominantly the attribute of *buddhi*; *rajas* is *cāñcalya*—unsteadiness. This is predominantly the attribute of *manas*; *tamas* is *āvaraṇa* covering, concealing. This is the attribute of *ahaṁkāra* inasmuch as it conceals the nature of the real Self.

Therefore the statement that *ātmā* clings to *sattva*, *rajas* and *tamas* signifies the fact that it uses *buddhi*, *manas* and *ahaṁkāra* for its expression in the lower planes.

2. *Aṇu* : minute, atomic, a mere point, The universal consciousness limits itself to a Point. Hence the individual self is known as *aṇu*.

EXPOSITION

Āṇavopāya or *Āṇava Yoga* is concerned with *aṇu*—a mere Point or the empirical self. The first *sūtra*, therefore, defines the nature of *aṇu*.

Cit or universal consciousness during the course of manifestation becomes reduced to *Citta* which consists of *buddhi*, *manas*, and *ahaṁkāra*. The *citta* becomes conditioned by its desire for the pleasure of the objects of sense. The constituent of *buddhi* is primarily *sattva*, that of *manas* is *rajas* and that of *ahaṁkāra* is *tamas*. It is this *citta* which is *aṇu*. This *citta* or *aṇu* is called *ātmā* in this context. Using *buddhi*, *manas* and *ahaṁkāra* it moves about (*atati*) from one form of existence to another. *Citta* is *aṇu* or ātmā i.e. the individual self in this context. Therefore, *āṇavopāya* is concerned with *buddhi*, *manas* and *ahaṁkāra*. Bhāskara gives a different interpretation of this *Sūtra*. According to him, *citta* and *manas* are synonymous, when *manas* is extroverted, then mentation is called *saṁkalpa*; when *manas* is introverted and it reflects on the Self, its reflection is known as *mantra*. When *manas* is turned inward, it can grasp the real nature of Self. This interpretation does not seem to be borne out by the wordings of the *Sūtra*.

INTRODUCTION TO THE 2nd SŪTRA

TEXT

अस्य चित्तस्वरूपस्य अण्वात्मनः––

TRANSLATION

Of this limited self whose nature is citta.

SŪTRA—2

ज्ञानं बन्धः ॥ २ ॥

Jñānam bandhaḥ.

ज्ञानं =knowledge which is the product of *citta*;

बन्धः—source of bondage.

"(Of this limited, empirical self) mind-born knowledge is a source of bondage."

COMMENTARY

TEXT

सुखदुःखमोहमयाध्यवसायादिवृत्तिरूपं तदुचितभेदावभासनात्मकं यत् ज्ञानं, तत्बन्धः। तत्पाशितत्वादेव हि अयं संसरति। तदुक्तं श्रीतन्त्रसद्भावे

'सत्त्वस्थो राजसस्थश्च तमस्थो गुणवेदकः ।
एवं पर्यटते देही स्थानात्स्थानान्तरं व्रजन् ॥'

इति । एतदेव

'तन्मात्रोदयरूपेण मनोऽहंबुद्धिवर्तिना ।
पुर्यष्टकेन संरुद्धस्तदुत्थं प्रत्ययोद्भवम् ॥
भुङ्क्ते परवशो भोगं तद्भावात्संसरेत् .... ।'

इत्यनेनानूदितम् ।

....................,अतः ।
संसृतिप्रलयस्यास्य कारणं संप्रचक्ष्महे ॥'

इत्येतत्प्रतिविधानाय स्पन्दशास्त्रे ॥ २ ॥

TRANSLATION

Modes of *buddhi* and *ahaṁkāra* which are full of pleasure, pain, and stupefaction and appearance of difference pertinent to the above modes are what constitute knowledge (*jñāna*) of the empirical self (*aṇu*). This (limited) knowledge is the source of bondage. Being bound by such knowledge, this empirical self (*aṇu*) leads a transmigratory existence. It has been said in *Tantrasadbhāva*.

"Confined to *sattva*, *rajas*, and *tamas* and knowing only what the senses can inform, the embodied one wanders about in existence, moving from one station to another."

The same idea has been repeated in the following verses of *Spandakārikā*.

"Being bound up by the *Puryaṣṭaka* that arises from *tanmātras* and by the modes of mind, the I-making principle and the determinative faculty, the empirical self experiences as a subservient creature pleasure and pain that result from the ideas which originate from the *puryaṣṭaka* and so he becomes subject to transmigratory existence because of the existence of that *puryaṣṭaka*. I shall, therefore, clearly explain what brings about the dissolution of the transmigratory existence of such an individual." (III, 17-18). The *Spandaśāstra* proposes the means for the annulment of this transmigratory existence.

NOTES

1. *Puryaṣṭaka* : Lit., the city of the group of eight i.e. the five *tanmātras*—five subtle forms of matter, viz., *śabdatanmātra*-sound-in-itself, *sparśa tanmātra*—touch-in-itself, *rūpa-tan-mātra*—form in-itself, *rasa-tanmātra*—taste-in-itself, *gandha-tanmātra*-smell-in-itself, and three psychic factors, viz., *buddhi, manas*, and *ahaṁkāra*. It is a synonym for *sūkṣma-śarīra* or subtle body.

2. *Pratyaya* means idea, but it is used in a technical sense here, verse No. 14. of *Niṣyanda* III in *Spandakārikā* defines 'pratyayaḥ' in the following words:

स च तन्मात्रगोचर: *Tanmātra-gocarah* has been explained as शब्दादिविषयविषय: It has been further defined as श्रोत्रादिद्वारेण विषयदर्शने ज्ञानोत्पत्ति: ।

Gathering up the various ideas, *pratyaya* may be defined as sense-born and word-governed ideas which lead a man towards enjoying objects of the external world. The word *pratyaya* also means *vikalpa*—thought-construct, fancy. It is impossible to find one word in English which can do justice to such a rich connotation.

EXPOSITION

The second *sūtra* says that the lower, limited knowledge of the embodied individual becomes the cause of his bondage.

This lower, limited knowledge becomes the cause of the individual's bondage in many ways.

Firstly, in practical life we have to do with particulars. Therefore, the empirical individual thinks that particulars are the sole truth of life. He is confined to differences and distinctions and is unable to grasp the Universal of which the particulars are only a limited expression. He misses the wood for the trees. He is unable to see 'the life that vibrates in every atom, the light that shines in every creature, the love that embraces all in oneness.' He is 'cabined, caged and confined' within his particular self and its needs and desires. Because he is unable to flow with the current of life, he remains bound, chained to transient pleasures.

Secondly, all the ideas of the individual are derived from sensori-motor perceptions, their images, and thought-constructs, imagination, and fancies of the mind and *Śabda-rāśi*—the stock of words that he has gathered by experience and study. He becomes a play-thing of the *Mātṛkā-cakra*. He is unable to believe that there can be any supersensuous reality. So he builds a prison for himself in which he takes the utmost delight to live.

Thirdly he considers his mind-body complex, his psycho-physical organism to be his Self. He does not care to know that these are only instruments for the life of the Ātmā—his real Self on the material plane. So he indulges in gross physical pleasures. The desire for them becomes so strong that he becomes their victim. He does not enjoy them; they enjoy him.

As Bhagavadgītā puts it;

ये हि संस्पर्शजा भोगा दुःखयोनय एव ते ।
आद्यन्तवन्तः कौन्तेय न तेषु रमते बुधः ॥ (V, २२)

"Pleasures born of contact are only sources of pain. O son of Kunti, they have a beginning and an end (i.e. they are transient). The wise man does not indulge in them."

He does not realize that the residual traces (vāsanās) of all his strong desires and cravings are deposited in his *puryaṣṭaka*, his subtle body and by the law of forces of desire they drag him down again in the next life to a body in which those desires and cravings can be satisfied. As *Kṣemarāja* puts it in his commentary on the 1st verse of the 3rd *Niṣyanda* in *Spandakārikā*:

तस्य पुर्यष्टकस्य भावादेव पुनः पुनरुद्बोधितविचित्र-वासनः संसरेत् तत्तद्भोगोचितभोगायतनानि शरीराण्यर्जयित्वा गृह्णाति ।

"The various desires of such a person are awakened by the force of his subtle body, and he wanders from life to life by acquiring suitable bodies in which these desires can be suitably satisfied."

So the lower, limited knowledge of the individuals becomes a source of bondage in many ways.

INTRODUCTION TO THE 3rd SŪTRA

TEXT

ननु च

'ज्ञानं प्रकाशकं लोके आत्मा चैव प्रकाशकः ।

अनयोरपृथग्भावाज्ज्ञाने ज्ञानी प्रकाशते ॥'

इति-श्रीविज्ञानभैरवोक्तदृष्ट्या ज्ञानमपि प्रकाशमयमेव, इति कथमस्य बन्धरूपत्वम् । सत्यमेतत्, यदि परमेश्वरप्रसादादेवं प्रत्यभिज्ञायेत, यदा तु तन्मायाशक्तितो नैवं विमर्शस्तदा—

TRANSLATION

A doubt may arise regarding *jñāna*. In *Vijñāna-bhairava*, it is said:

"In the world, knowledge is light that reveals, and Ātmā is the universal light that reveals. As both *jñāna* (knowledge) and *Ātmā* are light and there is no difference between them, it is the knower himself that is revealed in knowledge."

In view of this statement of *Vijñānabhairava*, even limited knowledge is light itself, then how can limited knowledge be said to be the cause of bondage. This is true if through God's grace one could really realize its significance, but if through God's *māyā śakti* there is no realization like this, then:

SŪTRA—3

कलादीनां तत्त्वानामविवेको माया ॥ ३ ॥

Kalādīnāṁ tattvānām aviveko māyā.

कलादीनाम् = of *kalā* etc; तत्त्वानाम् of constitutive principles; अविवेक: non-discrimination.

The non-discrimination of the *tattvas* like kalā etc. is *māyā*.

COMMENTARY

TEXT

किञ्चित्कर्तृ तादिरूपकलादिक्षित्यन्तानां तत्त्वानां कञ्चुक-पुर्यष्टक-स्थूलदेहत्वेन अवस्थितानां योऽयमविवेकः, पृथक्त्वाभिमतानामेव अपृथगात्मत्वेन प्रतिपत्तिः, सा माया तत्त्वाख्यातिमयः प्रपञ्चः । तदुक्तं श्रीतन्त्रसद्भावे

'कलोद्वलितचैतन्यो विद्यादर्शितगोचरः ।
रागेण रञ्जितात्मासौ बुद्ध्यादिकरणैर्युतः ॥
एवं मायात्मको बन्धः प्रोक्तस्तस्य दरात्मकः ।
तदाश्रयगुणो धर्मोऽधर्मश्चैव समासतः ॥
तत्रासौ संस्थितः पाश्यः पाशितस्तैस्तु तिष्ठति ।'

इति । स्पन्दे तु

'अप्रबुद्धधियस्त्वेते स्वस्थितिस्थगनोद्यताः ।'

इत्यनेन एतत् भङ्ग्या उक्तम् ॥३॥

TRANSLATION

Māyā is non-discrimination (*aviveka*) i.e. taking as identical those which are considered to be separate. 'Those' refers to the *tattvas* (constitutive principles) from *kalā* which brings about limited doership or efficacy upto the earth, which are arranged in the form of Kañcukas (coverings of Māyā) and subtle and gross bodies. In other words, *Māyā* is only an extension of the primal ignorance of Reality. The same thing has been said in *Tantrasadbhāva*:—

"The consciousness of the empirical individual is reduced to limited efficacy by *kalā* (limited doership), the objects of sense are exhibited to him in attractive light by *vidyā* (limited knowledge), he is emotionally affected by *rāga* (desire for particular things); he is endowed with organs of sense-perception and organs of action. Thus arises bondage due to Māyā. This bondage is terrible for him (*darātmakaḥ*).

In brief, the *guṇas* (*sattva*, *rajas* and *tamas*) depend on it (*māyā*) and also the righteous and evil activities depend on it. Imbued with them, he is subject to bondage, and remains bound by these." In Spandakārikā also, the same idea has been expressed in another way in the following verse.

"These (the particular *spandas*), always intent on concealing the experient's real nature, push down people of unawakened (unenlightened) mind into the terrible ocean of worldly existence which is hard to cross." (I, 20)

EXPOSITION

The second *sūtra* says that limited knowledge is the cause of bondage. The third *sūtra* elaborates the idea contained in the second. Limited knowledge is due to *Māyā.* The word *Māyā* is used in three senses in this system—*Māyā śakti, Māyā tattva* and *Māyā granthi.* *Māyā śakti* is an aspect of Śiva's *Svātantrya* (absolute freedom); it is His power of manifestation in different ways. *Māyā tattva* is the constitutive principle which gives rise to limited objective experience. It is the material cause of *Prakṛti* and insentiency.

Māyā-granthi is the knot of insentiency and sentiency into oneness brought about by Māyā. Due to this, the constitutive elements of the psycho-physical organism are taken to be the Self; the *kalā, vidyā, rāga* etc. the *kañcukas* of Māyā, the *puryaṣṭaka* (the subtle body), and the physical body which are *pṛthak*—separate from the Self are considered to be *apṛthak* i.e. identical with the Self. It is in the sense of *Māyā-granthi* that the word Māyā has been used in this *Sūtra.* The knowledge (*jñāna*) brought about by *Māyā granthi* is the cause of bondage and *māyāgranthi* means taking kalā etc. which are not-self as Self.

INTRODUCTION TO THE 4th SŪTRA

TEXT

अतश्च एतत्प्रशमाय—

TRANSLATION

Therefore in order to put an end to the bondage brought about by Māyā—

SŪTRA—4

शरीरे संहारः कलानाम् ॥ ४ ॥

Śarīre Saṁhāraḥ Kalānām.

कलानाम् = of the various parts; संहारः = dissolution शरीरे in the body.

Dissolution of the various parts of the *tattvas* in the body (gross, subtle, and causal) should be practised by *bhāvanā*.

COMMENTARY

TEXT

महाभूतात्मकं, पुर्यष्टकरूपं, समनान्तं यत् स्थूलं, सूक्ष्मं, परं शरीरं, तत्र याः पृथिव्यादिशिवान्ततत्त्वरूपाः कला भागाः, तासां संहारः, स्वकारणे लयभावनया दाहादिचिन्तनयुक्त्या वा ध्यातव्यः, इति शेषः । यदुक्तं श्रीविज्ञान-भैरवे

'भुवनाध्वादिरूपेण चिन्तयेत्क्रमशोऽखिलम् ।
स्थूलसूक्ष्मपरस्थित्या यावदन्ते मनोलयः ॥'

इति । तथा

'कालाग्निना कालपदादुत्थितेन स्वकं पुरम् ।
प्लुष्टं विचिन्तयेदन्ते शान्ताभासः प्रजायते ॥'

इति । एवमादि च सर्वागमेष्वस्ति । अत एव

'उच्चारकरणध्यानवर्णस्थानप्रकल्पनैः ।
यो भवेत्स समावेशः सम्यगाणव उच्यते ॥'

इति-श्रीपूर्वशास्त्रे ध्यानादि एव आणवत्वेन उक्तम् । एतच्च स्थूलत्वात् शाक्तोपायप्रकाशात्मनि स्पन्दशास्त्रे न संगृहीतम् । यत्तु अत्र पर्यवसानभङ्ग्या शाक्तादि अस्ति, तत् अस्माभिः अत्रापि स्पन्दग्रन्थात् संवादितं; संवादयिष्यते च किंचित् ॥४॥

TRANSLATION

By *śarīra* (body) is meant the gross body consisting of the five gross elements, the subtle body (consisting of the five *tanmātrās*, *manas*, *buddhi* and *ahaṁkāra*) and the highest or the causal body consisting of prāṇa and subtle *manas* upto *samanā*.[1] In this body (i.e. in the physical, subtle, and causal body) dissolution has to be contemplated upon (*dhyātavyaḥ*) of all the constitutive parts from the earth upto Śiva into the preceding causes by *bhāvanā*[2] or by the device of burning etc. This should be taken as the remaining part of the *sūtra*.

As has been said in *Vijñānabhairava:*

"One should contemplate successively by means of Bhuvana adhvā etc. from gross to subtle and subtle to para or causal till at last the mind is completely dissolved."[3] (Verse 56)

Also:

"One should think of one's body being burnt by kālāgni[4] arising from the toe of the right foot. At last there is the realization of light which is *śānta*, i.e. in which there is not the slightest trace of difference.[5] (Verse 52)

In this way, there is the description of dissolution in all the *āgamas*. Therefore :

"The full *samāveśa* which occurs by means of *uccāra*,[6] *karaṇa*[7] *dhyāna*[8] *varṇa*[9], and *sthāna-kalpana*[10] is known as *āṇava samāveśa*". (Mālinī-Vijaya II, 21).

Thus dhyāna (meditation) etc. has been described in Mālinī-vijaya as *āṇava upāya.*

This *upāya* being gross has not been adopted in *Spanda-śāstra* because it deals mainly with *Śāktopāya*. Whatever of *Śāktopāya* has been used here as a concluding means has been supported by me by quoting parallel ideas from *Spanda-śāstra* and shall be supported further also.

NOTES

1. *Samanā* : When the *unmanā śakti* of *Śiva* displays herself in the form of the universe from *śūnya* upto the earth as thought, she is known as *Samanā.*

2. *Bhāvanā* : directing one's thought in a particular way, imagining oneself to be in a particular mode.

3. Dissolution of the mind is known as *layībhāvanā*—the technique of dissolution which is a kind of Śākta technique.

4. Kālāgni Rudra is the deity full of tejas i.e. burning light. In the human body, his place is supposed to be the toe of the right foot. One has to meditate that Kālāgni is arising from that place and burning the entire body.

5. This is *dāha-bhāvanā* which is again a kind of Śākta technique.

6. *Uccāra* : holding the mind at rest on *prāṇa*.

7. *Karaṇa* : This is a technical practice of this *yoga*. The word *Karaṇa* does not mean sense in this context. It has been used in an abstract sense. *Kṛtiḥ iti karaṇam-bhāvārthe*. *Karaṇam* here means doing, operation. It has been used here in the sense of 'Yogic or mystic operation or practice.' In *āṇavopāya*, this

practice is used in a technical sense. It is the body which is made the object of the meditative practice. The aspirant imagines the body as the representative of the entire universe, then admires the glory of the divine in this universe, and finally considers it all as the divine Self within. The word 'body' in this context has to be taken in the sense of the physical gross body, the subtle and also the causal body. Mudrā which means certain postures of the body indicative of certain inward states is also used in *karaṇa-yoga.*

8. *Dhyāna*—meditation, what has to be meditated on is the foundational divine light of consciousness inherent in all the *tattvas* or constitutive principles. This *dhyāna* is the same as defined by Patañjali, viz. *pratyaikatānatā dhyānam* i.e. the continuous uninterrupted flow of the mental mode.

9. *Varṇa*—The word *varṇa* literally means letter or sound of a letter. Here it is the unification or assimilation of all the sounds which is known as *nāda*. In the subtle *prāṇa* inside the body, there is always an unstruck vibration (*anāhata nāda*) which is the seed of creativity and dissolution (*Sṛṣṭi-saṁhāra bīja*). Concentration on the *nāda* is another variety of *āṇava yoga*. This kind of *yoga* is also known as *nādānusandhāna* in other systems of *yoga*.

Abhinavagupta says :

एको नादात्मको वर्णः सर्ववर्णाविभागवान ।
सोऽनस्तमितरूपत्वाद् अनाहत इहोदितः ॥

"There is one *varṇa* in the form of *nāda* which pervades all the *varṇas*. It never ceases i.e. is eternal and is called *anāhata* i.e. unstruck, natural, uncaused. The aim in *varṇa prakalpanā* is to concentrate finally on this inner *nāda*.

10. *Sthāna-Kalpanā*. The word *sthāna* means station, i.e. place of concentration in this context, The stations of concentration are mainly three, viz; (1) the body (2) the *prāṇa-vāyu* (the breath) and (3) anything external i.e. outside the body.

1. The following are the stations or the places in the body on which concentration is to be made. (1) *Trikoṇa* or *mūlādhāra* (ii) navel (iii) the heart (iv) throat (v) the central place between the two eye-brows. This is what is called *dhāraṇā* in a limited sense in Patañjali's *yoga*.

Deśabandhaś-cittasya dhāraṇā—fixing of the mind on a particular spot is *dhāraṇā*.

2. *Prāṇavāyu—sthāna-kalpanā.* This refers to concentration on *prāṇa* i.e. on the expiration and inspiration of breath from the centre of the body up to a distance of twelve fingrs in the external space. The mind has to be concentrated on the starting point of the breath from the centre and the ending point at a distance of twelve fingers from the centre which is known as (the end of *dvādaśānta* the distance of twelve fingers). The external distance is known as *bāhya dvādaśānta*, and the internal (the starting point) is known as *antar dvādaśānta*. One has to concentrate on the points where the expiring and inspiring breaths stop for a split second.

3. Anything external, i.e. image of a deity etc.

INTRODUCTION TO THE FIFTH SŪTRA

TEXT

एवं ध्यानाख्यमाणवमुपायं प्रदर्श्य, तदेकयोगक्षेमान् प्राणायाम-धारणा-प्रत्याहार-समाधीन् प्रदर्शयति—

TRANSLATION

Thus after describing the *dhyāna* aspect of *āṇavopāya* the formulation of the *sūtras* now describes *prāṇāyāma*, *dhāraṇā*, *pratyāhāra*, and *samādhi* which serve as means for the acquisition and maintenance of *dhyāna* (meditation).

SŪTRA—5

नाडीसंहार-भूतजय-भूतकैवल्य-भूतपृथक्त्वानि ॥ ५ ॥

Nāḍī-saṁhāra-bhūtajaya-bhūtakaivalya-*bhūtapṛthaktvāni*.

नाडी संहार—dissolution of the *prāṇa* flowing in the channel; भूतजय—conquest i.e. control of the elements भूत कैवल्य—withdrawal of the mind from the elements; भूतपृथक्त्व—separation from the elements.

"Dissolution of the flow of *prāṇa* in the nerve channels into the *suṣumnā*, control over the elements. withdrawal of the mind from the elements and separation from the elements (are to be brought about by the *yogī* by means of *bhāvanā*).

COMMENTARY

TEXT

योगिना भावनीयानि इति शेषः । नाडीनां प्राणापानादिवाहिनीनां सुषीणां संहारः, प्राणापानयुक्त्या एकत्र उदानवह्न्यात्मनि मध्यनाड्यां विलीनतापादनम् । यदुक्तं श्रीमत्स्वच्छन्दे

'अपसव्येन रेच्येत सव्येनैव तु पूरयेत् ।
नाडीनां शोधनं ह्येतन्मोक्षमार्गपथस्य च ॥
रेचनात्पूरणाद्रोधात्प्राणायामास्त्रिधा स्मृताः ।
सामान्या बहिरेते तु पुनश्चाभ्यन्तरे त्रयः ॥
आभ्यन्तरेण रेच्येत पूर्येताभ्यन्तरेण तु ।
निःस्पन्दं कुम्भकं कृत्वा कार्याश्चाभ्यन्तरास्त्रयः ॥'

इति । भूतानां पृथिव्यादीनां जयो धारणाभिर्वशीकारः । यथोक्तं तत्रैव

'वायवी धारणाङ्गुष्ठे आग्नेयी नाभिमध्यतः ।
माहेयी कण्ठदेशे तु वारुणी घण्टिकाश्रिता ॥
आकाशधारणा मूर्ध्नि सर्वसिद्धिकरी स्मृता ।'

इति । भूतेभ्यः कैवल्यं, चित्तस्य ततः प्रत्याहरणम् । यदुक्तं तत्रैव

'नाभ्यां हृदयसंचारान्मनश्चेन्द्रियगोचरात् ।
प्राणायामश्चतुर्थस्तु सुप्रशान्त इति स्मृतः ॥'

इति । हृदयान्नाभौ प्राणस्य, विषयेभ्यो मनसश्च तत्रैव संचारणादित्यर्थः । भूतेभ्यः पृथक्त्वं, तदनुपरक्तस्वच्छन्दचिदात्मता । यदुक्तं तत्रैव

'भित्त्वा क्रमेण सर्वाणि उन्मनान्तानि यानि च ।
पूर्वोक्तलक्षणैर्देवि त्यक्त्वा स्वच्छन्दतां व्रजेत् ॥'

इति । 'भूतसंधानभूतपृथक्त्वविश्वसंघट्टाः' (१–२०) इति यत् पूर्वमुक्तम्, तत् शाम्भवोपायसमाविष्टस्य अयत्नतो भवति । इदं तु आणवोपायप्रयत्नसाध्यमिति विशेषः ॥ ५ ॥

"Should be brought about by the *yogī* by contemplation"—this has been left to be supplied. *Nāḍīnām* means the channels which carry *prāṇa*, *apāna* etc. *Saṁhāraḥ*[1] means bringing about their dissolution into the middle *nāḍī* which is of the form of *udāna* fire[2] by the device of *prāṇāpāna* i.e. by stopping their outer and inner flow in order to bring them together in the middle or *suṣumnā nāḍī*. As has been said in *Svacchanda*.

"One should breathe in through the left (nose) and breathe out through the right.[3] This brings about cleansing of the *nāḍīs* (channels) and of the middle *nāḍī* which is the path to liberation. By breathing out, by breathing in, and by restraining or stopping the breath, there are said to be three types of *prāṇāyāma*.[4] They are all common and external. There are also three types of internal *prāṇāyāma*. By the internal one has to perform the *recaka*, by the internal one has to perform the *pūraka* and by the internal one has to perform tremorless *kumbhaka*. Thus the three internal *prāṇāyāmas* should be performed." (VII, Verse 294-296)

The conquest of the elements like earth, etc. means control over them by means of *dhāraṇā*.[5] As has been said in the same book:

"Concentration on air at the place of the toe of the left foot, on fire in the middle of the navel, on earth in the throat, on water in the uvula, on *ākāśa* (ether) on the top of the head brings about all supernormal powers" (VII 299-300)

Bhūta-kaivalya means *pratyāhāra* or the withdrawal of the mind from the elements.[6] As has been said in the same book:

"The transition of *prāṇa* from the heart to the navel, and checking it there, the withdrawal of the mind from sense-objects and its transition to the navel (by the device of *pratyāhāra*) this is the fourth *prāṇāyāma*[7] known as the calm or tranquil one" (*supraśānta*)" (VII, 297)

The meaning of the verse is that there should be transition of *prāṇa* from the heart to the navel, and withdrawal of the mind from objects and its transition also to the navel.

Bhūtapṛthakatva means detachment of the mind from the elements and thus its assuming the nature of pure and free Self. As has been said there itself (i.e. *Svacchanda Tantra* itself) "O goddess having pierced through all the knots, such as the heart, the throat etc. right up to *unmanā* by the aforesaid means, and abandoning them altogether, one can attain to the state of the highest freedom of spirit, i.e. Bhairava aspect" (VII, 327) *Bhūta-sandhāna-bhūta-pṛhaktva-viśva-saṃghaṭṭāḥ* which has been mentioned before (in I, 20) happens effortlessly as it has been included in *śāmbhavopāya*. This coming under *āṇavopāya* has to be acquired with effort. This is the difference.

1. *Nāḍī-saṁhāra* or dissolution of the prāṇa and apāna into *suṣumnā* is brought about by *Prāṇāyāma.*

2. *Udāna*-fire—*Udāna* is also a kind of *prāṇa.* It is called fire figuratively, because *prāṇa* and *apāna* are dissolved in it.

3. Usually *apasavya* means right and *savya* means left, but when *apasavya* is used as an indeclinable i.e. as *apasavyam* or *apasavyena,* it means 'to or on the left', and so also *savyam* or *savyena* means 'to or on the right'. This is how *Kṣemarāja* interprets it in his commentary on *Svacchanda Tantra.*
सव्येन दक्षनासापथेन अपसव्येन वामेन । This interpretation is confirmed by Svāmī Lakṣamaṇa Joo also.

4. *Prāṇāyāma* means breath control. *Pūraka* means inhaling the breath, *recaka* means exhaling it, and *kumbhaka* means retaining it.

5. The word *dhāraṇā* has been used here in the same sense in which it is used in Patañjali's *yoga,* viz., *Deśabandhaścittasya dhāraṇā* i.e. fixing of the mind on a particular spot is known as dhāraṇā. *Bhūta-jaya* or control over the elements is brought about by *dhāraṇā.*

6. *Bhūta-kaivalya* is brought about by *pratyāhāra* which means both withdrawal of the mind from its object and withdrawal of the senses from their objects.

7. This is how Kṣemarāja has interpreted the verse आभ्यन्तरेण मध्यपथेन रेचनं द्वादशान्ते, पूरणं हृदि, निष्कम्पं कुम्भकमिति निरायासं प्रशान्तकुम्भकमित्यर्थः ।

"By the internal means 'through the middle nāḍī' i.e. *suṣumnā,* the *recana* (exhalation) has to be done up to *dvādaśānta* (a distance of 12 fingers) and the inhalation has to be done towards the heart i.e. the centre of the body. *Niṣkampa* means effortless or calm, free from agitation." This is a *pratyāhāra prāṇāyāma.*

This is called the fourth *prāṇāyāma* in relation to the earlier one which has three aspects, viz., *pūraka, recaka,* and *kumbhaka,*

8. *Unmanā*—अनुत्तरपरमशिवः अविचलप्रकाशात्मा यदा स्वेच्छया प्रसरति सा शक्तिः उन्मना शिवादभिन्नेव इत्युच्यते ।
When the supreme *Śiva* who is of the nature of changeless light moves forth by His Will, such Śakti, inseparable from Him, is called Unmanā. Literally, the word means above the mind.

It is a supramental power. How the various *granthis* have to be crossed through has been described under *Praṇavādhikāra* in *Svacchanda Tantra.* *Svacchanda Tantra* saya that after *unmanā śakti* has been acquired, one develops the power of entering another body. संक्रामेत्परदेहेषु क्षुत्तृष्णाभ्यां न बाध्यते ।

(VII, 329)

EXPOSITION

Prāṇāyāma, *Dhāraṇā*, *Pratyāhāra* and *Samādhi* come, according to this system, under *āṇavopāya.* This *sūtra* says how by using these techniques of *āṇavopāya* certain, supernormal powers (*siddhis*) are obtained.

By *prāṇāyāma*, there can be dissolution of *prāṇa* and *apāna* in *Suṣumnā.* By *dhāraṇā*, the *yogī* can acquire control over the elements; by *pratyāhāra*, he can withdraw his mind from the elements. Cases have been known of *yogīs* undergoing operation of certain parts of the body without chloroform. They withdraw their consciousness from the particular part and hence do not feel any pain. By perfection in *Samādhi*, the *yogī* can detach himself completely from his body and enter another body if he so desires.

INTRODUCTION TO THE 6th SŪTRA

TEXT

एवं देहशुद्धि-भूतशुद्धि-प्राणायाम-प्रत्याहार-धारणा-ध्यान-समाधिभिर्या तत्त-त्तत्त्वरूपा सिद्धिर्भवति सा मोहावरणात्, न तु तत्त्वज्ञानादित्याह—

TRANSLATION

Thus the various supernormal powers accrue to the *yogī* by means of purification of the body, purification of the elements, *prāṇāyāma*, *pratyāhāra*, *dhāraṇā*, *dhyāna* and *samādhi.* All such powers are due to a veil drawn by ignorance, and not to the highest knowledge of reality. Therefoe, the next *sūtra* says:

SŪTRA—6

मोहावरणात्सिद्धिः ॥ ६ ॥

Mohāvaraṇāt siddhiḥ

मोहावरणात्—due to a veil of ignorance; सिद्धिः: supernormal power.

"Supernormal power is due to a veil drawn by ignornce."

COMMENTARY

TEXT

मोहयति इति मोहो, माया, तत्कृतादावरणात् प्रोक्तधारणादिक्रमसमासादिता तत्तत्तत्त्वभोगरूपा सिद्धिर्भवति । न तु परतत्त्वप्रकाशः। यदुक्तं श्रीमल्लक्ष्मी-कौलार्णवे

**'स्वयम्भूर्भगवान्देवो जन्मसंस्कारवर्जितः ।
निर्विकल्पं परं धाम अनादिनिधनं शिवम् ॥
प्रत्यक्षं सर्वजन्तूनां न च पश्यति मोहितः ।'**

इति । विगलितमोहस्य तु

**'मध्यमं प्राणमाश्रित्य प्राणापानपथान्तरम् ।
आलम्ब्य ज्ञानशक्तिं च तत्स्थं चैवासनं लभेत् ॥
प्राणादिस्थूलभावं तु त्यक्त्वा सूक्ष्ममथान्तरम् ।
सूक्ष्मातीतं तु परमं स्पन्दनं लभ्यते यतः ॥
प्राणायामः स निर्दिष्टो यस्मान्न च्यवते पुनः ।
शब्दादिगुणवृत्तिर्या चेतसा ह्यनुभूयते ॥
त्यक्त्वा तां परमं धाम प्रविशेत्तत्स्वचेतसा ।
प्रत्याहार इति प्रोक्तो भवपाशनिकृन्तनः ॥
धीगुणान्समतिक्रम्य निर्ध्येयं परमं विभुम् ।
ध्यात्वा ध्येयं स्वसंवेद्यं ध्यानं तच्च विदुर्बुधाः ॥
धारणा परमात्मत्वं धार्यते येन सर्वदा ।
धारणा सा विनिर्दिष्टा भवपाशनिवारिणी ॥
स्वपरस्थेषु भूतेषु जगत्यस्मिन्समानधीः ।
शिवोऽहमद्वितीयोऽहं समाधिः स परः स्मृतः ॥'**

इति श्रीमन्मृत्युजिद्भट्टारकनिरूपितनीत्या धारणादिभिरपि परतत्त्वसमावेश एव भवति, न तु मितसिद्धिः ॥ ६ ॥

TRANSLATION

That which deludes is *moha*; in other words it is *Māyā*. There occurs supernormal power in the form of control and enjoyment of the various things brought about by *dhāraṇā*, etc—in succession which have been mentioned above owing to the veil drawn by *māyā*.[1] This power does not denote the manifestation of the highest reality. As has been said in *Lakṣmī-Kaulārṇava*:

"The Lord, the divine who is self-existent, and without the residual effect of any previous life, being deluded (by His own Māyā śakti) does not perceive Śiva who is beyond all thought-constructs, who is the highest abode (of all), who is without beginning and without end and who is obvious to all beings (as their innermost Self)

What follows applies to the person whose delusion has melted away:

"One should resort to the middle *prāṇa* (*udāna* in *suṣumnā*) in between the passages of *prāṇa* and *apāna*, and resorting to *jñānaśakti*,[2] and having established himself there (i.e. in *jñāna-śakti*), he should take his *āsana* (seat) there.

Inasmuch as the highest pulsation (of consciousness) is obtained beyond the subtle *prāṇāyāma* after abandoning the gross *prāṇāyāma* (consisting of *pūraka*, *recaka*, *kumbhaka*), and also the subtle one that is carried on inside the *suṣumnā*, therefore this is the *prāṇāyāma* prescribed as the best from which there is no fall of the aspirant any more.[3]

Leaving aside even subtle supernormal sound etc which are modes of sensation caused by the *guṇas* of *Prakṛti* and are experienced by the mind, one should enter the highest state with full I-consciousness (without any thought-construct). This is said to be (real) *pratyāhāra*.[4] This cuts away the noose of transmigratory existence.

The highest Reality is all-pervasive and cannot be meditated on[5] in any objective form. Transcending the attributes of the mind, one should meditate on the universal consciousness as the Light experienced within oneself as the *pramātā* or knower. This is what the wise know as meditation.

When the Highest Self is always held in consciousness by the aspirant, that is defined as the *dhāraṇā* which sets at naught the fetter of transmigratory existence.

In this world, whether in oneself or in other creatures, if one maintains the idea of sameness i.e. if one experiences in everything the same secondless *Śiva* as I, that is known as *Samādhi*."[6] (VIII, 11-18) Therefore as defined by *Mṛtyujit* (Netratantra), there can be *samāveśa* in the highest Reality, also by Dhāraṇā, etc., in a higher sense, not merely the attianment of limited supernormal powers.

NOTES

1. The word 'Māyā' has been used here in the sense of illusory or deceptive power.

2. The *prāṇa* in the middle path (*suṣumnā*) is *udāna*. *Udāna-śakti*, developed at its highest turns into *jñāna-śakti*, or errorless *prajñā* or knowledge. Kṣemarāja in his commentary on this verse says.
मध्यनाड्यां भवं प्राणमित्यूर्ध्वंगामिनमुदानमाश्रित्य, ततश्च प्राणीयव्याप्तिनिमज्जनेन चिद्व्याप्तिमुन्मज्जनात् ज्ञानशक्तिमुन्मिषत् स्फुरत्तारूपां संविदमालम्ब्य i.e. when *prāṇa* and *apāna* are submerged in the middle channel i.e. *suṣumnā*, then *udāna* begins to function within it. With the submergence of the function of *prāṇa* and the emergence of *cit*, the function of *jñānaśakti* emerges which is the manifestation of higher consciousness, the yogī should then resort to this *jñāna-śakti*.
Therefore, the word *jñāna-śakti* has been used here.

3. 'There is no fall' means that he no more loses the sense of being the *Cit-pramātā* i.e. the central consciousness being the subject in him.

4. Pratyāhāra is *prati*+*āhāra*. *Prati* means *pratīpa* i.e. in a reverse direction, *āhāra*=taking away. So *pratyāhāra* is taking away the senses or the mind in a reverse (inverted) direction. In the present context, it is taking the individual mind in a reverse direction. *Kṣemarāja* rightly says in his commentary चितिभ्रमेः प्रसृतस्य चित्तस्य तत्प्रतीपप्रापणात्मा प्रत्याहारः i.e. *Pratyāhāra* is turning back the individual mind to the universal consciousness from which it has wandered away.

5. Unmeditable or *nirdhyeyam* (not an object of meditation) has been used for the highest Reality, because what any one meditates on is an object, but the highest Reality can never be reduced to the position of an object. It is the eternal subject, and it is present in every body as the metaphysical subject apart

from the psychological subject. Therefore, the next line adds ध्येयं स्वसंवेद्यम् i.e. what one should meditate on can be experienced within oneself (as the ever-present Subject).

6. The verse says that real समाधि is समानधीः i.e. the idea of sameness in all, the idea that everything is *Śiva* or I. It is impossible to bring out this significant play on the word समानधीः in the translation.

EXPOSITION

The fifth *sūtra* says that *prāṇāyāma*, *dhāraṇā*, *pratyāhāra* and *samādhi* are all *āṇavopāya*, all *kriyā-yoga*, disciplinary practices which the *aṇu* or the individual can adopt and by means of these disciplinary practices certain supernormal powers are obtained.

The sixth *sūtra* warns that the individual should not aim at the attainment of such limited, inferior powers. His aim should be genuine Self-realization which is *Śiva*-realization. It then points out that *āsana*, *prāṇāyāma*, *dhāraṇā*, *dhyāna* and *samādhi* which are the usual techniques of *yoga* can all be taken in a higher mystic sense and not simply in the usual sense of mechanical, disciplinary practices which they are at the level of *āṇavopāya*. The higher senses of these practices pertain to *Śāktopāya* and the *sūtra* hints that *āṇavopāya* should lead to *Śāktopāya*.

Bhāskara in his *Vārttika* interprets this *sūtra* differently. He says that *moha* etc. only veil the essential nature of Self, it is only by concentrating on the Highest that one acquires Supernormal powers like omniscience and omnipotence. In this interpretation, there does not seem to be any connexion between mohāvaraṇāt and siddhiḥ. Kṣemarāja's interpretation appears to be better.

INTRODUCTION TO THE 7th SŪTRA

TEXT

तदाह—

TRANSLATION

The *sūtrakāra* says this (i.e. what happens by conquering moha):

SŪTRA—7

मोहजयादनन्ताभोगात्सहजविद्याजयः ॥ ७ ॥

Mohajayād anantābhogāt sahajavidyājayaḥ.

मोह—delusive Māyā; मोहजयात्—conquest of delusive Māyā; अनन्त—boundless, infinite; आभोग —expansion, extension अनन्ताभोगात् whose extension is boundless i.e. which pervades to an unlimited extent; सहजविद्या—natural inherent knowledge; सहजविद्याजयः =mastery of natural, inherent knowledge.

"By an all pervasive conquest of delusive Māyā is there mastery of the natural, inherent knowledge of Reality."

COMMENTARY

TEXT

मोहस्य, अख्यात्यात्मकसमनान्तपाशात्मनो मायाया जयाद्, अभिभवात् । कीदृशात् ? अनन्तः, संस्कारप्रशमपर्यन्तः आभोगो विस्तारो यस्य तादृशात्

'वेदनानादिधर्मस्य ....।'

इत्यादिना निरूपितरूपायाः सहजविद्याया जयो लाभो भवति । आणवोपायस्यापि शाक्तोपायपर्यवसानादित्युक्तत्वात् । तथा च श्रीस्वच्छन्दे

'समनान्तं वरारोहे पाशजालमनन्तकम् ।'

इत्युपक्रम्य

'पाशावलोकनं त्यक्त्वा स्वरूपालोकनं हि यत् ।
आत्मव्याप्तिर्भवत्येषा शिवव्याप्तिस्ततोऽन्यथा ॥
सार्वज्ञादिगुणा येऽर्था व्यापकान्भावयेद्यदा ।
शिवव्याप्तिर्भवत्येषा चैतन्ये हेतुरूपिणी ॥'

इति-ग्रन्थेन आत्मव्याप्त्यन्तस्य मोहस्य जयात् उन्मनाशिवव्याप्त्यात्मनः सजह-विद्यायाः प्राप्तिरुक्ता । यदुक्तं तत्रैव

'आत्मतत्त्वं ततस्त्यक्त्वा विद्यातत्त्वे नियोजयेत् ।
उन्मना सा तु विज्ञेया मनः संकल्प उच्यते ।
संकल्पात्क्रमतो ज्ञानमुन्मनं युगपत्स्थितम् ।
तस्मात्सा च परा विद्या यस्मादन्या न विद्यते ॥

न्दतेविद्ध्यत्र युगपत् सार्वज्ञादि गुणान्परान् ।
वेदनानादिधर्मस्य परमात्मत्वबोधना ॥
वर्जनापरमात्मत्वे तस्माद्विद्येति चोच्यते ।
तत्रस्थो व्यञ्जयेत्तेजः परं परमकारणम् ॥'

इति ॥ ७ ॥

TRANSLATION

By conquest means by subjugation of *moha* (delusion) i.e. of *Māyā* which is a bond extending up to *samanā*, a bond of the nature of primal ignorance. By what kind of conquest ? Of that kind of conquest which is boundless i.e. which extends up to the annulment of even the residual traces of ignorance.

By such conquest is there mastery i.e. acquisition of inherent knowledge defined in the verse "Because she brings about the investigation of the beginningless characteristic of *Śiva* etc."

The mastery of *sahaja Vidyā* or inherent knowledge has been spoken of in the context of *āṇavopāya* because even *āṇavopāya* must terminate in Śāktopāya. So in *Svacchanda Tantra*, beginning with 'O fair one, there is an endless network of bonds stretching up to *samanā*' and ending with the following verses, the acquisition of *sahaja vidyā* has been spoken of—*sahajavidyā* which is of the nature of *unmanā* inhering in *Śiva* and which comes about by the conquest of delusion that extends up to the final inherence in Self.

"Abandoning identification of Self with bonds existing up to *samanā* one views the essential nature of oneself as pure consciousness. This, however, only amounts to inherence in Self (*ātmavyāpti*).[1] Inherence in *Śiva*[2] (*Śiva-vyāpti*) is different from this.

When desired objects like omniscience etc. are contemplated upon within oneself as pervading everything, there is inherence in *Śiva*. This becomes an effective means for the development of *caitanya* or consciousness as *Svātantrya* (absolute freedom)" (IV, 434-435).

As has been said in *Svacchanda* itself,

"Therefore abandoning merely pure consciousness or merely inherence in Self (*ātma-vyāpti*) (as the aim), one should attach oneself to *vidyā tattva*. This *vidyā tattva* should be known as *unmanā*. Manas is only a notion in the heart. Such a kind of knowledge is only gradual, proceeding step by step, by degrees while *unmanā* is knowledge in one sweep and perennial. Because there is no other *vidyā* (knowledge) like this, therefore is it the highest *vidyā*[3]. By this knowledge one attains the highest qualities like omniscience, etc. simultaneously. It is called *Vidyā,* because it brings about the investigation of the beginningless characteristic of Śiva, viz., *Svātantrya-Śakti,* because it brings about the knowledge of the Highest Self and because it dispels all that is not the Highest Self. Established in that (*unmanā*), one can manifest the highest light (light of consciousness-*cit-jyoti*) the highest cause (i.e. Highest Śiva the source of all manifestation) (IV, 393-397).

NOTES

1. Pervasion of inherence in Self or *ātma-vyāpti* (also called *ātma-tattva* in *this context*) is a technical term. When *ātmā* (Self) is established in itself as pure consciousness, this state of being confined only to its being pure consciousness is termed *ātma-vyāpti.* This is considered to be an inferior state of realization in this system, because in this realization the Self is isolated from everything else and because the Self is considered to be only consciousness without *Kriyā-śakti* (the power of activity). When *ātmā* enters the state of *Śiva,* then only is it considered to be the highest realization, because there is no sense of *bheda* or difference now inasmuch as those things from which the Self was isolated are also now known as Śiva and because there is *svātantrya śakti* in *Śiva.*

2. Pervasion or inherence in Śiva or *Śiva-vyāpti* is another technical term. As Kṣemarāja puts it अस्यैव आत्मन उन्मनापदारोहेण चिदानन्दघनपरतत्त्वव्याप्तिरूपा शिवव्याप्तिः

(Svacchanda Tantra IV, p. 246)

When ātmā by rising to *unmanā* enters the state of the highest consciousness-bliss of Śiva, that state is known as *Śiva-Vyāpti* .

3. Kṣemarāja in his commentary on this *vidyā* in Svacchanda Tantra warns that this *vidyā tattva* should not be confused with the *vidyā tattva* which includes the experients from Vijñānakāla, upto Mantramaheśvara. This *vidyā tattva* is different. It is *unmanā* identified with Śiva-consciousness.

EXPOSITION

The seventh *sūtra* says that *moha* has to be conquered to such an extent that even its residual traces (*saṁskāra*) are completely annulled. It is only then that one acquires *Sahaja vidyā*—knowledge inherent in Reality. *Sahaja vidyā* is only another name of *unmanā*. There are many stages between *aṇu* (the limited empirical individual) and Śiva. Upto *Samanā*, there is the reign of *manas* or mind. By conquering *moha* upto *samanā*, one may be able to acquire *ātma-vyāpti*, the stage of pure consciousness. But this is the aim of *Sāṁkhya* and *Vedānta*. According to Śaiva philosophy, one should not rest content with *ātma-vyāpti*. The aim of this system is not only *ātma-vyāpti*, but *Śiva-vyāpti* or *Śivatva-yojanā*. This is possible only when the aspirant crosses the boundary of *Samanā*. *Samanā* is the highest expression of mind, but upto *samanā*, there is still the reign of mind, of *saṁkalpa-vikalpa*, of thought-construct and desire. The aspirant has to mount to the stage of *Sahaja vidyā* or *unmanā* where mental consciousness ceases and pure divine consciousness begins. It is only at this stage that one can experience *cidānanda ghana* massive consciousness bliss, and *svātantrya śakti* and thus *Śivavyāpti* or *Śiva's* inherent state of being.

Such a high state of realization is not possible by *āṇavopāya*. It is possible only by *Śāktopāya*. But *āṇavopāya* is only a stepping stone to *Śāktopāya*. It is not an end in itself. It has to end in *Śāktopāya*.

INTRODUCTION TO THE 8th SŪTRA

TEXT

एवमयमासादितसहजविद्यः—

TRANSLATION

Thus this one who has attained to *Sahaja vidyā*.

SŪTRA-8

जाग्रद्द्वितीयकरः ॥ ८ ॥

Jāgrat-dvitīya-karaḥ.

जाग्रत् —awake, watchful; द्वितीय the second one i.e. the world; करः an effulgence of light.

"(He is) one who is always awake i.e. who is always at-onement with *unmanā* and in whom the world appears as his effulgence of light.

COMMENTATY

TEXT

लब्ध्वापि शुद्धविद्यां तदैकध्यव्याप्तौ जागरूकः, पूर्णविमर्शात्मकस्वाहन्तापेक्षया यत् द्वितीयमिदन्तावमृश्यं वेद्यावभासात्मकं जगत्, तत् करो रश्मिर्यस्य तथाविधो भवति । विश्वमस्य स्वदीधितिकल्पं स्फुरति इत्यर्थः । यथोक्तं श्रीविज्ञानभैरवे

'यत्र यत्राक्षमार्गेण चैतन्यं व्यज्यते विभोः ।
तस्य तन्मात्रधर्मित्वाच्चिल्लयाद्भरितात्मता ॥'

इति । श्रीसर्वमङ्गलायामपि

'शक्तिश्च शक्तिमांश्चैव पदार्थद्वयमुच्यते ।
शक्तयोऽस्य जगत्कृत्स्नं शक्तिमांस्तु महेश्वरः ॥'

इति ॥ ८ ॥

TRANSLATION

Having obtained the pure *vidyā* (*unmanā*), and having obtained perfect identification with it, he is ever awake[1] (*jāgrat*). In relation to his full consciousness of I, that which appears as the second i.e. that which is considered as this, viz., the world appearing as an object is his effulgence of light. Such is he. The sense is that the world appears like his own light.[2] As has been said in 'Vijñānabhairava' "In whichever thing the consciousness of the universal Being is manifested through the senses, consciousness alone is the substratum of that appearance. Realizing this, one is dissolved in *cit* or consciousness (which is the substratum of the universe) and thus, experiences the entire fulness of being i.e. there is full aspect of *bhairava* in him". (Verse 117).

In *Sarvamaṅgalā* also, it is said:

"There are only two entities, *Śakti* (energy, power) and the possessor of that *śakti*. The possessor of the *Śakti* is the great Lord, and His *śakti* constitutes the whole world."

NOTES

1. Jāgrat = One who is awake : This has been used here figuratively. It means that having attained the *unmanā* state, he always lives in that condition. He has become a divinized man.

2. It is not only the I-consciousness which is divine. The world in his case is not a mere this—something separate from him, but a ray of his inward light. Dualism in his case has disappeared.

Bhāskara interprets this *sūtra* differently. According to him, *jāgrat* here means *jñāna-śakti*—the power of knowledge. By *kara* he means 'hand'. *jñāna-Śakti* is that which grasps the entire world as non-different from *jñāna*.

INTRODUCTION TO THE 9th SŪTRA

TEXT

ईदृशश्चायं सर्वदा स्वस्वरूपविमर्शाविष्टः—

TRANSLATION

Such a one is always immersed in the consciousness of his essential nature.

SŪTRA—9

नर्तक आत्मा ॥ ९ ॥

Nartaka ātmā.

नर्तक = dancer on the world-stage, actor, आत्मा = self.

"Such a one who has realized his essential spiritual nature is a Self that is only an actor (on the world stage)."

COMMENTARY

TEXT

नृत्यति, अन्तर्विगूहितस्वस्वरूपावष्टम्भमूलं तत्तज्जागरादिनानाभूमिकाप्रपञ्चं स्वपरिस्पन्दलीलयैव स्वभित्तौ प्रकटयति इति नर्तक आत्मा । तदुक्तं श्रीनैश्वासदेवीमहेश्वरनर्तकाख्ये सप्तमपटले देवीकृतस्तवे

'त्वमेकांशेनान्तरात्मा नर्तकः कोशरक्षिता ॥'

इति । भट्टश्रीनारायणेनापि

'विसृष्टाशेषसद्वीजगर्भं त्रैलोक्यनाटकम् ।
प्रस्ताव्य हर संहर्तुं त्वत्तः कोऽन्यः कविः क्षमः ॥'

इति । सर्वागमोपनिषदि श्रीप्रत्यभिज्ञायाम्

'संसारनाटचप्रवर्तयिता सुप्ते जगति जागरूक एक एव परमेश्वरः ॥'

इति ॥ ९ ॥

TRANSLATION

Dances i.e. he exhibits in himself by his playful movements varied roles of his waking etc which are based on his essential nature that is concealed within. Hence his *ātmā* is (like) a dancer[1] or actor. As has been said in the laudatory verse uttered by the goddess in the seventh section of *Naiśvāsyatantra* entitled 'Goddess and God as dancer':

"In one aspect you are the inner Self, a dancer, (in another aspect) you are preserver of your essential nature as the Highest Self."[2]

Bhaṭṭa Śrīnārāyaṇa also says in his *Stavacintāmaṇi*:

"O Śiva, you have produced a three-world drama which has in its interior *Māyā* as the source of all the existents. You have presented the introductory portion of the drama. Where is the creative artist other than yourself who can bring about its conclusion"[3] (Verse 59).

In *Īśvara-pratyabhijñā* also which contains the secret of all *āgamas*, it has been said,

"When the whole world is asleep only the highest Lord, the producer of the world-drama is awake."

NOTES

1. The *nartaka* in the Sanskrit drama is both a dancer and actor.

2. In one aspect, viz, as the individual self with its inner subtle and causal body, you play different roles in the world in repeated births i.e. in one aspect, you are immanent in the world. In another aspect, you abide always in your essential nature as the Divine and are not identified with the psychological individual

who plays different roles in the world drama. You are both in the world drama and above it.

3. This verse is full of *double entendre*. It is not possible to bring out all its implications in the translation. *Bīja* in the case of a drama is the source of the plot; *bīja* in the case of the world-drama is *Māyā*. In the drama, the source of the plot is the seed out of which all the events in the drama grow. In the world-drama, it is *Māyā* that is the origin of all the events of the world. A drama has its prologue or introductory portion known as *Prastāva* and its concluding portion known as *saṁhāra*. The poet says "You have presented the *prastāva* or prologue of the drama, who else excepting yourself can bring about its *saṁhāra* i.e. who else can bring about the liberation of the characters that are involved in it. Again there is a play on the word *kaḥ* which means both 'who' and 'prajāpati', the creator of beings. The poet says "Where is the Prajāpati other than yourself who can bring about the conclusion i.e. the dissolution of the plot of the drama?"

EXPOSITION

One who has attained to *sahaja vidyā* and has risen to the *unmanā* level does not retire to a forest or a cave, but accepts his role in the cosmic drama and carries on the duties of life. Just as an actor in a drama plays the part of a certain character but is neither affected nor deluded by the assumption of a particular role, so the Self on the world-stage is not affected by the events in which he participates in life. Inwardly, he is always detached.

INTRODUCTION TO THE 10th SŪTRA

TEXT

एवंविधस्य अस्य जगन्नाटचनर्तकस्य भूमिकाग्रहण-पदबन्धस्थानरङ्ग-माह—

TRANSLATION

The next *sūtra* now speaks about the stage on which this actor in the world drama plants his feet and plays his part.

SŪTRA—10

रङ्गोऽन्तरात्मा ॥ १० ॥

Raṅgo'ntarātmā.

अन्तरात्मा—the inner self i.e. the subtle and causal aspects which contain the inner life of the individual; रंग : —the stage.

The inner soul constitutes the stage (of the Self that is the actor).

COMMENTARY

TEXT

रज्यतेऽस्मिन् जगन्नाटचक्रीडाप्रदर्शनाशयेनात्मना इति रङ्गः, तत्तद्भूमिका-ग्रहणस्थानम् ; अन्तरात्मा , संकोचावभाससतत्त्वः शून्यप्रधानः प्राणप्रधानो वा पुर्यष्टकरूपो देहापेक्षया अन्तरो जीवः । तत्र हि अयं कृतपदः स्वकरणपरिस्पन्दक्रमेण जगन्नाटचमाभासयति । उक्तं च श्रीस्वच्छन्दे

'पुर्यष्टकसमावेशाद्विचरन्सर्वयोनिषु ।
अन्तरात्मा स विज्ञेयः ··········॥'

इति ॥ १० ॥

TRANSLATION

The place where the Self takes delight with the intention of exhibiting the world drama is the *raṅga* or the stage i.e. the place where the Self adopts the various roles.

Antarātmā is the inner soul of the subtle form (*puryaṣṭaka rūpa*) that has a contracted manifestation with the main constituent being either the void or *prāṇa*. The word inner i.e. *jīva* is used relatively to the external body. Having planted his feet on that stage of the inner soul, this actor (Self) displays the world drama by means of the active movements of his inner sense[1]" (*Karaṇa*).

It has been said in *Svacchanda Tantra* also "Entering into the *puryaṣṭaka* and moving about in all forms of existence[2], he (the self) is to be known as *antarātmā* (the inner soul), bound by the residual traces of good and evil deeds" (XI, 85)

NOTES

1. Here again there is *double entendre* in the word *karaṇa.* It means both *sense* and *dance pose with particular position of the fingers.* In the context of life, *Karaṇa* means sense; in the context of dance, it means a pose.

2. The *vāsanās* (impressions) of the *karmas* (good or evil deeds) are deposited in the *puryaṣṭaka* and they determine the course of future life. So the individual moves from one form of existence to another.

INTRODUCTION TO THE 11th SŪTRA

TEXT

इत्थमन्तरात्मरङ्गे नृत्यतोऽस्य—

TRANSLATION

In this way, of this one acting on the stage of the inner soul.

SŪTRA—11

प्रेक्षकाणीन्द्रियाणि ॥ ११ ॥

Prekṣakāṇi indriyāṇi.

प्रेक्षकाणि—spectators; इन्द्रियाणि the senses.

The senses (of the yogī) are the spectators (of his acting).

COMMENTARY

TEXT

योगिनश्चक्षुरादीनि इन्द्रियाणि हि संसारनाटयप्रकटनप्रमोदनिर्भरं स्वस्वरूपम् अन्तर्मुखतया साक्षात्कुर्वन्ति, तत्प्रयोगप्ररूढ्या विगलितविभागां चमत्काररससंपूर्णतामापादयन्ति । यच्छ्रुतिः

'कश्चिद्धीरः प्रत्यगात्मानमैक्षद् आवृत्तचक्षुरमृतत्वमश्नन् ॥'

(कठोपनिषदि अ० २ । व० ४ । मं० १) ।

इति ॥ ११ ॥

TRANSLATION

The senses like eyes etc. of the *yogī* witness inwardly their inmost Self full of the delight in exhibiting the world drama. By the development of the performance of the drama, they provide to the *yogī* fulness of aesthetic rapture in which the sense of difference has disappeared. As the *Upaniṣad* says:

"Some wise man, wishing to taste immortality with reverted eyes (i.e. introspectively) beholds the immanent Self." (Kaṭha II, 4, 1).

EXPOSITION

The senses of the ordinary person are extroverted and drag down the person towards the pleasures of worldly objects. The senses of the accomplished *yogī* who has attained *unmanā* do not lead him to worldly pleasures; they become introverted, and present to the *yogī* only the glory, the beauty and the delight of the cosmic actor. The senses of the *yogī* only reveal the inmost actor and no longer conceal Him as they do in the case of the ordinary folk.

INTRODUCTION TO THE 12th SŪTRA

TEXT

अस्य च—

TRANSLATION

And of such a *yogī*.

SŪTRA—12

धीवशात्सत्त्वसिद्धिः ॥ १२ ॥

Dhīvaśāt Sattva-siddhiḥ.

धीवशात्—through the higher, spiritual intelligence; सत्त्वसिद्धिः—realization of the inner Light of the Self.

"Through the higher spiritual intelligence, there is the realization of the Light of the Self."

COMMENTARY

TEXT

धीः, तात्त्विकस्वरूपविमर्शनविशारदा [विशदा] धिषणा तद्वशात् सत्त्वस्य स्फुरत्तात्मनः सूक्ष्मस्य आन्तरपरिस्पन्दस्य सिद्धिरभिव्यक्तिर्भवति । नाटचे च सात्त्विकाभिनयसिद्धिर्बुद्धिकौशलादेव लभ्यते ॥ १२ ॥

TRANSLATION

Dhī means the intelligence proficient in the awareness of the essential nature. Through it, there is the realization of the *sattva* which means the subtle, inner throb of the Light of the Self. In drama also the acting of the inner mental condition is achieved through talent.

EXPOSITION

In the commentary on this sūtra also, there is *double entendre* in *Sattva* and *dhī*. *Sattva* in this context does not refer to the constituent of *Prakṛti*, but the throb of the perfect I-consciousness and *dhī* does not mean mere intelligence but *ṛtambharā prajñā*, inward awakening laden with truth. The Yogī realizes the *Sattva* (the light of the essential nature of Self) through *dhī* (the spiritual intuition), just as the actor can act out the *sattva* (mental state) only through *dhī* (talent).

INTRODUCTION TO THE 13th SŪTRA

TEXT

एवं स्फुरत्तात्मकसत्त्वासादनादेव अस्य योगिनः—

TRANSLATION

Thus through the realization of the subtle inner throb of the Light of the Self, in the case of the Yogī.

SŪTRA—13

सिद्धः स्वतन्त्रभावः ॥ १३ ॥

Siddhaḥ svatantrabhāvaḥ.

सिद्ध: —is achieved; स्वतंत्रभाव: —the state of being Free; Freedom.

Freedom is achieved.

COMMENTARY

TEXT

सिद्धः संपन्नः ; स्वतन्त्रभावः, सहजज्ञत्व-कर्तृत्वात्मकम् अशेषविश्ववशीकारि स्वातन्त्र्यम् । यदुक्तं श्रीश्रीनाथपादैः

'श्रयेत्स्वातन्त्र्यशक्तिं स्वां सा श्रीकाली परा कला ।'

इति । श्रीस्वच्छन्देऽपि

'सर्वतत्त्वानि भूतानि मन्त्रवर्णाश्च ये स्मृताः ।
नित्यं तस्य वशास्ते वै शिवभावनया सदा ॥'

इति ॥ १३ ॥

TRANSLATION

Siddhaḥ means 'is achieved'; *svatantrabhāvaḥ* means 'Freedom which is of the form of inherent knowledge and activity and can bring the entire universe under its control'. As has been said by Śrī Nāthapāda (Śrī Avatārakanātha):

"One should resort to one's *Svātantrya Śakti* (the power of Absolute Freedom). She (*Svātantrya Śakti*) is *Kālī*, the *parā kalā*.[1]

In *svacchanda Tantra* also, it has been said,

"All the *tattvas*, all the *living beings*,[2] all the *mantras* and letters that are known are always under the control of one who has realized himself as non-different from *Śiva*." (VII, 245).

NOTES

1. *Parā* is derived from the root of the 9th conjugation which means 'to nourish' and 'to fill'. Because Kālī nourishes and fills the universe both internally and externally, therefore, she is called *parā*.

She is called *Kalā* because she projects the universe (the root 'kala' means 'to project'—*kala kṣepe*), because she knows the universe in its different aspects, ('Kala' also means 'to know', *kala Saṁkhyāne*), because she makes a reckoning of the world ('kala', means also 'to count, *kala*, *gaṇane*) because, she knows the universe as herself (*parāmṛśati*, *kala śabde*).

2. *Bhūtāni*—Living beings are of 14 kinds—eight kinds of *devas* or gods, 5 kinds of animals and 1 kind of man. (8+5+1=14).

EXPOSITION

This *Yogī* acquires *Svātantrya*—full freedom of knowledge and action and acquires control over everything in the universe.

INTRODUCTION TO THE 14th SŪTRA

TEXT

एष स्वतन्त्रभावोऽस्य—

TRANSLATION

His state of being Free i.e. his freedom.

SŪTRA—14

यथा तत्र तथान्यत्र ॥ १४ ॥

Yathā tatra tathā anyatra.

यथा —as; तत्र there, in the body; तथा so; अन्यत्र elsewhere.

As he (the *Yogī*) can manifest Freedom in his own body, so can he elsewhere.

COMMENTARY

TEXT

यत्र देहे योगिनः स्वाभिव्यक्तिर्जाता तत्र यथा, तथा अन्यत्र सर्वत्र सदावहितस्य सा भवति । यथोक्तं श्रीस्वच्छन्दे

'स्वच्छन्दश्चैव स्वच्छन्दः स्वच्छन्दो विचरेत्सदा ।'

इति । श्रीस्पन्देऽपि

'लभते, तत्प्रयत्नेन परीक्ष्यं तत्त्वमादरात् ।
यतः स्वतन्त्रता तस्य सर्वत्रेयमकृत्रिमा ॥'

इति ॥ १४ ॥

TRANSLATION

As the *Yogī* can manifest himself in his own body, so this

power of manifestation of the ever vigilant Yogī can prevail elsewhere also.

As is said in *Svacchanda:*

"He (*Yogī*) rambles about free of will in the beginning, free of will in the middle, free of will towards the end."[1] (VII, 260).

In *Spandakārikā* also, it is said,

"That divine Spanda principle should be carefully and faithfully examined (by which this class of senses alongwith its inner group, though inconscient acts as conscious and acquires the power of going forth towards an object, maintaining it in perception and withdrawing). This freedom of the Spanda principle is natural and prevalent everywhere."[2] (I, 6-7).

NOTES

1. He had freedom of will in the past, has into the present and future, i.e. constantly.

2. Through the power of Spanda, even senses which are believed to be unconscious can operate as conscious entities. So if one develops *Svātantrya Śakti*, one can acquire many powers including the power of entering another body.

INTRODUCTION TO THE 15th SŪTRA

TEXT

न चैवमपि उदासीनेन अनेन भाव्यम् अपि तु—

TRANSLATION

He (the *Yogī*) should not (by acquiring the above powers) become indifferent but rather

SŪTRA—15

बीजावधानम् ॥ १५ ॥

Bījāvadhānam

बीज—seed, the source of the world,
अवधानम् —attentiveness.

"He should give full attention to the active Light of consciousness, the source of the world."

COMMENTARY

TEXT

कर्तव्यमिति शेषः । बीजं विश्वकारणं स्फुरत्तात्मा परा शक्तिः । यदुक्तं मृत्युजिद्भट्टारके

'सा योनिः सर्वदेवानां शक्तीनां चाप्यनेकधा ।
अग्नीषोमात्मिका योनिस्ततः सर्वं प्रवर्तते ॥'

इत्यादि । तत्र परशक्त्यात्मनि बीजे, अवधानं भूयो भूयश्चित्तनिवेशनं कार्यम् ॥ १५ ॥

TRANSLATION

Kartavyam—'should be paid' which has been left out should be supplied (i.e. attention should be paid).

Bījam means the source of the universe—the active Light of consciousness, the highest *Śakti*.

As has been said in *Mṛtyujit* (*Netra Tantra*)

"She (the *Parā Śakti*) is the source of all the gods, and of the various *Śaktis* in many ways. This Source is of the nature of fire and moon. From it proceeds everything." (VII, 40).

The *Yogī* should direct his attention again and again to *parā śakti* which is the source of the universe.

NOTES

1. *Parā Śakti* and *parā vāk* are the same.
2. Fire and moon—*agnī-somātmikā*. This symbolism applies to *pramāṇa-prameya*, *prakāśa-vimarśa*, *jñāna-kriyā*, etc.

INTRODUCTION TO THE 16th SŪTRA

TEXT

एवं हि सति असौ योगी—

TRANSLATION

This being so, this *Yogī*

SŪTRA—16

आसनस्थः सुखं ह्रदे निमज्जति ॥ १६ ॥

Āsanasthaḥ sukhaṁ hrade nimajjati.

आसनस्थः: —established in the highest power of Śakti; सुखं — —easily; ह्रदे lit, in the lake, here —in the ocean of immortality; निमज्जति —is steeped in, is plunged.

"Established in the highest power of divine Śakti, he is, with ease, steeped in the ocean of immortality."

COMMENTARY

TEXT

आस्यते, नित्यमैकात्म्येन स्थीयते अस्मिन् इति आसनं, परं शाक्तं बलम्; यस्तत्र तिष्ठति, परिहृतपरापरध्यानधारणादिसर्वक्रियाप्रयासो नित्यमन्तर्मखतया तदेव परामृशति यः, स सुखमनायासतया, ह्रदे, विश्वप्रवाहप्रसरहेतौ स्वच्छोच्छलत्तादियोगिनि परामृतसमुद्रे निमज्जति, देहादिसंकोचसंस्कारब्रोडनेन तन्मयीभवति । यदुक्तं श्रीमृत्युजिद्भट्टारके एव

'नोर्ध्वे ध्यानं प्रयुञ्जीत नाधस्तान्न च मध्यतः ।
नाग्रतः पृष्ठतः किञ्चिन्न पार्श्वे नोभयोरपि ॥
नान्तः शरीरसंस्थं तु न बाह्ये भावयेत्क्वचित् ।
नाकाशे बन्धयेल्लक्ष्यं नाधो दृष्टिं निवेशयेत् ॥
न चक्षुर्मीलनं किञ्चिन्न किंचिद्दृष्टिबन्धनम् ।
अवलम्बं निरालम्बं सालम्बं नैव भावयेत् ॥
नेन्द्रियाणि न भूतानि शब्दस्पर्शरसादयः ।
एवं त्यक्त्वा समाधिस्थः केवलं तन्मयीभवेत् ॥
सावस्था परमा प्रोक्ता शिवस्य परमात्मनः ।
निराभासं पदं तत्तु तत्प्राप्य विनिवर्तते ॥'

इति ॥ १६ ॥

TRANSLATION

That on which he (the *yogī*) sits with a sense of full identification (with the Divine) is *āsana*[1] or seat.[1] The 'seat' in this context is the power of the highest *Śakti.* 'He sits there' means 'leaving all kinds of higher and lower practices involving effort like meditation, concentration etc., he is always mindful of that Power in an introverted way'.

Such a one is with ease (*sukham*) steeped (*nimajjati*) (i.e. is identified with the ocean of immortality) by drowning all impressions of the limitation of the body etc. in the most exquisite limpid ocean of immortality (*hrade*) which has the characteristic of springing up (*ucchalattā yoginī*) and is the source of the expansion of the world-process. As has been said in Mṛtyujit (*Netra Tantra*).

"Neither meditate on something above[2], nor on the middle, nor on something down below, neither in front, nor at the back, nor at both the sides, neither on something within the body, nor should one meditate on something outside. Neither one should fix one's gaze on the sky, nor on something down below. Neither one should close one's eyes nor should one keep the eyes open without blinking. Neither one should meditate on something as a support (*avalambam*) (like image, picture etc.) nor on a negation of support (*nirālambam*) nor on a support over and over again (*sālambam*)[3] nor on the senses, nor beings, nor on sense-perceptions like sound, touch, taste etc. Thus leaving aside every support, established in *samādhi*,[4] one should only abide identified with the Highest. That has been said to be the highest state of *Śiva*, that verily is the seat of the Highest Ātmā which is without any external appearance. If one attains this state, he does not return any more (i.e. he is freed of transmigratory existence)." (VIII, 41-45).

NOTES

1. *Āsana* here is not physical seat, but mental. So *āsanasthaḥ* means 'one who is mentally established in *parāśakti*, one who is always mindful of her'.

2. High and lower (*parāpara dhyāna*) refers to *Śākta* and *āṇava* practices.

3. *Avalambam* is a support like an image, an idol, a portrait etc. *Nirālambam*—negation of support. When the mind thinks of negation of support, the idea of support crops up within it. The difference between *avalamba* and *sālamba* is that in *avalamba*,

the mind lays hold of a support to start with and it continues, in *sālamba*, the support slips and the mind has to seize it over and over again.

4. *Samādhi* in this context has been thus interpreted by *Kṣemarāja* in his commentary—*Udyota*:

"अकिञ्चिच्चिन्तकत्वेन स्वस्वरूपविमर्शनप्रवणस्तन्मय:"

i.e. not thinking of any thing, only being mindful of one's essential nature and thus being identified with it.

EXPOSITION

The 15th *Sūtra* says that the *Yogī* should constantly maintain awareness of Parā Śakti, the primal cause and source of the world process. The 16th *Sūtra* says that if he is fully established in the awareness of *parā Śakti*, then he need not go through any formal process of concentration or meditation anymore. By completely setting aside all notion of the body etc. being identified with the Self, he will be steeped in the bliss of immortality.

INTRODUCTION TO THE 17th SŪTRA

TEXT

तदेवं नाडीसंहाराद्याणवोपायक्रमासादितमोहजयोन्मज्जच्छुद्धविद्यात्मक-शाक्तबलासादनप्रकर्षाद् आत्मीकृतपरामृतह्रदात्मकशाम्भवपदो योगी—

TRANSLATION

There comes about the conquest of delusion by means of *āṇava* technique such as dissolution of the flow of *prāṇa* (in the *suṣumnā*) etc. Through that emerges the power of *Śakti* in the form of *Śuddha Vidyā*. When this power reaches a high degree of excellence, the *Yogī* acquires the *Śāmbhava* state of being immersed in the most exquisite ocean of immortality. Such a *Yogī*—

SŪTRA—17

स्वमात्रानिर्माणमापादयति ॥ १७ ॥

Svamātrānirmāṇam āpādayati.

स्वमात्रा—The measure of Consciousness i.e. that aspect of Consciousness which coagulates. निर्माणं—production, creation, fabrication, formation. आपादयति—effects, brings about, produces. "He can bring about forms in accordance with that measure or aspect of consciousness which is creative and in which he is established."

COMMENTARY

TEXT

स्वस्य चैतन्यस्य संबन्धिनी मात्रा चिद्रसाश्यानतात्मा अंशः, तद्रूपं यथेष्ट-वेद्यवेदकावभासात्मकं निर्माणमापादयति, निर्मितत्वेन दर्शयति । यदुक्तं श्रीस्वच्छन्दे

'तदेव भवति स्थूलं स्थूलोपाधिवशात्प्रिये ।
स्थूलसूक्ष्मविभेदेन तदेकं संव्यवस्थितम् ॥'

इति : प्रत्यभिज्ञायामपि

'आत्मानमत एवायं ज्ञेयीकुर्यात्पृथक्स्थिति ।
ज्ञेयं न तु ························॥'

इति । आगमेऽपि

'जलं हिमं च यो वेद गुरुवक्त्रागमात्प्रिये ।
नास्त्येव तस्य कर्तव्यं तस्यापश्चिमजन्मता ॥'

इति अनेनैव आशयेन उक्तम् । एतदेव

'इति वा यस्य संवित्तिः क्रीडात्वेनाखिलं जगत् ।
स पश्यन्सततं युक्तो जीवन्मुक्तो न संशयः ॥'

इति—अनेन स्पन्दे प्रतिपादितम् ॥ १७ ॥

TRANSLATION

Svamātrā means the measure pertaining to his consciousness i.e. the aspect of the essence of consciousness that coagulates i.e. that creates.

In accordance with that measure of the creativity of Consciousness, he produces forms of objects or beings as desired by him i.e. he brings them to view by producing them. As has been said in *Svacchanda*—

"That[1] alone exists as gross, O dear one, owing to its desire to appear as gross. That alone gets settled differently as gross or subtle" (IV, 295).

In *Īśvara-pratyabhijñā* also, it has been said—

"Because of the power of creative thought (*vimarśa śakti*), He (the foundational Self) makes Himself as the object of knowledge. The object has no separate existence of its own. If He were to depend upon an object[2] (something outside Himself) for creation, His absolute freedom would be violated." (I, 5, 15).

In the *āgama* also, the following has been said with the same purport in view:

"O dear one, one who knows from the mouth of his spiritual director that water and ice are (essentially) the same (is liberated). He has no further obligation to discharge. He will have no further birth."

The same point of view has been expounded in the following verse of Spandakārikā—

"He who knows thus (viz., that there is nothing which is not *Śiva*), regarding the whole world as the play (of the Divine), is ever united (with the universal consciousness), and is, without doubt, liberated even while alive." (II, 5).

NOTES

1. 'That' refers to *prakāśa* or *Caitanya*—the Light of Consciousness having absolute freedom.

2. Objects are determined by Consciousness, not vice versa. If consciousness were to be determined by the objects, the absolute freedom of the Lord cannot be maintained. There would be a break in His absoluteness of freedom so far as objects are concerned.

EXPOSITION

When the *Yogī* acquires the power of *Śuddha Vidyā*, he is established in Creative Consciousness, and in accordance with the measure of that Consciousness, he can create creatures and objects (vedaka and vedya).

The doubt that an object is entirely different from the subject, then how can the Yogī create an object is unfounded, for the Supreme Consciousness itself appears as both subject and object.

When the power of *Parā Śakti* is attained, there can be no difficulty in appearing either as Subject or object, for consciousness is both.

INTRODUCTION TO THE 18th SŪTRA

TEXT

न चैवं स्वशक्तिनिर्मितभूतभावशरीरवतोऽस्य जन्मादिबन्धः कश्चिदित्याह—

TRANSLATION

It cannot be said that there is the possibility of the bondage of birth etc. for the *Yogī* who has created a gross body consisting of the five elements and a mental body consisting of perceptions, emotions etc. In order to emphasize this point, the next *sūtra* says:

(He cannot undergo rebirth, because he does not create according to the Law of *Karma*, but purely out of *Icchā Śakti*. Rebirth is associated with *Karma*).

SŪTRA—18.

TEXT

विद्याऽविनाशे जन्मविनाशः ॥ १८ ॥

Vidyā-avināśe janma-vināśaḥ.

विद्या—*Sahaja Vidyā*; अविनाशे—So long as the vidyā does not disappear; जन्मविनाशः—there is disappearance (of the possibility) of another birth.

"So long as *Śuddha vidyā* does not disappear, the possibility of another birth for him vanishes completely."

COMMENTARY

TEXT

प्रोक्तायाः सहजविद्याया अविनाशे सततोन्मग्नतया स्फुरणे, जन्मनः अज्ञानसहकारिकर्महेतुकस्य दुःखमयस्य देहेन्द्रियादिसमुदायस्य, नाशो विध्वंसः संपन्न एव । यदुक्तं श्रीकण्ठ्याम्

'सप्रपञ्चं परित्यज्य हेयोपादेयलक्षणम् ।
तृणादिकं तथा पर्णं पाषाणं सचराचरम् ॥
शिवाद्यवनिपर्यन्तं भावाभावोपबृंहितम् ।
सर्वं शिवमयं ध्यात्वा भूयो जन्म न प्राप्नुयात् ॥'

इति । श्रीस्वच्छन्दे

'स्वनिर्वाणं परं शुद्धं गुरुपारम्परागतम् ।
तद्विदित्वा विमुच्येत गत्वा भूयो न जायते ॥'

इति । श्रीमृत्युजित्यपि

'तत्त्वत्रयविनिर्मुक्तं शाश्वतं त्वचलं ध्रुवम् ।
दिव्येन योगमार्गेण दृष्ट्वा भूयो न जायते ॥'

इति ॥ १८ ॥

TRANSLATION

So long as the *sahaja* or *śuddha vidyā* does not disappear i.e. in the event of its constant appearance as an emergent reality, the cessation of (another) birth consisting of the multitude of the body, the senses etc. full of misery, and brought about by one's deeds (*karma*) together with the co-operation of ignorance (in the form of *āṇava* and *māyīya* mala) is fully accomplished. It has been said in *Śrī-Kaṇṭhī*,

"If leaving the world with its expanse of phenomena acceptable or rejectable, straw, leaf, stone, together with the mobile and immobile existents, right from *Śiva*[1] down to earth accompanied by positive and negative entities, one meditates over all as *Śiva*, one will not have to undergo birth again."

In *Svacchanda* also, it has been said,

"One's liberation acquired through a tradition of spiritual teachers is excellent and pure. Having realized it, one becomes liberated while alive, and after passing away from the world is not born again."

In *Mṛtyujit Tantra* also, it is said,

"If one realizes what is free of the three *tattvas*[2] what is eternal, changeless, and permanent by means of divine *Yoga*,[3] one is never born again." (VIII, 26-27).

NOTES

1. Taking *Śiva* as an object is also ignorance. This mentality has also to be given up. *Śiva* is the eternal Subject and should not be considered to be an object.

2. The three *tattvas* are *nara*, *Śakti*, and *Śiva*. *Nara tattva* is *bhedapradhāna*, predominantly associated with difference. It is objective. *Śakti tattva* is *bhedābhedapradhāna*. It posits *abheda* or identity in difference. It is cognitive. *Śiva tattva* is *abheda-pradhāna*, predominantly concerned with non-difference. These *tattvas* are only aspects of temporal manifestation; they do not belong to eternity.

3. The divine *Yoga* is *avikalpa vimarśa* i.e. awareness without thought-construct.

Bhāskara adopts the reading *vidyā vināśe* instead of 'vidyā-avināśe'. He interprets *vidyā* as lower, impure *vidyā* pertaining to objects, and says that with the disappearance of this *vidyā*, there is no further birth.

INTRODUCTION TO THE 19th SŪTRA

TEXT

यदा तु शुद्धविद्यास्वरूपम् अस्य निमज्जति तदा—

TRANSLATION

When the *Śuddha vidyā* of this *Yogī* sinks down, then—

SŪTRA—19

कवर्गादिषु माहेश्वर्याद्याः पशुमातरः ॥ १९ ॥

Kavargādiṣu māheśvaryādyāḥ paśu-mātaraḥ.

माहेश्वर्याद्याः —*Māheśvarī* and other deities कवर्गादिषु —in the 'ka' group and other groups of letters पशुमातरः—who are the mothers of the limited, empirical beings.

Māheśvarī and others who have their field of operation in 'ka' group and other groups of letters and are the mothers of limited beings (become their governing deities).

COMMENTARY

TEXT

अधिष्ठात्र्यो भवन्ति इति शेषः ।

'या सा शक्तिर्जगद्धातुः कथिता समवायिनी ।
इच्छात्वं तस्य सा देवि सिसृक्षोः प्रतिपद्यते ।
सैकापि सत्यनेकत्वं यथा गच्छति तच्छृणु ॥
एवमेतदिति ज्ञेयं नान्यथेति सुनिश्चितम् ।
ज्ञापयन्ती जगत्यत्र ज्ञानशक्तिर्निगद्यते ॥
एवं-भूतमिदं वस्तु भवत्विति यदा पुनः ।
जाता तदैव तत्तद्वत्कुर्वत्यत्र क्रियोच्यते ॥
एवं सैषा द्विरूपापि पुनर्भेदैरनन्तताम् ।
अर्थोपाधिवशात्प्राप्ता चिन्तामणिरिवेश्वरी ॥
तत्र तावत्समापन्नमातृभावा विभिद्यते ।
द्विधा च नवधा चैव पञ्चाशद्धा च मालिनी ॥
बीजयोन्यात्मकाद्भेदाद् द्विधा बीजं स्वरा मताः ।
कादिभिश्च स्मृता योनिर्नवधा वर्गभेदतः ॥
बीजमत्र शिवः शक्तिर्योनिरित्यभिधीयते ।
वर्गाष्टकविभेदेन माहेश्वर्यादि चाष्टकम् ॥
प्रतिवर्णविभेदेन शतार्धकरणोज्ज्वला ।
रुद्राणां वाचकत्वेन तत्संख्यानां निवेशिता ॥'

इति-श्रीमालिनीविजयनिरूपितनीत्या पारमेश्वरी परावाक् प्रसरन्ती, इच्छा-ज्ञान-क्रियारूपतां श्रित्वा, बीजयोनि-वर्ग-वर्ग्यादिरूपा शिव-शक्ति-माहेश्वर्यादि वाचक-आदि-क्षान्तरूपां मातृकात्मतां श्रित्वा, सर्वप्रमातृषु अविकल्पक-सविकल्पक-तत्तत्संवेदनदशासु, अन्तःपरामर्शात्मना स्थूलसूक्ष्मशब्दानुवेधनं विदधाना, वर्ग-वर्ग्यादिदेवताधिष्ठानादिद्वारेण स्मय-हर्ष-भय-राग-द्वेषादिप्रपञ्चं प्रपञ्चयन्ती, असंकुचितस्वतन्त्रचिद्घनस्वस्वरूपमावृण्वाना संकुचितपरतन्त्र-देहादिमयत्वमापादयति । तदुक्तं श्रीतिमिरोद्घाटेपि

'करन्ध्रचितिमध्यस्था ब्रह्मपाशावलम्बिकाः ।
पीठेश्वर्यो महाघोरा मोहयन्त्यो मुहुर्मुहुः ॥'

इति पूर्वमपि संवादितम् । 'ज्ञानाधिष्ठानं मातृका' (१--४--) इति सामान्येन उक्तम्, इदं तु प्राप्ततत्त्वोऽपि प्रमाद्यन् माहेश्यादिभिः पशुजनाधिष्ठातृभूताभिरपि शब्दानुवेधद्वारेण मोह्यते इत्याशयेन इति विशेषः ॥ १९ ॥

TRANSLATION

"Become their governing deities" is to be supplied—

"That *Śakti* (in the form of I-consciousness) of the Creator of the world who is said to be constantly co-inhering in Him—becomes *Icchā* (will power) when He wants to create. Listen, how She, though one, becomes many. 'This object is like this, not otherwise'—announcing this positively, she is said to be *jñāna śakti* (the power of knowledge) in this world. When *Icchā Śakti* appears in the form 'well, let this thing now become' and then making that thing like that (i.e. according to the decision), she is said to be *kriyā-Śakti* (the Power of execution). Thus being of two kinds, she undergoes innumerable changes according to the desired objects. This goddess becomes like *Cintāmaṇi*[1] (a thought-gem). Then when she assumes the aspect of mother[2], she is divided in two ways, nine ways, and becomes a wearer of a garland of fifty letters.

With the division of *bīja* and *yoni*, she is of two kinds. The vowels are considered to be the *bīja* (seed). With *ka* and other letters she is said to be *yoni* (consonants). According to the division of the groups of the consonants, she is of nine kinds.

In this context *bīja* (the vowel) is called Śiva and *yoni* (the consonant) is called *Śakti*.

According to the division of eight groups of letters, there is a group of eight deities[3], such as Māheśvarī and others. According to letter by letter division, she shines with the rays of fifty (letters), Being the indicator of *Rudras*, she is established in the same number as *Rudras* (i.e. fifty) (Mālinī-Vijaya III, 5-13).

Thus as ascertained in *Mālinī-vijaya*, the Divine *Parāvāk* expands, having recourse to the forms of *icchā* (will) *jñāna* (knowledge) and *kriyā* (action); assuming the forms of vowel and consonant, group and the letters pertaining to the groups, Śiva, Śakti, Māheśī and other deities, she becomes *mātṛkā* in the form of letters from 'a' to 'kṣa'. In all the experients, she brings about, on the occasion of knowledge with thought-constructs and knowledge without thought-constructs, the application of gross and subtle words by means of inner awareness. By means of the deities presiding over the groups and the letters denoted by those groups, she exhibits in various ways wonder, joy, fear, attraction, aversion etc., and by concealing the unlimited independent nature of consciousness, she brings about limited, dependent embodiment. It is said in *Timirodghāṭa* also.

"The *Mahāghorā*[4] *Śaktis* who hover about the consciousness in *Brahmarandhra*[5] with a terrible noose of Brahmā, and who are the deities of the *pīṭhas*[6], delude people constantly."

This has been quoted previously also in support of a similar statement. *Mātṛkā* has been spoken of in a general way in *Sūtra* 4 under the first section. Here *mātṛkā* has been mentioned with the intention of showing that even if a person has realized the truth, he is, if he happens to be heedless, deluded by Māheśī and other deities governing the limited individuals by means of the application of words that influence his mind. This is the difference between the two.

NOTES

1. *Cintāmaṇi* or thought-gem is a fabulous gem supposed to yield its possessor all desires.
2. Mother—She is called *mātā* (mother) because she brings about the world consisting of words and objects (*vācaka-vācya jagat*).
3. Vide note No. 4 under the *sūtra* 4 in the 1st Section.
4. Vide note No. 1 under the Sūtra 4 in the 1st Section.
5. *Brahmarandhra* is the psychic centre above the head.
6. *Pīṭhas*—Vide note No. 2 under the sūtra four in the 1st Section.

EXPOSITION

Sūtra 18 says that if the *Sahaja Vidyā* that has appeared in the *Yogī* continues unabated, he is freed of rebirth.

Sūtra 19 says that the *Yogī* should not become heedless after he has acquired *Sahaj Vidyā*. Until all the residual traces of his life are completely wiped out, there is always a possibility of fall from the high pedestal he has risen to. There are always attractions of the ordinary course of life couched in words. If he comes under their influence, he is bound to be ruined spiritually. There are certain dark forces in the world carrying out their designs through words which have a tremendous influence on the minds of people. The *Yogī* should, therefore, be always on the alert and should not fall a victim to the solicitation of sense-pleasure.

INTRODUCTION TO THE 20th SŪTRA

TEXT

यत एवम् अतः शुद्धविद्यास्वरूपमुक्तयुक्तिभिरासादितमपि यथा न नश्यति, तथा सर्वदशासु योगिना सावधानेन भवितव्यम् इत्याह—

TRANSLATION

As this is so (i.e. as there is always likelihood of a fall), therefore the *Yogī* should be careful under all circumstances that the *Śuddha Vidyā* that he has acquired by the aforesaid means should not be lost. Therefore, the next *sūtra* says:

SŪTRA—20.

त्रिषु चतुर्थं तैलवदासेच्यम् ॥ २० ॥

Triṣu caturthaṁ tailavad āsecyam.

चतुर्थम्—the fourth one (the Ātmic state of consciousness) त्रिषु —in all the three states of consciousness viz., waking, dreaming, and deep sleep; तैलवत्—Like (uninterrupted flow of) oil; आसेच्यम् —should be poured into.

The fourth state of Ātmic consciousness should be poured like (uninterrupted flow of) oil in the three states (of waking, dreaming and deep sleep).

COMMENTARY

TEXT

त्रिषु जागरादिषु पदेषु, चतुर्थं शुद्धविद्याप्रकाशरूपं तुर्यानन्दरसात्मकं धाम, तैलवदिति, यथा तैलं क्रमेण अधिकमधिकं प्रसरद् आश्रयं व्याप्नोति तथा आसे-

च्यम् । त्रिष्वपि पदेषु उन्मेषोपशान्त्यात्मकाद्यन्तकोटचोः परिस्फुरता तुर्यरसेन मध्यदशामपि अवष्टम्भयुक्त्या व्याप्नुयात्, येन तन्मयीभावमाप्नुयात् । 'जाग्रत्स्वप्नसुषुप्तेषु तुर्याभोगसंभवः' (१–७) इत्यनेन उद्यम-शक्तिचक्रानुसंध्यवष्टम्भभाजः स्वरसप्रसरज्जागरादिपदेषु सत्तामात्रं तुर्यस्योक्तम् । 'त्रितयभोक्ता वीरेशः' (१–११) इति शाम्भवोपायानुगुणहठपाकयुक्त्या जागरादिसंहारो दर्शितः । अनेन तु सूत्रेण आणवोचितावष्टम्भयुक्त्या दलकल्पं जागरादित्रयं तुर्यरसासिक्तं कार्यम् इत्युक्तम्; इति विशेषः ॥

TRANSLATION

Triṣu means the three states of waking, etc. *Caturtham* means the fourth state of bliss which consists of the light of *śuddha vidyā*. *Tailavat* means 'as oil gradually spreading more and more pervades its receptacle, so should the fourth one be poured so that the lustrous elixir of the fourth state which appears at the initial and the final point may pervade the intervening state also by the device of firm grip so that the triad of the waking, dreaming and deep sleep state may acquire the condition of complete identification with it.

In the seventh *Sūtra* under the first Section, only the existence of the fourth state was stated whose elixir spreads in the waking condition etc. in the case of those in whom it occurs either as spontaneous emergence or by a firm grip of the awareness of the collective whole of *Śaktis*. In *sūtra* 11 under the 1st section, the dissolution of the waking and other states was shown by the device of *haṭhapāka*[1] in accordance with *Śāmbhava* technique. By means of the present *sūtra*, it has been stated that by the technique of firm hold appropriate to *āṇava yoga*, the three states of waking etc. should become like the sheath of a sword which may be saturated with the elixir of *turya*.[9] This is the difference between these *sūtras*.

NOTES

1. *Haṭhapāka* means assimilation of an experience to the consciousness of the experient by a single obstinate, forcible grip.

2. Just as a sheath is different from the sword but can hold it completely within itself so the three states are different from the fourth, but can be completely saturated with its elixir.

EXPOSITION

This *Sūtra* says that the fourth state which is the natural state of *ātmic* consciousness should be maintained in all the three states of waking, dreaming and deep sleep. What usually happens in the case of the acquisition of the fourth state by *āṇava* means is that the awareness of the fourth state occurs only at the initial and final stages of waking, dreaming and deep sleep, but is missed in the intervening condition. The present *sūtra* exhorts the *Yogī* to be on the alert and not lose his hold on the 4th state so that it may permeate the three states in all the stages—initial, intervening and final.

INTRODUCTION TO THE 21st SŪTRA

TEXT

अत्रोपायमाह—

TRANSLATION

In the matter of saturating the waking states, etc. with the fourth, the next *sūtra* describes the means.

SŪTRA—21

मग्नः स्वचित्तेन प्रविशेत् ॥ २१ ॥

Magnaḥ svacittena praviśet.

मग्नः —plunged; स्वचित्तेन—with the mind of the inner I without any thought-construct; प्रविशेत् should enter.

"One should enter it by being plunged into it with an awareness of the inner I without a thought-construct".

Bhāskara reads *svacitte* instead of *svacittena* and interprets *svacitte* as *svātmani*—in one's essential Self. According to him, the *sūtra* means one should (mentally) plunge into one's essential self.'

COMMENTARY

TEXT

'प्राणादिस्थूलभावं तु त्यक्त्वा सूक्ष्ममथान्तरम् ।
सूक्ष्मातीतं तु परमं स्पन्दनं लभ्यते यतः ॥'

इत्युपक्रम्य

.... प्रविशेत्तत्स्वचेतसा ॥'

इति श्रीमृत्युजिद्भट्टारकनिरूपितनीत्या प्राणायाम-ध्यान-धारणादिस्थूलोपायान् परित्यज्य, स्वचित्तेन, अविकल्पकरूपेण अन्तर्मुखान्तरविमर्शचमत्कारात्मना संवेदनेन, प्रविशेत् समाविशेत् । कीदृक् सन् ? मग्नः, शरीरप्राणादिप्रमातृतां तत्रैव चिच्चमत्काररसे मज्जनेन प्रशमयन् । तदुक्तं श्रीस्वच्छन्दे

'व्यापारं मानसं त्यक्त्वा बोधरूपेण योजयेत् ।
तदा शिवत्वमभ्येति पशुर्मुक्तो भवार्णवात् ॥'

इति । श्रीविज्ञानभट्टारकेऽपि

'मानसं चेतना शक्तिरात्मा चेति चतुष्टयम् ।
यदा प्रिये परिक्षीणं तदा तद्भैरवं वपुः ॥'

इति । एतदेव ज्ञानगर्भे स्तोत्रे

'विहाय सकलाः क्रिया जननि मानसीः सर्वतो
विमुक्तकरणक्रियानुसृतिपारतन्त्र्योज्ज्वलम् ।
स्थितैस्त्वदनुभावतः सपदि वेद्यते सा परा
दशा नृभिरतन्द्रितासमसुखामृतस्यन्दिनी ॥'

इत्यनेन महागुरुर्भिनिबद्धम् ॥ २१ ॥

TRANSLATION

Mṛtyujit says, beginning with "One should give up gross *prāṇāyāma* and even the inner subtle one and thus the highest pulsation of consciousness which is beyond even the subtle *prāṇāyāma* is obtained" and ending with 'enter the highest state with one's mind as a knower" (VIII, 12).

In accordance with the process pointed out by *Mṛtyujit*, one should, giving up gross means like *Prāṇāyāma*, meditation, concentration etc, enter it (i.e. get immersed in the fourth consciousness) with one's mind i.e. with an awareness without thought-construct, and of the nature of an introverted inner joy of I-consciousness. In what way ? By plunging into it i.e. *by extinguishing the idea of the body, prāṇa etc. as being the knower in the elixir of the joy of I-consciousness.*

It has been said in *Svacchanda.*

"Giving up all mental activity, one should be united to *Śiva* only with *bodha*[1] (i.e. an awareness without any thoughtconstruct'). Then one acquires the status of *Śiva* (i.e. is identified with Śiva), and the limited empirical self is liberated from the ocean of transmigratory form of existence." (IV, 437)

In *Vijñānabhairava* also it has been said,

"O dear one, when the *mānasa*[2] *cetana*[3] *śakti*[4] and *ātmā*[5]—these four are dissolved, then one acquires the essential nature of *Bhairava*". (Verse, 138).

The same idea has been emphasized in the following laudatory verse Cf Jñānagarbha :

"When, O Mother, men renounce all mental activities and are poised in a pure state, being free from the bondage of the pursuit of sense activities,[6] then by thy grace is that supreme state realized at once which rains down the nectar of unlimited and unparalleled happiness.

This has been composed by the great teacher.[7]

NOTES

1. *Bodharūpeṇa*—'in the form of only *bodha*, In his commentary on Svacchanda, Kṣemarāja interprets it thus : "अविकल्प संवित्स्पर्शनेनैव" i.e. only 'with a touch of awareness freed of all thought-construct'. Wherever here is *vikalpa* or thought-construct, there is mental activity. When there is no thought-construct, the mind is reduced to utter silence. It is with such a mind that one can be united to Śiva.

2. *Mānasa*—*Mānasa* means the mind full of desire and thought-construct.

3. *Cetanā* here means *buddhi*, the ascertaining intellect.

4. *Śakti* here means *prāṇa*.

5. Ā*tmā* here means the limited empirical self, conditioned by *manas*, *buddhi* and *ahaṁkāra*.

6. *Karaṇa-Kriyā* means sense-activities. It may also mean the activities of *karaṇa*—one of the forms of *āṇavopāya*.

7. The great teacher referred to is *Pradyumnabhaṭṭapāda*, a pupil of *Kallaṭa*.

EXPOSITION

The 20th sūtra mentions an *āṇava upāya* of maintaining an awareness of the 4th or the central *ātmic* consciousness by means of *dhāraṇā, dhyāna*, etc.

The 21st sūtra suggests *Śāktopāya*. By means of this, one takes a direct plunge into the 4th State by silencing the mind, by detaching oneself from the body, *prāṇa*, etc. by the sheer awareness of the pure I-consciousness. The aspirant enters the secret chamber of the transcendental consciousness with a spontaneous immediacy of feeling as the baby slips into its mother's arms.

INTRODUCTION TO THE 22nd SŪTRA

TEXT

इत्थं च परमपदप्रविष्टस्य अस्य वस्तुस्वाभाव्यात् यदा पुनः प्रसरणं भवति तदा—

TRANSLATION

Thus in the case of this *Yogī* who has entered the highest state, when there is a spreading out of the consciousness as is its nature, then,

SŪTRA—22

प्राणसमाचारे समदर्शनम् ॥ २२ ॥

Prāṇa-samācāre samadarśanam

प्राण — of the *prāṇa* (the vital breath); समाचारे—on the occasion of proper and slow spreading out; समदर्शनम्—awareness of all being the same.

When the *prāṇa* of the *Yogī* properly and slowly spreads out (then) he has an awareness of all being the same i.e. he has unity-consciousness.

In *Bhāskara*, there is a difference in the order of the *sūtras*. The 23rd *sūtra* of *Kṣemarāja* is the 22nd *sūtra* of *Bhāskara*, and the 22nd *sūtra* of *Kṣemarāja* is the 23rd *sūtra* of *Bhāskara*. *Bhāskara* thus interprets this sūtra. Prāṇa here means the power of omniscience and omnipotence. This manifests itself as the highest *nāda* which enters letters, words, and the empirical individuals and experiences identity with them. This is what is meant by *samadarśana*.

COMMENTARY

TEXT

परस्फुरत्तात्मकशाक्तपरिमलसंस्कृतस्य प्राणस्य, सम्यक् इति विकसित-समग्रग्रन्थ्यात्मकान्तरावष्टम्भबलात्, आ ईषत् बहिर्मन्दमन्दं चारे प्रसरणे, समं चिदानन्दघनात्मतया एकरूपं, दर्शनं संवेदनम्, अर्थात् सर्वदशासु अस्य भवति इत्यर्थः । उक्तं च श्रीमदानन्दभैरवे

"उत्सृज्य लौकिकाचारमद्वैतं मुक्तिदं श्रयेत् ।
स समं सर्वदेवानां तथा वर्णाश्रमादिके ॥
द्रव्याणां समतादर्शी स मुक्तः सर्वबन्धनैः ।"

इति । अत एव श्रीप्रत्यभिज्ञायाम्

'बुद्धिप्राणप्रसरेऽपि बाह्यदेशाद्युपादानानाहितसंकोचानां
विश्वात्मस्वरूपलाभ एव ॥'

इत्युक्तम् ॥ २२ ॥

TRANSLATION

Prāṇasya[1] means 'of the prāṇa' consecrated by the aroma of *Śakti* which is the radiance of the Highest. *Sama* in *samācāra* means *Samyak* i.e. by the force of a firm hold on the inner nature whose all the complexes have become evolved i.e. have been brought fully under control. *Ācāre* means on the spreading out a little slowly externally. *Samadarśanam* means 'awareness of every thing uniformly as a mass of the bliss of *Cit* (the central divine consciousness)'. This is what he experiences in all conditions[2]. It has been said in *Ānandabhairava*:

"Giving up customary practices, one should resort to non-dualism which brings about liberation. Then his attitude towards all the gods becomes the same, and also towards all the castes and *āśramas*. He looks upon all things as the same. He is free from all bonds."

Therefore, it has been said in the commentary on *Īśvara-pratyabhijñā*:

"In the case of those who are free from the limitations caused by the assumption of external space, time and form; even when *buddhi* and *prāṇa* are active (i.e. in the normal course of life), they have the experience of the entire universe as the Self."[3]

NOTES

1. When the *Yogī* is fully plunged in the fourth state, his vital breaths—*prāṇa* and *apāna* i.e. exhaling and inhaling breaths are dissolved in the middle *nāḍī* i.e. the *suṣumnā*. When he wakes up to the usual, normal consciousness, his *prāṇa* and *apāna* breaths resume their usual course of breathing out and breathing in. This is what is meant by *prāṇasamācāra*.

2. The experience of the delight and unity consciousness of the 4th State does not vanish when the *Yogī* wakes up to normal consciousness. It persists even in the normal consciousness and the *Yogī* feels that he and everything else in the universe are the expression of the same universal consciousness.

3. They experience *jagadānanda*—the bliss of the Divine made visible in the form of the world.

EXPOSITION

The 21st *Sūtra* suggests that when an aspirant has advanced far enough in *Yoga* by *āṇavopāya*, he is led into *śāktopāya* and enters the transcendental consciousness. The 22nd *sūtra* says that when the aspirant is sufficiently steeped in the fourth state or transcendental consciousness, he rises to *Śāmbhava* state; the experience of the transcendental consciousness persists even in the normal course of life; he acquires cosmic consciousness. To him the whole world is apparelled in celestial light—a visible symbol of the bliss of Divine Consciousness.

INTRODUCTION TO THE 23rd SŪTRA

TEXT

यदा तु अन्तर्मुखतुर्यविधानावष्टम्भप्रकर्षलभ्यं तुर्यातीतपदम् एवमयं न समाविशति, अपि तु पूर्वापरकोटिसंवेद्यतुर्यचमत्कारमात्रे एव संतुष्यन्नास्ते, तदा अस्य—

TRANSLATION

When, however, he (the *Yogī*) does not enter the *turyātīta* state which is attainable by the intensity of the awareness of the inner *tūrya*, but is rather content only with the delight of the fourth state experienced at the initial and final point of the waking, dreaming state etc. then his (i.e. in his case)

SŪTRA—23

मध्येऽवरप्रसवः ।२३॥

Madhye'vara-prasavaḥ

मध्ये—in the intervening stage, अवर—inferior; प्रसवः :—generation or arising (of states).

'In the intervening stage, there arise inferior states of mind.'

COMMENTARY

TEXT

पूर्वापरकोटचोस्तुर्यरसमास्वादयतो, मध्ये मध्यदशायाम्, अवरः अश्रेष्ठः, प्रसवो व्युत्थानात्मा कुत्सितः सर्गो जायते । न तु 'विद्यासंहारे तदुत्थस्वप्न-दर्शनम्' (२–१०) इत्युक्तसूत्रार्थनीत्या सदा व्यामुह्यति इत्यर्थः । उक्तं श्रीमालिनीविजये

'वासनामात्रलाभेऽपि योऽप्रमत्तो न जायते ।
तमनित्येषु भोगेषु योजयन्ति विनायकाः ॥
तस्मान्न तेषु संसक्तिं कुर्वीतोत्तमवाञ्छया ।'

इति प्रागपि संवादितम् ॥ २३ ॥

TRANSLATION

In the case of the *Yogī* who has enjoyed the delight of the transcendental consciousness at the initial and final stages of waking, dream etc., inferior stages of mind characteristic of the normal course of life arise in the intervening stage.

As is the case of the *Yogī* described in *Sūtra* ten of the 2nd section, he is not permanently deluded: It has been said in *Mālinīvijaya:*

"Even when one has obtained some impression of the transcendental state, if one is not on the alert, then the *vināyakas* induce him to transient pleasures. Therefore one who desires to obtain the highest state should not have any attachment for these (transient pleasures)." This I have quoted as an authority previously also.

INTRODUCTION TO THE 24th SŪTRA

TEXT

एवमेव प्रसवेऽपि प्रवृत्ते यदि तुर्यरसावष्टम्भेन मध्यपदं सिञ्चति पुनरपि, तदा—

TRANSLATION

Even when inferior states arise, if the *Yogī* sprinkles the intervening stage with the elixir of the tightly-gripped fourth state, then :

SŪTRA—24

मात्रास्वप्रत्ययसंधाने नष्टस्य पुनरुत्थानम् ॥ २४ ॥

Mātrā-svapratyaya-sandhāne naṣṭasya punarutthānam.

मात्रा—objects; स्वप्रत्ययसंधाने—on the union of the real I-consciousness; नष्टस्य—of the lost; पुनरुत्थानम्—rising again.

"When the real I-consciousness is joined to the objects, the transcendental state of consciousness which had disappeared appears again".

COMMENTARY

TEXT

मात्रासु पदार्थेषु स्वप्रत्ययसंधानम् ।

'चक्षुषा यच्च संधानं वाचा वा यश्च गोचरः ।
मनश्चिन्तयते यानि बुद्धिश्चैवाध्यवस्यति ॥
अहङ्कृतानि यान्येव यच्च वेद्यतया स्थितम् ।
यश्च नास्ति स तत्रैव त्वन्वेष्टव्यः प्रयत्नतः ॥'

इति-श्रीस्वच्छन्दनिरूपितनीत्या 'विश्वमिदम् अहम्, इति चिद्घनात्मरूपतां सर्वत्र अनुसंदधतः, पूर्वोक्तावरप्रसवात् नष्टस्य, अपहारिततुर्यैकघनचमत्कारमयस्वभावस्य, पुनरुत्थानम् उन्मज्जनं तदैक्यसंपत्संपूर्णत्वं योगिनो भवति इत्यर्थः । तदुक्तं श्रीस्वच्छन्दे

'प्रसह्य चञ्चलीत्येव योगिनामपि यन्मनः ।'

इत्युपक्रम्य

'यस्य ज्ञेयमयो भावः स्थिरः पूर्णः समन्ततः ।
मनो न चलिते तस्य सर्वावस्थागतस्य तु ॥
यत्र यत्र मनो याति ज्ञेयं तत्रैव चिन्तयेत् ।
चलित्वा यास्यते कुत्र सर्वं शिवमयं यतः ॥'

इति ।

'विषयेषु च सर्वेषु इन्द्रियार्थेषु च स्थितः ।
यत्र तत्र निरूप्येत नाशिवं विद्यते क्वचित् ॥'

इति च ॥ २४ ॥

TRANSLATION

Mātrāsu means 'in objects'; joining of the real I-consciousness.

"Whatever is perceived through the eye, whatever becomes an object of consciousness through word, whatever the mind thinks of (viz., pleaure, gain etc.), whatever the intellect ascertains, whatever is appropriated to the empirical I-consciousness, whatever exists as an object of consciousness, even what does not exist (and is only a matter of imagination or fancy), the Light of Consciousness or *Śiva* should be assiduously investigated in all these." (XII, 163-164).

Thus in accordance with what has been pointed out in *Svacchanda-tantra*, in the case of the *Yogī* who over and over again thinks of his compact consciousness in every case in the form "I am this universe", there is again reappearance or emergence of the delight of the fourth state of consciousness which had disappeared on account of the appearance of inferior states of mind mentioned before. In other words the *Yogī* experiences complete fulfilment in his identification with that fourth state of consciousness. It has been said in *Svacchanda-tantra*, beginning with,

"As the mind even of *Yogīs* forcibly runs (after, objects of enjoyment)"

and ending with,

"Whose mind is chock-full of the highest reality (that being the sole object of knowledge), steady, fully contented (i.e., without any desire) in all cases, his mind does not deviate (from its fixed aim), even when he passes through all sorts of circumstances.

Wherever his mind moves, he should think of *Śiva* (the object of his knowledge) there itself. As everything is *Śiva*, where else shall his mind go to ?

In the apprehension of all objects, in all sense-enjoyments—in whichever condition the *Yogī* may happen to be placed, wherever he may investigate, there is no place where *Śiva* does not exist." (IV, 311-314).

INTRODUCTION TO THE 25th SŪTRA

TEXT

इत्थमासादितप्रकर्षो योगी—

TRANSLATION

Thus the *yogī* who has obtained pre-eminence in transcendental consciousness.

SŪTRA—25

शिवतुल्यो जायते ॥ २५ ॥

Śiva-tulyo jāyate

शिवतुल्यः :—like *Śiva*; जायते—becomes.

(Such a Yogi) becomes like *Śiva.*

COMMENTARY

TEXT

तुर्यपरिशीलनप्रकर्षात् प्राप्ततुर्यातीतपदः परिपूर्णस्वच्छस्वच्छन्दचिदानन्दघनेन शिवेन भगवता तुल्यो, देहकलाया अविगलनात् तत्समो जायते। तद्विगलने साक्षाच्छिव एव असौ इत्यर्थः। तथा च श्रीकालिकाक्रमे

'तस्मान्नित्यमसंदिग्धं बुद्ध्वा योगं गुरोर्मुखात्
अविकल्पेन भावेन भावयेत्तन्मयत्वतः ॥
यावत्तत्समतां याति भगवान्भैरवोऽब्रवीत् ।'

इति ॥ २५ ॥

TRANSLATION

With the intensive practice of remaining in the *turya* state, he obtains the *turyātīta* state and thus becomes like God Śiva who is perfectly pure, absolutely free, and a mass of consciousness and bliss. So long as the body-aspect[1] does not vanish, he is like *Ś*iva. When the body perishes, he is veritable *Śiva.*

In *Kālikā-krama*, it has been said similarly :

"Therefore, having understood always and without doubt from the mouth of the spiritual director the means of union with *Śiva*, one should contemplate over Him without any thought-construct, with unshakable zeal and with a sense of identification with Him till one becomes identified with Him.[2] This is what Lord Bhairava has said.

NOTES

1. So long as he is a *jīva*, so long as there is the flow of *prāṇa* and *apāna* in him.

2. The identification with *Śiva* is, to start with, only mental. Finally, it is actual.

INTRODUCTION TO THE 26th SŪTRA

TEXT

एवमपि च 'येनेदं तद्धि भोगतः' इत्याद्युक्तरीत्या उपनतभोगातिवाहनमात्रप्रयोजनात् देहस्थितिः अस्य न अतिक्रमणीया इत्याह—

TRANSLATION

Even thus (i.e. even when he is like *Śiva*), in accordance with the principle laid down in the scriptures viz., 'since there is this body, it should be ended only with full use of the objects of experience determined for the particular life', the purpose of the continuance of the body is to carry on with the objects of experience falling to one's share. Therefore, its continuance should not be neglected. This is what the next *sūtra* says.

SŪTRA—26

शरीरवृत्तिर्व्रतम् ॥ २६ ॥

Śarīravṛttir Vratam

शरीरवृत्तिः—remaining in the body, retaining the body; व्रतम् —observance of pious act.

Remaining in the body is all his observance of a pious act (*vratam*).

COMMENTARY

TEXT

प्रोक्तदृशा शिवतुल्यस्य योगिनः शिवाहंभावेन वर्तमानस्य, शरीरे वृत्तिर्वर्तनं यत्, तदेव व्रतम्; स्वस्वरूपविमर्शात्मकनित्योदितपरपूजातत्परस्य नियमेन अनुष्ठेयम् अस्य। तथा च श्रीस्वच्छन्दे

'सुप्रदीप्ते यथा वह्नौ शिखा दृश्येत चाम्बरे।
देहप्राणस्थितोऽप्यात्मा तद्वल्लीयेत तत्पदे ॥'

इत्युक्त्या देहप्राणाद्यवस्थितस्यैव शिवसमाविष्टत्वमुक्तम्। न पुनस्तस्य देहस्थितिव्यतिरिक्तं व्रतमुपयुक्तम्। यदुक्तं श्रीत्रिकसारे

'देहोत्थिताभिर्मुद्राभिर्यः सदा मुद्रितो बुधः।
स तु मुद्राधरः प्रोक्तः शेषा वै अस्थिधारकाः ॥'

इति। श्रीकुलपञ्चाशिकायामपि

'अव्यक्तलिङ्गिनं दृष्ट्वा संभाषन्ते मरीचयः।
लिङ्गिनं नोपसर्पन्ति अतिगुप्ततरा यतः ॥'

इति ॥ २६ ॥

TRANSLATION

As described before 'of the *Yogī* who is like *Śiva* i.e. who exists with the consciousness that I am *Śiva*', remaining in the body is his observance of a pious act. In other words, the regular observance of a pious act in the case of this *Yogī* consists in his being engaged in the worship of the ever-present Supreme in the form of the awareness of one's essential nature.

It has been said in *Svacchanda-tantra.*

"As in a well-kindled fire, the flame is seen in the sky: so like that the Self (*ātmā*) though existing in the body and *prāṇa* is merged in the state of *Śiva*."[1] (IV, 398).

In accordance with this, it has been declared that though the *Yogī* is still existing in the body, *prāṇa* etc. his self is immersed in the state of Śiva.

No other observance of a pious act apart from the maintenance of the body is appropriate for him. As has been said in Trikasāra:

"The wise man is always marked with higher modes of yogic poses that arise *from* the body (i.e., while the body is retained). He alone is the (real) holder of yogic poses; the rest who only maintain certain gross poses *of* hands and the body are only holders of bones."

In *Kulapañcāśikā* also, it has been said—

"The (higher) powers[2] (lit., rays of light) converse only with those who do not put on any perceptible (religious) mark. They do not come near those who put on visible marks of piety, for they are very occult beings."

NOTES

1. In this verse, *deha* or body has been compared to wood, *mantra* has been compared to *araṇi*—a piece of wood used for kindling fire by friction; *prāṇa* has been compared to fire. *śikhā* or flame has been compared to *ātmā* (Self) ; *ambara* or sky has been compared to Śiva.

When prāṇa is kindled by means of *mantra* used as *araṇi*, fire in the form of *udāna* arises in *suṣumnā*, and then just as flame arises out of kindled fire and gets dissolved in the sky, so also *ātmā* (Self) like a flame having burnt down the fuel of the body, gets absorbed in *Śiva*.

2. When there is realization of Reality, *Śakti-cakra* (host of powers) according to *Śaivāgama*, appears to the *Yogī*. The verse says that these powers never appear to one who believes only in outward marks of piety but is spiritually bankrupt. They appear only to one who has inward realization and does not believe in a show of piety by putting on an outward mark.

INTRODUCTION TO THE 27th SŪTRA

TEXT

एवं-विधस्य अस्य—

Translation

Of this sort of *Yogī*.

SŪTRA—27

कथा जपः ॥ २७ ॥

Kathā japaḥ.

कथा—conversation; जप: muttering prayer or sacred formula. ('His) conversation constitues muttering of prayer.'

COMMENTARY

TEXT

'अहमेव परो हंसः शिवः परमकारणम् ।'

इति-श्रीस्वच्छन्दनिरूपितनीत्या नित्यमेव पराहंभावनामयत्वात् ।

'तस्य देवातिदेवस्य परबोधस्वरूपिणः ।
विमर्शः परमा शक्तिः सर्वज्ञा ज्ञानशालिनी ॥'

इति-श्रीकालिकाक्रमनिरूपितनीत्या महामन्त्रात्मकाकृतकाहंविमर्शारूढस्य यद्यदालापादि तत्तदस्य स्वात्मदेवताविमर्शानवरतावर्तनात्मा जपो जायते । यदुक्तं श्रीविज्ञानभैरवे

'भूयो भूयः परे भावे भावना भाव्यते हि या ।
जपः सोऽत्र स्वयं नादो मन्त्रात्मा जप्य ईदृशः ॥'

इति । तथा

'सकारेण बहिर्याति हकारेण विशेत्पुनः ।
हंस-हंसेत्यमुं मन्त्रं जीवो जपति नित्यशः ॥
षट्शतानि दिवारात्रौ सहस्राण्येकविंशतिः ।
जपो देव्या विनिर्दिष्टः सुलभो दुर्लभो जडैः ॥'

इति ॥ २७ ॥

TRANSLATION

As he is always full of the Supreme I-consciousness, as indicated in the following verse of *Svacchanda-tantra*,

"I am the highest *ātmā*; I am *Śiva*, the highest cause", even an ordinary conversation of his amounts to the muttering of a prayer.

As expounded in the following verse of Kālikākrama:

"Of that God who is greater than all the gods and who is supreme consciousness itself, the highest *Śakti* is I-consciousness which is omniscient, full of wisdom." I-consciousness is the highest *Śakti* of this *Yogī*. Whatever conversation etc. there may be of the *Yogī* who has attained to the natural I-consciousness which is of the nature of the highest *mantra*, all that amounts to *japa* (utterance of a prayer) whose essential characteristic is ceaseless repetition of the awareness of the deity which is one's own Self.[1]

As has been said in *Vijñānabhairava*:

"That contemplation which is made over and over again on the highest state (i.e. on the Supreme I-consciousness) is in this subtle teaching a *japa*. Such an inner automatic Sound (of I) which is of the nature of a *mantra* should be pondered over again and again. This is the kind of subtle *japa* that the *yogī* should perform." (Verse 145).

Again it has been said :

"The breath is exhaled with the sound *sa* and inhaled again with the sound *ha*. Therefore, the empirical individual always repeats the mantra *Haṁsaḥ*.[2] Throughout the day and night, he repeats this mantra 21,600 times.[3] Such a *japa* of the goddess (*Gāyatrī*) has been prescribed which is quite easy for the wise, but difficult for the ignorant."

NOTES

1. Awareness of I which is being sounded inwardly automatically without anybody's utterance is the occult *japa*. Since the *Yogī* never loses his hold on this I-consciousness even while he is chatting with others, therefore even ordinary conversation is a *japa* on his part. The word *japa* is here taken as an anacrostic word—'ja' standing for *jani* meaning birth, creation, and *pa* standing for *pālana* meaning protection. *Japa*, therefore, means that which protects created beings.

2. The *mantra haṁsaḥ* is repeated automatically by the *jīva* in every round of expiration—inspiration. It is known as *haṁsa mantra*. This is also known as *ajapājapa* i.e. automatic *japa*. The *ha* of this *mantra* represents *Śakti* and *saḥ* represents *Śiva*. *Am* in *haṁsaḥ* represents the *jīva*. The *apāna* or incoming breath represents *Śakti* and *prāṇa*, the outgoing breath represents *Śiva*. This is known as *trika-mantra* also as it includes in itself the three realities of *Śiva*, *Śakti* and *nara* (*jīva*). The aspirant has to concentrate on *am* which is the junction point of *ha* and *saḥ*.

3. One round of inspiration-expiration takes 4 seconds. So there is automatic *japa* of *haṁsaḥ* (I am He) 15 times in a minute. In one hour, there would be (15×60) 900 repetitions of this *japa*. In a full day and night, there would be (900×24) 21,600 repetitions of this *japa*.

INTRODUCTION TO THE 28th SŪTRA

TEXT

ईदृग्जपव्रतवतोऽस्य चर्यामाह—

TRANSLATION

The next *sūtra* describes the daily life and conduct of the *Yogī* who practices this kind of *japa* and *vrata*.

SŪTRA—28

दानमात्मज्ञानम् ॥ २८ ॥

Dānam ātmajñānam.

दानम्—charity; gift; आत्मज्ञानम्—knowledge of Self.

'Knowledge of Self is the gift that he disseminates (all round)'

COMMENTARY

TEXT

प्रोक्तचैतन्यरूपस्य आत्मनो यत् ज्ञानं, साक्षात्कारः, तत् अस्य दानम् ; दीयते परिपूर्णं स्वरूपम्, दीयते खण्डयते विश्वभेदः, दायते शोध्यते माया-स्वस्वरूपम्, दीयते रक्ष्यते लब्धः शिवात्मा स्वभावश्च अनेन इति कृत्वा ।

अथ च दीयते इति दानम् आत्मज्ञानमेव अनेन अन्तेवासिभ्यो दीयते ।

तदुक्तम्

'दर्शनात्स्पर्शनाद्वापि वितताद्भवसागरात् ।
तारयिष्यन्ति योगीन्द्राः कुलाचारप्रतिष्ठिताः ॥'

इति ॥ २८ ॥

TRANSLATION

As described before, *ātmā* is universal consciousness. Its *jñāna* means its realization. *Dānam*[1] means gift derived from the root *da* of the 3rd conjugation, the meaning accordingly would be—the perfect essential mature is given as a gift.

The word *dānam* can also be derived from the root *do* of the 2nd conjugation which means 'to cut, to divide'. In this sense, *dānam* indicates that the difference of the universe (from Śiva) is cut asunder.

The word *dānam* can be derived also from the root 'dai' of the 1st conjugation; meaning 'to purify', to cleanse'. This would indicate that *Māyā* is cleansed, purified by knowledge of the Self.

The word *dānam* may also be derived from the root 'dī' of the 2nd conjugation which means 'to preserve', suggesting that the Śiva-nature acquired by him is well preserved.

The main meaning of the *Sūtra* is that Self-knowledge is disseminated by him among his pupils. It has been rightly said:

"The great *Yogīs* who are well-established in *kulācāra* will enable people to cross the extensive ocean of worldly existence by their sight or touch."

NOTES

1. The word *dānam* is derived in various ways in Sanskrit. Each derivation suggests a certain aspect of the *Yogī's* self-realization.

2. *Kulācāra* means *trikācāra*—the unity of *nara* (jīva) *Śakti* and *Śiva.*

EXPOSITION

Vrata—observance of a pious act like fasting on a particular sacred day, *japa*—recitation of a *mantra, dāna,* giving alms in charity may well begin as *āṇavopāya*, as *kriyā-yoga*, but the *Sūtras* 26, 27, and 28 say that when the *anu* or empirical self is advanced in *yoga* and has realized Self, then *vrata, japa,* and *dāna* are converted into *Śāktopāya,* then they are lifted from ordinary, routine rituals to the status of mystic practices where they are not merely external routine observances but expressions of *jñāna* or Self-realization.

INTRODUCTION TO THE 29th SŪTRA

TEXT

यथोक्तनीत्या शिवतुल्यतया नित्यमेवं व्रतजपचर्यानिष्ठत्वात् निजशक्तिचक्रारूढः स एव तत्त्वत उपदेश्यानां प्रतिबोधक इत्याह—

TRANSLATION

In accordance with what has been described, he becomes similar to *Śiva.* As he is always devoted to *vrata, japa* and religious practice and has acquired mastery over his group of *śaktis,* he alone is competent to enlighten the seekers about Reality. Therefore, the next *sūtra* says:

SŪTRA—29

योऽविपस्थो ज्ञाहेतुश्च ॥ २९ ॥

Yo'vipastho jñāhetuśca.

यः—who; अविपस्थ—is established in *Śakti Cakra*; ज्ञाहेतुः—(he) is the means, agency of wisdom; च —indeed, surely.

"He who is established in the group of *śaktis* (who has acquired mastery over the *śaktis*) serves, indeed, as an agency of wisdom."

COMMENTARY

TEXT

अवीन् पशून् पाति इति अविपं 'कवर्गादिषु माहेश्वर्याद्याः पशुमातरः' (३-१९) इत्यभिहितदृशा माहेश्वर्यादिशक्तिचक्रं, तत्र तिष्ठति विदितस्वमाहात्म्यत्वात् प्रभुत्वेन यः प्रतपति, संज्ञाहेतुः; जानाति इति ज्ञा ज्ञानशक्तिः, तस्या हेतुः, उपदेश्यान् ज्ञानशक्त्या प्रतिबोधयितुं क्षमः । अन्यस्तु शक्तिचक्रपरतन्त्रीकृतत्वात् स्वात्मनि अप्रभविष्णुः कथमन्यान् प्रबोधयेत् । यच्छब्दापेक्षया सूत्रेऽत्र तच्छब्दोऽध्याहार्यः । च शब्दो ह्यर्थे । योऽयमविपस्थः स यस्मात् ज्ञानप्रबोधनहेतुस्तस्माद्युक्तमुक्तम् 'दानमात्मज्ञानम्' (३-२८) इति ।

अन्ये तु 'अक्षरसारूप्यात् प्रब्रूयात्' इति निरुक्तस्थित्या 'यो' इति योगीन्द्रः, 'वि' इति विज्ञानम्, 'प' इति पदम्,'स्थ' इति पदस्थः इत्यस्य अन्त्यमक्षरम् । 'ज्ञ' इति ज्ञाता, 'हे' इति हेयः, 'तु' इति तुच्छता, विसर्जनीयेन विसर्गशक्तिः, चकारेण अनुक्तसमुच्चयार्थेन कर्ता परामृश्यते इत्याश्रित्य, यो योगीन्द्रो विमर्शशक्त्या स्वरूपात्मविज्ञानपदस्थः, स ज्ञाता कर्ता च अवगन्तव्यः; तदा च अस्य हेयतां तुच्छतां निःसारतां, न तु उपादेयतामासादयति इति व्याचक्षते । एतच्च न नः प्रतिभाति, पदार्थसङ्गतेर्नातिचारुत्वात्; प्रतिसूत्रं च ईदृशव्याख्याक्रमस्य सहस्रशो दर्शयितुं शक्यत्वात् ॥ २९ ॥

TRANSLATION

Avipasthaḥ — (*avi* — *pa* — *sthaḥ*)—*Avi* means 'animal'; *pa* means 'protector'; *Avipa*, therefore, means the protector of animals i.e. those who look after limited individuals i.e. the deities *Māheśvarī* etc. presiding over the group of letters like *ka* etc., who are *paśu-mātaraḥ* as stated in the 19th *sūtra* of the 3rd section, i.e. mothers of empirical individuals *Sthaḥ* means he is seated there i.e. being aware of his pre-eminence: he shines in all his glory as the lord of those *śaktis*. *Jñā* means *jñānaśakti*—the power of wisdom. So *Jñāhetuḥ* means the source or agency of wisdom i.e. he is competent to awaken the seekers (from their sleep of ignorance) through his *jñāna-śakti* (power of wisdom). How can any body else who is under the sway of *śakti-cakra* and is thus incompetent to awaken himself enlighten others ? With reference to *yaḥ* (who) in the *sūtra, saḥ* (he) should be supplied (to complete the sense). The word *ca* in this *sūtra* has been used in the sense of 'indeed'.

Since he has acquired control over the group of *śaktis* and is thus an instrument in enlightenment, it has been rightly said in the 28th *Sūtra* that he disseminates knowledge of Self.

Others from the point of view of hermenia which maintains that interpretation should be made in accordance with every letter interpret this *sūtra* thus: *Yo* suggests *Yogīndra*—a *yogī par excellence*, *vi* suggests *vijñāna*—special knowledge, *pa* suggests *pada* or state. So *pa* and *sthaḥ* which is the final word together make up *padasthaḥ* which means 'established in the state'.

Jña suggests *jñātā* or knower; *he* suggests *heya*—rejectable: *tu* suggests *tucchatā*—worthlessness; the *visarga* suggests *visarga-śakti*—creative energy; the word *ca* which should not be taken in the sense of 'and' refers to the agent (since an agent is needed). So they interpret the whole *sūtra* thus:

'The great *Yogī* through the power of Self-awareness is established in the state of the wisdom of his essential nature. He should be considered to be both knower and doer; 'hetu' stands for the rejectibility and worthlessness or unacceptibility of this world. This interpretation does not appeal to us, for it is not very agreeable from the point of view of consistency of the words of the *sūtra*. Such an interpretation of every *sūtra* can be given in a thousand ways.

INTRODUCTION TO THE 30th SŪTRA

अस्य च—

TRANSLATION

And of this *Yogī*.

SŪTRA—30

स्वशक्तिप्रचयोऽस्य विश्वम् ॥ ३० ॥

Svaśakti-pracayo'sya viśvam.

स्व—his; शक्ति—power; प्रचयः—elaboration; unfoldment; विश्वम्—the universe.

"The universe is the unfoldment of his power."

COMMENTARY

TEXT

यतोऽयं शिवतुल्य उक्तस्ततो यथा

'शक्तयोऽस्य जगत्कृत्स्नम् .... ।'

इत्याद्याम्नायदृष्ट्या शिवस्य विश्वं स्वशक्तिमयं, तथा अस्यापि स्वस्याः संविदात्मनः शक्तेः, प्रचयः क्रियाशक्तिस्फुरणरूपो विकासो, विश्वम् । यदुक्तं श्रीमृत्युजिति

'यतो ज्ञानमयो देवो ज्ञानं च बहुधा स्थितम् ॥
नियन्त्रितानां बद्धानां त्राणं तन्नेत्रमुच्यते ॥'

कालिकाक्रमेऽपि

'तत्तद्रूपतया ज्ञानं बहिरन्तः प्रकाशते ।
ज्ञानादृते नार्थसत्ता ज्ञानरूपं ततो जगत् ॥
न हि ज्ञानादृते भावाः केनचिद्विषयीकृताः ।
ज्ञानं तदात्मतां यातमेतस्मादवसीयते ॥
अस्तिनास्तिविभागेन निषेधविधियोगतः ।
ज्ञानात्मता ज्ञेयनिष्ठा भावानां भावनाबलात् ॥
युगपद्वेदनाज्ज्ञानज्ञेययोरेकरूपता ।'

इति ॥ ३० ॥

TRANSLATION

From the point of view of the scriptures which maintain that 'the entire world is *Śiva's śakti*', this world is only a form of His *śakti*. As the Yogi has been described to be like *Śiva*, therefore the universe is *pracaya* i.e. expansion of Consciousness

—power. In other words, it is the unfoldment of his *kriyā-śakti* (creative power). As has been said in *Mṛtyujit* "As the Lord is *jñānamaya*[1] or sheer consciousness and His *jñāna* or consciousness-power exists in multitudinous forms,[2] and as He saves the restrained (limited) and therefore bound beings, therefore is He called *Netra*."[3] (IX, 12)

In Kālikākrama also it is said,

"Consciousness shines in various external and internal forms.[4] There is no existence of objects apart from consciousness. Therefore, the world is simply a form of consciousness. Objects are not known by anybody without consciousness. It is consciousness that has assumed the forms of objects. It is through consciousness that objects are ascertained. Through the application of affirmation and negation, there is division of existents either as positive or negative. The objectivity of existents through the operation of consciousness is only a form of consciousness itself. As knowledge and the known i.e. its objects are apprehended together, therefore are they (knowledge and its object) one and the same."[5]

NOTES

1. *Jñānamaya* here means, as Kṣemarāja in his commentary on *Netratantra* says, *Cinmātra-paramārthaḥ*—sheer consciousness as the highest Reality.

2. It exists in multitudinous forms through contraction or compression.

3. *Netra* in its *nairuktic* or etymological interpretation means *niyantritānāṁ trāṇam*—the saviour of the restrained or limited beings. The letter *na* (न) of *netra* (नेत्र) stands for नियंत्रितानां and the letter *tra* (त्र) stands for त्राणम् It is impossible to bring this out in translation. *Śiva* is called *netra* (lit. eye), not because He is the physical eye, but because it is He who through His grace reveals His concealed being to them who turn towards Him. It is He alone who both conceals and reveals Himself.

4. Consciousness appears in the external form as a jar or blue, etc., and in its internal form as pleasure, pain, thought, emotion etc.

5. The world, according to this philosophy, is only a congealed form of consciousness.

EXPOSITION

The advanced *Yogī* becomes like *Śiva*. His consciousness is now the consciousness of *Śiva*. As the world is simply a congealed form of the consciousness of *Śiva*, and as the *Yogi's* consciousness is the same as that of *Śiva*, the world in his case also is an unfoldment of his consciousness.

INTRODUCTION TO THE 31st SŪTRA

TEXT

न केवलं सृष्टिदशायां निजशक्तिविकासोऽस्य विश्वं, यत् तत्पृष्ठपातिनौ—

TRANSLATION

Not only is the universe an unfoldment of his power in the state of its creation, but also in the states following it.

SŪTRA—31

स्थितिलयौ ॥ ३१ ॥

Sthiti-layau

स्थिति—maintenance (of manifestation); लयः reversion to a potential state.

"Maintenance of the manifested state and its reabsorption are also an unfoldment of his power."

COMMENTARY

TEXT

'स्वशक्तिप्रचयः' इत्यनुवर्तते । क्रियाशक्त्या भासितस्य विश्वस्य तत्तत्प्रमात्रपेक्षं कंचित्कालं बहिर्मुखत्वावभासनरूपा या स्थितिः, चिन्मयप्रमातृविश्रान्त्यात्मा च यो लयः, तावेतौ एतस्य स्वशक्तिप्रचय एव; तत्तद्वेद्यं हि आभासमानं विलीयमानं च निजसंविच्छक्त्यात्मकमेव, अन्यथा अस्य संवेदनानुपपत्तेः । अत एव श्रीकालिकाक्रमे

'अस्तिनास्तिविभागेन··········।'

इत्यादि स्थितिलयपरत्वेनोक्तम् । तथा

'सर्वं शुद्धं निरालम्बं ज्ञानं स्वप्रत्ययात्मकम् ।
यः पश्यति स मुक्तात्मा जीवन्नेव न संशयः ॥'

इति ॥ ३१ ॥

TRANSLATION

"Unfoldment of his power" should follow the *sūtra*. *Sthiti* or maintenance (of the manifested world) means external appearance for some time, with reference to the various experients, of the universe which has come into appearance in consequence of *kriyā-śakti* (creative power). *Laya* means resting in the experient who is sheer consciousness. These two (*sthiti* and *laya*) are only an unfoldment of his (*yogī's*) *śakti* or creative power. The various knowable objects which appear and finally revert to their potential state are only a form of his (*yogī's*) consciousness-power, otherwise (i.e. without assuming consciousness-power), the apprehension of the world would be impossible. Therefore in *Kalikākrama* 'through the division of existence and nonexistence' has been spoken of only with reference to *sthiti* and *laya*. So,

"He who experiences that consciousness which is entirely pure, not depending on any support (i.e. object) and is of the same form as one's deeper I-consciousness is liberated while alive; there is no doubt about it."

INTRODUCTION TO THE 32nd SŪTRA

TEXT

नन्वेवं सृष्टिस्थितिलयावस्थासु अन्योन्यभेदावभासमयीषु अस्य स्वरूपान्यथात्वमायातम्! इत्याशङ्काशान्त्यर्थमाह—

TRANSLATION

A doubt arises here, viz., the awareness of the *Yogī* which is oriented towards objects would suffer a break in the states of manifestation, maintenance of manifestation and dissolution which differ from one another in the matter of appearance. In order to remove this doubt, the next *sūtra* says:

SŪTRA—32

तत्प्रवृत्तावप्यनिरासः संवेत्तृभावात् ॥ ३२ ॥

Tat pravṛttau api anirāsaḥ Saṁvetṛ-bhāvāt.

तत्प्रवृत्तावपि—in spite of the occurrence of manifestation etc. अनिरास—no break or shift. संवेतृभावात्—because of the state of the knower.

"In spite of the maintenance and dissolution of the world occurring one after another, there cannot be break in the awareness of the *Yogī*, because of his being the knower or Subject."

COMMENTARY

TEXT

तेषां सृष्टयादीनां प्रवृत्तावपि उन्मज्जनेऽपि, नास्य योगिनः संवेत्तृभावात् तुर्यचमत्कारात्मकविमर्शमयात् उपलब्धृत्वात्, निरासश्चलनम्; तन्निरासे कस्यचिदप्यप्रकाशनात् । यदुक्तं तत्रैव

'नाशेऽविद्याप्रपञ्चस्य स्वभावो न विनश्यति ।
उत्पत्तिध्वंसविरहात्तस्मान्नाशो न वास्तवः ॥
यतोऽविद्या समुत्पत्तिध्वंसाभ्यामुपचर्यते ।
यत्स्वभावेन नष्टं न तन्नष्टं कथमुच्यते ॥'

इति । एतदेव स्पन्दे

'अवस्थायुगलं चात्र कार्यकर्तृत्वशब्दितम् ।
कार्यता क्षयिणी तत्र कर्तृत्वं पुनरक्षयम् ॥'

तथा ।

'कार्योन्मुखः प्रयत्नो यः केवलं सोऽत्र लुप्यते ।
तस्मिंल्लुप्ते विलुप्तोऽस्मीत्यबुधः प्रतिपद्यते ॥
न तु योऽन्तर्मुखो भावः सर्वज्ञत्वगुणास्पदम् ।
तस्य लोपः कदाचित्स्यादन्यस्यानुपलम्भनात् ॥'

इत्यनेनोक्तम् ॥ ३२ ॥

TRANSLATION

In spite of the occurrence i.e. emergence of manifestation, etc. there cannot be a break of or shift in the awareness of the *Yogī* because of his being a knower full of the delightful awareness of the fourth state of consciousness, for if there be a break in knowership, nothing whatsoever can appear.[1]

As has been said there itself i.e. in *Kālikākrama*.

"With the disappearance of phenomena brought about by *avidyā* (nescience), the nature of consciousness does not disappear. As consciousness or awareness is free of appearance or disappearance, there cannot be a real disappearance of knowership.

Since it is *avidyā* itself which is spoken of as appearing or disappearing figuratively, how can that (i.e. *saṁvit* or consciousness or knowership) be said to disappear which by nature never disappears."[2]

The same point has been made out in the following verses of *Spandakārikā*:

"In the highest reality known as Ātmā (the transcendental Self), there are two aspects called *kartā*[3] (subject) and *kārya*[4] (object). Of these two, the object is perishable, the subject is imperishable. Only the effort directed towards an object ceases. On its cessation, only an ignorant chap thinks "I am ruined".[5]

Because of the disappearance of another (the object) there can never be the disappearance of the inner nature (subject) which is the substratum of omniscience." (I, 14-16).

NOTES

1. With the change in manifestation, there is no change in Consciousness, or the Experient, for even change cannot be experienced without an unchanging principle.

2. There can be appearance or disappearance of *avidyā*—the primal ignorance only, not of foundational Consciousness which is indispensable for an awareness of both appearance and disappearance. With the appearance or disappearance of objects, there cannot be any change in the nature of Reality which is ever present and changeless.

3. *Kartā* means the Subject, experient, knower, doer, independent conscious I.

4. *Kārya* means the object, experienced, knowable, inconscient, dependent on something else.

5. There can be only cessation of the effort directed towards an object, there can never be a cessation of the subject whose effort it is. Even cessation of effort only means resting of the effort in the subject.

EXPOSITION

In spite of changes in the form of appearance and disappearance of manifestated objects, there is no change in the nature of Reality which is Experience, Awareness, Eternal Subject. As the *Yogi's* consciousness is that central Awareness, he abides as the Eternal changeless subject.

INTRODUCTION TO THE 33rd SŪTRA

TEXT

अस्य योगिन :—

Of this *yogī.*

SŪTRA—33

सुखदुःखयोर्बहिर्मननम् ॥ ३३ ॥

Sukha-duḥkhayor bahirmananam.

सुखदुःखयोः—of pleasure and pain; बहिर्मननं considering as external.

'This yogī considers pleasure and pain as something external'.

COMMENTARY

TEXT

वेद्यस्पर्शजातयोः सुखदुःखयोर्बहिरिव नीलादिवत् इदन्ताभासतया मननं संवेदनं, न तु लौकिकवत् अहन्तास्पर्शनेन; अस्य हि 'स्वशक्तिप्रचयोऽस्य विश्वम्' (३–३०) इत्युक्तसूत्रार्थनीत्या सर्वम् अहन्ताच्छादितत्वेन स्फुरति, न तु नियतं

सुखदुःखाद्येव, इत्येवंपरमेतत् । योगी हि प्रशान्तपुर्यष्टकप्रमातृभावः कथं सुख-दुःखाभ्यां स्पृश्यते । तथा च श्रीप्रत्यभिज्ञासूत्रविमर्शिन्याम् ।

'ग्राहकभूमिकोत्तीर्णानां वास्तवप्रमातृदशाप्रपन्नानां तत्तत्स्वहेतूपस्थापित-सुखदुःखसाक्षात्कारेऽपि न तेषां सुखदुःखादि, नोत्पद्यत एव वा सुखादि हेतुवैकल्यात्, सहजानन्दाविर्भावस्तु तदा स्यात् ॥'

इत्युक्तम् । अत एव

'न दुःखं न सुखं यत्र न ग्राह्यं ग्राहको न च ।
न चास्ति मूढभावोऽपि तदस्ति परमार्थतः ॥'

इति स्पन्दे निरूपितम् ॥ ३३ ॥

TRANSLATION

This *yogī* considers pleasure and pain born of contact with objects as a mere this—as something external to himself like blue etc. not like the common folk as something pertaining to the I.

When the *sūtra* 30 under the 3rd section says that the universe is an unfoldment of his *śakti* (creative power), it means that the *whole* universe appears as pervaded by his I-consciousness. It does not mean that particular experiences like pleasure and pain are identified with his I-consciousness. This is what this sūtra means to suggest. How can the *yogī*, whose identification with the subtle body as the subject has already been annulled, be affected with pleasure and pain ?[1] The same has been said in the following commentary of *Pratyabhijñā-sūtra-vimarśinī*.

"Those who have transcended the state of the limited subject[2] and entered the stage of a real subject[3] do not experience pleasure and pain even when they are presented by their respective causes. Rather pleasure and pain are not produced in their cases, for the causes of pleasure and pain are absent so far as they are concerned.[4] They have only the experience of the natural bliss of divine consciousness."

This truth has been clearly expounded in the following verse of Spandakārikā:

"When there is neither pleasure nor pain[5], nor object,[6] nor (limited) subject,[7] nor state of stupefaction or insentiency[8]—that is the state of Absolute Reality." (I, 5).

NOTES

1. Pleasure and pain are experiences of *antaḥkaraṇa*, the inner psychic apparatus. One who is identified with the psychic apparatus is bound to feel pleasure and pain. But the *yogī* who is completely detached not only from *antaḥkaraṇa* but also from the entire subtle mechanism of *puryaṣṭaka* (the five *tanmātrās*, *manas*, *buddhi* and *ahaṁkāra*) has risen to a state of consciousness where he cannot be affected by pleasure and pain. He has transcended the stage of the psychological individual.

2. Limited subject or *grāhaka* refers to *Māyā-pramātā*, the subject that is under the sway of *Māyā*.

3. The real subject is *Śiva-pramātā*—one who has acquired Śiva-Consciousness.

4. Pleasure is caused by *rāga* or attraction, personal interest in something; pain is caused by *dveṣa* or repulsion from something. The *yogī* has risen above *rāga* and *dveṣa*. So the causes of pleasure and pain are absent in his case.

5. Pleasure and pain are internal objects of experience.

6. Nor object refers to external object of experience like a colour, sound, jar etc.

7. *Grāhaka* or limited subject refers to *Māyā-pramātā*, not to the metempirical subject.

8. If there is no pleasure or pain etc. in that Reality, it does not mean that it is devoid of sentiency. It is the Absolute consciousness in itself.

EXPOSITION

The consciousness of the psychological individual is relational i.e. there is always relation of a subject to an object, a *grāhaka grāhya-bhūmi*—a subject-object duality. The transcendental consciousness is non-relational free from the duality of subject and object. The *Yogī* who has acquired transcendental consciousness is not affected by the psychological states of relational consciousness.

INTRODUCTION TO THE 34th SŪTRA

TEXT

यतश्च उत्तीर्णपुर्यष्टकप्रमातृभावस्य योगिनो नान्तः सुखदुःखसंस्पर्शः, अत एवासौ—

TRANSLATION

Since the *yogī* has transcended that stage in which the subject is identified with the subtle body and is unaffected by inner pleasure and pains, therefore he—

SŪTRA—34

तद्विमुक्तस्तु केवली ॥ ३४ ॥

Tadvimuktastu kevalī

तद्विमुक्तः :—Free from the influence of pleasure and pain; तु then, rather; केवली—established in his real Self.

"Being completely free from the influence of pleasure and pain, he is rather Alone—fully established in his real Self as sheer consciousness".

COMMENTARY

TEXT

ताभ्यां सुखदुःखाभ्यां विशेषेण मुक्तः संस्कारमात्रेणापि अन्तर् असंस्पृष्टः, केवली, केवलं चिन्मात्रप्रमातृतारूपं यस्य । तदुक्तं श्रीकालिकाक्रमे

'सुखदुःखादिविज्ञानविकल्पानल्पकल्पितम् ।
भित्त्वा द्वैतमहामोहं योगी योगफलं लभेत् ॥'

इति । तु-शब्दो वक्ष्यमाणापेक्षया विशेषद्योतकः, एवमुत्तरसूत्रगतोऽपि एतत्सूत्रापेक्षया ॥ ३४ ॥

TRANSLATION

Tat of the *sūtra* means (*tābhyām*) i.e. from pleasure and pain. *Vi-muktaḥ* means specially freed i.e. inwardly untouched even by the residual traces (of pleasure and pain). *Kevalī* means one whose knowership consists in sheer consciousness. The same has been said in Kālikākrama:

"The *Yogī* should obtain the fruit of *yoga* by shattering the barrier of the delusion of duality fabricated by the plethora of pleasure, pain etc., and the thought-constructs of various sorts of knowables."

The word *tu* (then, rather, but) in the *sūtra* has been used to show distinction with reference to the *sūtra* that is to follow; so also the word *tu* occurring in the following *sūtra* is used to show distinction with reference to the present one.

INTRODUCTION TO THE 35th SŪTRA

TEXT

यदाह—

TRANSLATION

So the next *sūtra* says:

SŪTRA—35

मोहप्रतिसंहतस्तु कर्मात्मा ॥ ३५ ॥

Mohapratisaṁhatas tu Karmātmā.

मोह—delusion; प्रतिसंहतः :—closely compacted
तु—but; कर्मात्मा—involved in good and evil deeds.

"But one who has become a compact mass of delusion is involved in good and evil deeds."

COMMENTARY

TEXT

मोहेन अज्ञानेन, प्रतिसंहतः तदेकघनः, तत एव सुखदुःखाश्रयो यः, स पुनः कर्मात्मा नित्यं शुभाशुभकलङ्कितः । तदुक्तं तत्रैव

'यदविद्यावृततया विकल्पविधियोगतः ।
शिवादीन्नैव झटिति समुद्भावयतेऽखिलान् ॥
ततः शुभाशुभा भावा लक्ष्यन्ते तद्वशत्वतः ।
अशुभेभ्यश्च भावेभ्यः परं दुःखं प्रजायते ॥'

इति ॥ ३५ ॥

TRANSLATION

Moha is to be interpreted, in the instrumental sense—*mohena* i.e. with delusion; *pratisaṁhataḥ* means has become a compact mass with it and thus becomes an abode of pleasure and pain, So he is one who is involved in *karma* (action) i.e. is always stained with good and evil deeds. The same has been said in the same treatise i.e. in *Kālikākrama*.

"When enveloped in *avidyā* (primal ignorance) and owing to the use of various thought-constructs, one does not immediately comprehend all the *tattvas* (principles) beginning with *Śiva* as his own Self, then good and evil states of mind appear and under the influence of *avidyā* intense misery accrues to him owing to evil deeds."

INTRODUCTION TO THE 36th SŪTRA

TEXT

एवमीदृशस्यापि कर्मात्मनो यदा अनर्गलमाहेशशक्तिपातवशोन्मिषितसहज-स्वातन्त्र्ययोगो भवति, तदा अस्य—

TRANSLATION

Even of such a one who is involved in *Karma*, when there is union with natural *svātantrya śakti* that blossoms forth owing to the unrestrained grace of *Maheśa* (Lord Śiva), there is

SŪTRA—36

भेदतिरस्कारे सर्गान्तरकर्मत्वम् ॥ ३६ ॥

Bheda-tiraskāre sargāntara-karmatvam.

भेद—difference; तिरस्कार removal, disappearance सर्ग—kingdom of Nature, variety of life; अन्तर another, कर्मत्वम्—performance, creation.

"On the disappearance of difference, there accrues (to the *yogī*) the capacity to create a different kingdom of Nature and variety of life."

COMMENTARY

TEXT

शरीरप्राणाद्यहन्ताभिमानात्मनः सकलप्रलयाकलादिप्रमात्रुचितस्य भेदस्य, तिरस्कारे स्थितस्यापि चिद्घनस्वभावोन्मज्जनाद् अपहस्तने सति, क्रमेण मन्त्र-मन्त्रेश्वर–मन्त्रमहेश्वरात्मकस्वमाहात्म्यावाप्तौ, सर्गान्तरकर्मत्वं यथाभिलषितनिर्मेयनिर्मातृत्वं भवति । तथा च श्रीस्वच्छन्दे

'त्रिगुणेन तु जप्तेन स्वच्छन्दसदृशो भवेत् ।'

इति स्वच्छन्दसादृश्येन भेदतिरस्कारमस्य उक्त्वा

'ब्रह्मविष्ण्विन्द्रदेवानां सिद्धदैत्योरगेशिनाम् ॥
भयदाता च हर्ता च शापानुग्रहकृद्भवेत् ।
दर्पं हरति कालस्य पातयेद्भूधरानपि ॥'

इत्युक्तम् ॥ ३६ ॥

TRANSLATION

Bheda connotes different fixed realms of experience appropriate to *sakala*, *pralayākala* etc. whose selves are identified with the body, *prāṇa* etc.[1] *Tiraskāre* means (difference) on being repelled with the emergence of compact consciousness and so on the acquisition gradually of the pre-eminence of *Mantra*; *Mantreśvara* and *Mantramaheśvara*[2], there accrues to him the capacity to create another world according to his desire.

So *Svacchanda-tantra* having declared in the following line his similarity to free-willed Bhairava inasmuch as he has dispelled all difference,

"With threefold *japa*,[3] the *yogī* would become similar to *svacchanda* (Free-Willed Bhairava)", has described further his wonderful power in the following lines:

"Of the gods Brahmā, *Viṣṇu*, and *Indra*, of *siddhas*, *daityas*, and kings of serpents, he becomes the creator of fear by his curse, and the dispeller of fear by his grace. He crushes the pride of death, and knocks down even mountains." (VI, 54-55).

NOTES

1. The experients referred to and their fields of experience are given below.

Experients	*Tattva*	*Field of Experience*
1. Vijñānākala	Mahāmāyā tattva	Experience of pure consciousness and all the pralayākalas and sakalas.
2. Pralayākala or Pralayakevalī or Śūnya-pramātā.	Māyā tattva	Mere Void.
3. Sakala (from the Devas upto the plants and minerals).	The remaining tattva upto the earth.	Full of three malas, bound by cause-effect relation and experiencing everything as different.

2. (i) Mantra is the experient who has realized *Śuddha Vidyā tattva.*

(ii) *Mantreśvara* is the experient who has realized *Īśvara tattva.*

(iii) *Mantra-Maheśvara* is the experient who has realized *Sadā-Śiva tattva.*

3. Three-fold *japa* is a technical term. It does not mean three times, but *japa* in a three-fold way as given below:

(1) *Śāmbhava japa*—In this, the aspirant has to concentrate on the junction-point of *prakāśa* and *vimarśa.* The three factors involved in this are—*prakāśa*, *vimarśa*, and their junction point.

(2) *Śākta japa*—In this, the aspirant has to concentrate on the junction point of *pramāṇa* and *prameya.* The three factors here are (i) *pramāṇa* (2) *prameya* and (3) the junction point from which *pramāṇa* and *prameya* arise.

(3) *Āṇava japa*—In this, the aspirant has to concentrate on the junction-point of *prāṇa* and *apāna.* The three factors here are (i) *prāṇa* (ii) *apāna* and (iii) their meeting point.

INTRODUCTION TO THE 37th SŪTRA

TEXT

न च एतदस्य असंभाव्यम्, यतः—

TRANSLATION

Such creation should not be considered to be impossible for him, because,

SŪTRA—37

करणशक्तिः स्वतोऽनुभवात् ॥ ३७ ॥

Karaṇaśaktiḥ svato'nubhavāt.

करणशक्तिः—the power to create. स्वतः—of one's own; अनुभवात् —from experience.

"One can realize the capacity of creativity from one's own experience."

COMMENTARY

TEXT

स्वतः स्वस्मादेवानुभवात् संकल्पस्वप्नादौ, करणशक्तिः तत्तदसाधारणार्थनिर्मातृत्वम् आत्मनः सिद्धमेव । अनेनैव आशयेन श्रीप्रत्यभिज्ञायाम्

'अत एव यथाभीष्टसमुल्लेखावभासनात् ।
ज्ञानक्रिये स्फुटे एव सिद्धे सर्वस्य जीवतः ॥'

इत्युक्तम् । तथासंभवात् यदि चैतत् गाढाभिनिवेशेन विमृशति, तदा सर्वसाधारणा अभीष्टार्थनिर्मातृतापि भवति । तदुक्तं तत्त्वगर्भे

'यदा तु तेऽपि सुव्यक्तस्वसामर्थ्यगुणोज्ज्वलाः ।
भवेद्दृढतराद्दूरदारिता दार्ढ्यदीनता ।
तदा च तेषां संकल्पः कल्पपादपतां व्रजेत् ॥'

इति ॥ ३७ ॥

TRANSLATION

From one's own experience in the matter of imagination and dreams one's capacity to create extraordinary things is well established. With this purport, it has been said in Pratyabhijñā:

"Therefore, from the power of conception (*avabhāsanāt*)[1] and execution (*samullekha*[2]) according to one's desire, i.e. the power of knowing and doing (*jñānakriyā*) of all living beings is clearly established." (I, VI, 11).

Such being the possibility, if he (the *Yogī*) is oriented towards creation with strong will, he can, according to his wish also create something common to all people.

This has been said in Tattvagarbha:

"When the *Yogīs* shine forth with manifest power of creativity, their want of firmness for creativity is firmly and immediately shattered, and then their Will power becomes a *Kalpataru*".[3]

NOTES

1. *Avabhāsana* denotes *jñānaśakti.*
2. *Samullekha* denotes *kriyāśakti.*
3. *Kalpataru* is a tree of *svarga* or *Indra's* paradise fabled to fulfil all desires; the wish-fulfilling tree.

INTRODUCTION TO THE 38th SŪTRA

TEXT

यतश्च करणशक्तिशब्दोक्त्या तुर्यात्मा स्वातन्त्र्यशक्तिरेव बोधरूपस्य प्रमातुः सारम्, अतो मायाशक्त्यपहस्तिततत्स्वरूपोत्तेजनाय—

TRANSLATION

Since the use of the word *Karaṇa-śakti*—the power of creating points to the fact that *svātantrya-śakti* (absolutic Will power) in the form of *turya* (the fourth state of consciousness) is the quintessence of the experient who is awareness personified, therefore in order to whet the nature of that *turya* which is suppressed by *māyāśakti*, the next *sūtra* says:

SŪTRA—38

त्रिपदाद्यनुप्राणनम् ॥ ३८ ॥

Tripad ādy anuprāṇanam.

त्रिपद—of the three states; आदि principal, pre-eminent, अनुप्राणनम् —enlivening,

"Of the three states, there should be enlivening by the main one (which is *svātantrya śakti* full of creative bliss)".

COMMENTARY

TEXT

त्रयाणां भावौन्मुख्यतदभिष्वङ्गतदन्तर्मुखीभावनामयानां सृष्टिस्थितिलय-शब्दोक्तानां पदानामवस्थानां, यद् आदि प्रधानं त्रिचमत्कृतित्वेन आनन्दघनं तुर्याख्यं पदं मायाशक्त्याच्छादितमपि तत्तद्विषयोपभोगाद्यवसरेषु विद्युद्वदाभासमानं तेन तत्तदवसरेषु क्षणमात्रोदितेनापि, अनुप्राणनम् अन्तर्मुखतद्विमर्शावस्थिति-तारतम्येन अनुगततया प्राणनम्, आत्मनस्तेनैव जीवितेनापि जीवितस्य उत्तेजनं कुर्यात् । तदुक्तं श्री विज्ञानभैरवे

'अन्तः स्वानुभवानन्दा विकल्पोन्मुक्तगोचरा ।
यावस्था भरिताकारा भैरवी भैरवात्मनः ।।
तद्वपुस्तत्त्वतो ज्ञेयं विमलं विश्वपूरणम् ।'

इत्याद्युपक्रम्य

'शक्तिसंगमसंक्षुब्धशक्त्यावेशावसानिकम् ।
यत्सुखं ब्रह्मतत्त्वस्य तत्सुखं स्वाक्यमुच्यते ।।
लेहनामन्थनाकोटैः स्त्रीसुखस्य भरात्स्मृतेः ।
शक्त्यभावेऽपि देवेशि भवेदानन्दसंप्लवः ।।
आनन्दे महति प्राप्ते दृष्टे वा बान्धवे चिरात् ।
आनन्दमुद्गतं ध्यात्वा तन्मयस्तल्लयीभवेत् ।।
जग्धिपानकृतोल्लासरसानन्दविजृम्भणात् ।
भावयेद्भरितावस्थां महानन्दस्ततो भवेत् ।।
गीतादिविषयास्वादासमसौख्यैकतात्मनः ।
योगिनस्तन्मयत्वेन मनोरूढेस्तदात्मता ।।'

इत्यादिना उपायप्रदर्शनेन प्रपञ्चितम् । एतच्च

'अतिक्रुद्धः प्रहृष्टो वा किं करोमीति वा मृशन् ।
धावन्वा यत्पदं गच्छेत्तत्र स्पन्दः प्रतिष्ठितः ।।' २२ [कारिका]

इत्यादिना

'.........प्रबुद्धः स्यादनावृतः ।।'

इत्यन्तेन प्रदर्शितम् । एतत् स्पन्दनिर्णये निराकांक्षं मयैव निर्णीतम् । 'त्रिषु चतुर्थम्.....' (३–२०) इति सूत्रेण जागरादौ तुर्यानुप्राणनमुक्तम् । अनेन

सर्वदशानुगतादिमध्यान्तेषु सृष्टिस्थितिसंहारनिरूपितया भङ्ग्या निरूपितेषु इति विशेषः ॥ ३८ ॥

TRANSLATION

Of the three states of manifestation (*sṛṣṭi*) maintenance of manifestation (*sthiti*) and reabsorption (*laya*) characterized by orientation towards objects, (*bhāvaunmukhya*) interest in the objects (*tadabhiṣvaṅga*) and inner assimilation of the objects (*antarmukhībhāvanāmaya*) that which is *ādi* i.e. the main one viz; *turya* (the transcendental state) is by infusion of its delight in all the three (viz., waking, dream, deep sleep) compact bliss. This transcendental bliss though veiled by *Māyā-śakti* appears (for an instant) like a flash of lightning on the occasion of the enjoyment of various objects of pleasure. Therefore though that bliss appears only for an instant on the various occasions, one should enliven oneself with it. *Anuprāṇanam* or enlivening oneself means vitalizing oneself by following more and more the awareness of that bliss which exists within. That is to say one should animate oneself with that vitality. The same has been said in *Vijñānabhairava*.

"She (*parāśakti*) is bliss that can be experienced within oneself, she can be known only when one is freed of all thought-constructs. She is a state of one's own Self that is Bhairava, hence she is known as Bhairavī, the Śakti of Bhairava. She is one whose essential nature is full of the delight of the unity of the entire universe. She is to be known essentially as the pure form filling (pervading) the entire universe." (Verse 15) and then elaborating with the following verses as a means of approach to her, it is said "At the time of sexual intercourse with a woman, an absorption into her is brought about by excitement, and the final delight that ensues at orgasm betokens the delight of Brahman. This delight is that of one's own Self. (It has not come from anything external. The woman is only an occasion for the manifestation of that delight). O goddess, even in the absence of a woman, there is a flood of delight, simply on account of memory[1] in full measure of sexual pleasure in the form of kissing, embracing, pressing etc. On the occasion of a great delight being obtained, or on the occasion of delight arising from seeing a friend or relative after a long time, one should meditate on the delight that has arisen and become absorbed in it, and identified with it.

When one experiences the expansion of the joy, delight and rapture of savour arising from the pleasure of eating and drinking, one should meditate on the perfect condition of this joy, and then one would become full of great bliss.

When a Yogī mentally becomes one with the incomparable joy of song and other objects, then of such a yogi, there is because of the exaltation of his mind identity with that (i.e. with the incomparable joy), because he becomes one with it."[2] (Verses 69-73).

The same point has been made out in Spandakārikā, beginning with,

"The *Spanda*[3] principle is established in that state in which is placed a man who is extremely exasperated or exceedingly delighted or is utterly bewildered, considering 'What am I to do' or runs to and fro (for the safety of his life)"[4] (I, 22) and ending with "One who is awake is unenveloped (in *avidyā*)" (I, 25) This has been conclusively discussed by me in *Spandanirṇaya* beyond the possibility of a doubt.

In the *sūtra Triṣu caturtham* (III, 20), it has been said that the three viz., waking, dream and deep sleep states should be vitalized with the fourth state; in the present *sūtra*, it has been said that in all conditions in the initial, intervening and the final states, in manifestation, maintenance of manifestation, and dissolution, there should be a vitalization of awareness with the elixir of the fourth state in the manner described above. This is the special point about this *sūtra*.

NOTES

1. Since the sexual pleasure is obtained only by memory even in the absence of a woman, it is evident that the delight is inherent within. It is this delight apart from any woman that one should meditate on in order to realize the bliss of the transcendental consciousness.

2. One can turn even a sensuous joy into a means of *Yoga*. In the above verses, examples of all sorts of sensuous joy have

been given. Joy of sexual intercourse is an example of *sparśa* (contact); joy at the sight of a friend is an example of pleasure of *rūpa* (visual perception); joy of delicious food is an example of *rasa* (taste); joy derived from a song is an example of the pleasure of *śabda* (sound).

3. *Spanda*=Cosmic pulsation—throb of the divine consciousness.

4. Whenever there is intensity of awareness, one should look for the divine principle of activity.

INTRODUCTION TO THE 39th SŪTRA

TEXT

एतच्च त्रिपदाद्यनुप्राणनमन्तर्मुखत्वावष्टम्भत्वदशायामेवासाद्य न संतुष्येत्, अपि तु—

TRANSLATION

The *yogī* should not rest content with the vitalization of the three normal states with the bliss of *turya* only in the condition of an inward grip of the *turya*, but also:

SŪTRA—39

चित्तस्थितिवच्छरीरकरणबाह्येषु ॥ ३९ ॥

Cittasthitivat śarīra-karaṇa-bāhyeṣu.

चित्तस्थिति=the state of mind, वत्=like शरीर=body, करण=organs of sense, बाह्य=external.

As in the case of the states of the mind, so also in the case of the body, organs of sense, and external things, there should be vitalization with the bliss of the transcendental consciousness.

COMMENTARY

TEXT

'त्रिपदाद्यनुप्राणनम्' इत्येव । यथा अन्तर्मुखरूपायां चित्तस्थितौ तुर्येणानुप्राणनं कुर्यात्, तथा शरीरकरणबाह्याभासात्मिकायां बहिर्मुखतायामपि आन्तर-

विमर्शावष्टम्भबलात् क्रमात्क्रमं तारतम्यभाजा तेन अनुप्राणनं कुर्यात् । यदुक्त श्रीविज्ञानभैरवे

'सर्वं जगत्स्वदेहं वा स्वानन्दभरितं स्मरेत् ।
युगपत्स्वामृतेनैव परानन्दमयो भवेत् ॥'

इति । एवं हि आनन्दात्मा स्वातन्त्र्यशक्तिः सर्वदशासु स्फुटीभूता सती यथेष्ट-निर्माणकारिणी भवति ॥ ३९ ॥

TRANSLATION

The previous *sūtra* (*tripadādyanuprāṇanam*) should be supplied to complete the sense.

As the *Yogī* should vitalize the inward states of mind with the bliss of the fourth (i.e. the transcendental consciousness), even so in the extroverted condition also, he should gradually, by degrees, vitalize, by means of the power acquired from the grip of internal awareness, the body, organs of sense, and the external objects, with the bliss of the transcendental consciousness.

The same has been said in *Vijñānabhairava:*

"One should consider the whole world or one's own body, as filled with the bliss of the Self. All at once with the nectar of one's own consciousness, he would be filled with the highest bliss." (Verse 65).

Thus the Absolute Power (*svātantrya śakti*) which is total bliss, when manifest in all states and conditions, can create anything as desired.

EXPOSITION

The 38th *sūtra* describes the technique of *Nimīlana Samādhi* or *Nimīlana Krama* i.e. introverted contemplation whereby the *citta*, the mental states are bathed in the bliss of the transcendental consciousness and thus purified. The 39th *sūtra* describes the technique of *Unmīlana samādhi* or *Unmīlana Krama* i.e. the extroverted contemplation whereby the whole world including one's body and the senses is filled with the bliss of the transcendental consciousness.

The *Yogī* not only feels *himself* full of that bliss, but also experiences the external *world* as full of that bliss.

Secondly when the *Yogī* reaches the state of highest *ānanda* (bliss), he experiences *svātantrya śakti*. *Ānanda* is, by nature, creative. And so the *Yogī* acquires the power of creating things according to his desire.

INTRODUCTION TO THE 40th SŪTRA

TEXT

यदा तु अयमेव आन्तरीं तुर्यदशाम् आत्मत्वेन न विमृशति, तदा देहादिप्रमातृताभावाद् अपूर्णमन्यतात्मकाणवमलरूपात्—

TRANSLATION

When, however, the *Yogī* does not feel the internal *turya* state as the state of Self, then owing to his sense of identification with the body etc., he becomes subject to *āṇavamala* which is characterized by the sense of imperfection and incompleteness, and on account of this—

SŪTRA—40

अभिलाषाद्बहिर्गतिः संवाह्यस्य ॥ ४० ॥

Abhilāṣāt bahirgatiḥ saṁvāhyasya.

अभिलाषात्=on account of feeling of want; बहिर्गतिः:—extroversion; संवाह्यस्य=the empirical individual who is carried forward from one form of existence to another.

"On account of a feeling of want and desire, there is extroversion of the empirical individual who is carried forward from one form of existence to another."

COMMENTARY

TEXT

शक्तिचक्राधिष्ठितैः कञ्चुकान्तःकरणबहिष्करणतन्मात्रभूतैः सह, संवाह्यते योनेर्योन्यन्तरं नीयते इति संवाह्यः, कर्मात्मरूपः पशुः तस्य ....अभिलाषो मलोऽत्र तु ।'

इति श्रीस्वच्छन्दोक्तनीत्या अपूर्णमन्यतात्मकाविद्याख्याणवमलरूपाद् अभिलाषाद्धेतोर्बहिर्गतिः, विषयोन्मुखत्वमेव भवति; न तु अन्तर्मुखरूपावहितत्वं जातुचित्। यदुक्तं कालिकाक्रमे

'यदविद्यावृततया विकल्पविधियोगतः ।
शिवादीन्नैव झटिति समुद्भावयतेखिलान् ॥
ततः शुभाशुभा भावा लक्ष्यन्ते तद्वशत्वतः ।
अशुभेभ्यश्च भावेभ्यः परं दुःखं प्रजायते ॥
अतथ्यां कल्पनां कृत्वा पच्यन्ते नरकादिषु ।
स्वोत्थैर्दोषैश्च दह्यन्ते वेणवो वह्निना यथा ॥
मायामयैः सदा भावैरविद्यां परिभुञ्जते ।
मायामयीं तनुं यान्ति ते जनाः क्लेशभाजनम् ॥'

इति ॥ ४० ॥

TRANSLATION

Saṁvāhya means a bound being involved in *Karma* who is, together with the coverings of Māyā, inner psychic apparatus, outer senses, *tanmātrās*, and the gross elements presided over by the group of *śaktis*, carried forward from one form of existence to another. Of such a being, as described by *Svacchandatantra* in the words, 'in such a case, desire is the limiting, tainting condition', there is extroversion on account of *āṇavamala* known as *avidyā* or primal ignorance consisting in the feeling of imperfection. *Bahirgatiḥ* or extroversion means that in him there is always an inclination towards and interest in external objects, and never an attentiveness to the inner nature. As has been said in *Kālikākrama*.

"Since one is involved in *avidyā* (primal ignorance) and so owing to the use of thought-constructs does not immediately comprehend all the *tattvas* beginning with *Śiva* as his own Self, therefore good and evil states of mind appear and under the influence of *avidyā*, intense misery accrues to him owing to evil deeds.

On account of false ideation, they are tormented in hell; they are burnt by their own vices just as bamboos are burnt by their own fire.

Owing to delusive ideas, these people reap the fruit of *avidyā*; they acquire a body which is the product of Māyā and suffer misery according to their deserts."

INTRODUCTION TO THE 41st SŪTRA

TEXT

यदा तु पारमेशशक्तिपातवशोन्मिषितं स्वं स्वभावमेव विमृशति, तदा अभिलाषाभावाद् न अस्य बहिर्गतिः, अपि तु आत्मारामतैव नित्यमित्याह—

TRANSLATION

When, however, he comprehends his own essential nature which has awakened owing to the grace of the highest Lord then owing to absence of desire, his extroversion ceases; rather he always takes delight in resting within his Self. Therefore the next *sūtra* says:

SŪTRA—41

तदारूढप्रमितेस्तत्क्षयाज्जीवसंक्षयः ॥ ४१ ॥

Tadārūḍhapramites tatkṣayāj jīvasaṁkṣayaḥ.

तदारूढप्रमितेः —of the one whose awareness is fully established in that (i.e. *turya* state); तत्क्षयात् =with the ending of that (i.e. desire); जीवसंक्षयः =the ending of the state of the empirical individual.

"Of the *Yogī* whose awareness is firmly established in the fourth state (*turya* or transcendental state), there is the ending of the state of the empirical individual with the ending of desire."

COMMENTARY

TEXT

तदिति पूर्वनिर्दिष्टसंवेत्रात्मनि तुर्यपदे, आरूढा तद्विमर्शनपरा, प्रमितिः संवित् यस्य योगिनस्तस्य । तदिति अभिलाषक्षयात्, जीवस्य संवाह्यात्मनः पुर्यष्टकप्रमातृभावस्य, क्षयः प्रशमः; चित्प्रमातृतयैव स्फुरति इत्यर्थः । यदुक्तं तत्रैव

'यथा स्वप्नानुभूतार्थान्प्रबुद्धो नैव पश्यति ।
तथा भावनया योगी संसारं नैव पश्यति ॥'

इति । तथा

'निरस्य सदसद्वृत्तीः संश्रित्य पदमान्तरम् ।
विहाय कल्पनाजालमद्वैतेन परापरम् ॥

यः स्वात्मनिरतो नित्यं कालग्रासैकतत्परः ।
कैवल्यपदभाग्योगी स निर्वाणपदं लभेत् ॥'
इति । कैवल्यपदभागिति इन्द्रियतन्मात्राभिरसंवाह्यः ॥ ४१ ॥

TRANSLATION

By the word *tat* is meant 'in the fourth state of the Subject or knower· indicated before.' *Ārūḍhapramiteḥ* means the *yogī* whose mind is intent on the awareness of that (fourth state) *Tat-Kṣayāt* means with the ending of desire. *Jīva-saṁkṣayaḥ* means the *kṣaya* or annulment of the identification with the *puryaṣṭaka* (subtle body) as the subject that is carried forward (from one form of existence to another). That is to say, he shines forth in the form of the foundational consciousness as the subject, It is said there itself (i.e. in *Kālikā-Krama*).

"As one who sees certain objects in dream, but does not see them when awake, so the *Yogī* contemplating over *Ātmā* as the sole reality does not see the world (as world)"[1]

Similarly:

"Rejecting mental modes like existents and non-existents,[2] by resorting to the middle position between the two, renouncing the fabrications of imagination such as different and non-different by means of the ascertainment of non-dualism, he—the *yogī* who is always devoted to his essential Self and is intent on destroying Death itself, and is devoted to the state of isolation, can acquire the state of Nirvāṇa".

Kaivalyapadabhāg (devoted to the state of isolation) means One who cannot be carried by his senses and *tanmātrās*."

NOTES

1. After realization, the previous experience of the world appears to the *yogī* as the experience of a dream. Now he sees the world in a different light—as the glory and splendour of Śiva.

2. The concepts of existence and non-existence, different and non-different are the products of the dichotomising activity of the mind, the fabrication of *vikalpa*. Freed of this limitation, the *yogī* sees reality as the background of all mind-made distincts, as lying in the middle of "either-or".

EXPOSITION

The 40th *sūtra* says that if the aspirant is attached to desires, he becomes extroverted and by the force of the residual traces of his desires inhering in his subtle body is carried forward from one form of existence to another. Attachment to objects of pleasure becomes an obstacle in the path of the aspirant who seeks liberation.

The 41st *sūtra* says that the aspirant is not doomed to be shuttle-cocked from one life to another. If he renounces desire and is rooted in the awareness of the transcendental state, he rises above the state of the limited empirical individual and becomes entitled to *Nirvāṇa*. *Nirvāṇa* in this system means *Śiva-śakti-sāmarasya*; the undifferentiated state of consciousness in which subject-object duality ceases for ever.

INTRODUCTION TO THE 42nd SŪTRA

TEXT

नत्वेवं जीवसंक्षये सति अस्य देहपातः प्राप्तः, न च असौ सुप्रबुद्धस्यापि देहिनः सद्य एव दृश्यते, तत्कथमयं तदारूढप्रमितिः ? इत्याशङ्क्याह—

TRANSLATION

A doubt arises here. The ending of the state of the empirical individual connotes the dissolution of the body. But this dissolution of the body is not noticed immediately even in the case of the perfectly awakened (enlightened) *yogī*. Then how can he be said to be rooted in the awareness of the transcendental state ? In order to remove this doubt, the next *sūtra* says:

SŪTRA—42

भूतकञ्चुकी तदा विमुक्तो भूयः पतिसमः परः ॥ ४२ ॥

Bhūta-Kañcukī tadā vimukto bhūyaḥ patisamaḥ paraḥ

भूतकञ्चुकी—one who uses the body of the gross elements as a mere covering; तदा—then; विमुक्तः — liberated; भूयः abundantly —pre-eminently; पतिसमः—like *Śiva*; परः —perfect.

"Then i.e. on the ending of desire, he uses the body of gross elements merely as covering and being liberated is pre-eminently like *Śiva*, the perfect reality.

COMMENTARY

TEXT

तदेति अभिलाषक्षयात्, जीवसंक्षये पुर्यष्टकप्रमातृताभिमानविगलने सति, अयं भूतकञ्चुकी, शरीरारम्भीणि भूतानि कञ्चुकमिव व्यतिरिक्तं प्रावरणमिव, न तु अहन्तापदस्पर्शीनि यस्य, तथाभूतः सन् विमुक्तो निर्वाणभाक्, यतो भूयो बाहुल्येन पतिसमः चिद्घनपारमेश्वरस्वरूपाविष्टः, तत एव परः पूर्णः, 'शरीरवृत्तिर्व्रतम्' (३–२६) इत्युक्तसूत्रार्थनीत्या दलकल्पे देहादौ स्थितोऽपि, न तत्प्रमातृतासंस्कारेणापि स्पृष्टः । तदुक्तं श्रीकुलरत्नमालायां

'यदा गुरुवरः सम्यक् कथयेत्तन्न संशयः ।
मुक्तस्तेनैव कालेन यन्त्रस्तिष्ठति केवलम् ॥
किं पुनश्चैकतानस्तु परे ब्रह्मणि यः सुधीः ।
क्षणमात्रस्थितो योगी स मुक्तो मोचयेत्प्रजाः ॥'

इति । श्रीमृत्युजित्यपि

'निमेषोन्मेषमात्रं तु तत्त्वं यद्युपलभ्यते ।
तदैव किल मुक्तोऽसौ न पुनर्जन्म चाप्नुयात् ॥'

इति । कुलसारेऽपि

'अहो तत्त्वस्य माहात्म्यं ज्ञातमात्रस्य सुन्दरि ।
श्रोत्रान्तरं तु संप्राप्ते तत्क्षणादेव मुच्यते ॥'

इति ॥ २ ॥

TRANSLATION

'Tadā' i.e. by the ending of desire, *Jīva-saṁkṣaya* means 'on the dissolution of the identification of the subject with the subtle body. Thus *bhūtakañcukī* means 'one whose gross elements that go to the formation of the body are like *kañcuka* i.e. like separate covering and do not even touch the state of 'I'. Such a one is liberated, is the enjoyer of *Nirvāṇa*.

Since he is pre-eminently (*bhūyaḥ*) like *Śiva* (*patisamaḥ*) i.e. possessed of the compact consciousness of the highest Lord, therefore is he perfect (*pūrṇaḥ*). In accordance with the *sūtra Śarīra-vṛttirvratam.* (III, 26), though hes till exists in the body which is to him like a mere sheath,[1] he is not touched even by a trace of the feeling of the body being the subject. It has been said in Kularatnamālā, "When the excellent *guru* (spiritual director) reveals to the disciple that mystery (of God-Consciousness) in its wholeness, then he (the disciple) is undoubtedly liberated at that very moment and afterwards remains in the body only like a machine.[2] How much more then the *yogī* of supreme understanding ! If he is established in the highest Brahman with one-pointedness even for a moment, he is liberated himself and liberates other people."

In *Mṛtyujit* also it has been said,

"If one realizes Reality even for the moment of a blink, he is verily liberated immediately and does not acquire another birth." (VIII, 8).

In *Kulasāra* also, the same idea has been expressed in the following verse:

"What a glorious eminence of this truth O fair one, if one has even intellectually assimilated it and imparts it to another (lit: to another ear), even that one is liberated instantly."

NOTES

1. Just as the sword is entirely separate from the sheath which is only a cover for it, even so the liberated one is entirely separate from the body. The body is only a physical covering for the spirit to carry on its function on the physical plane. The consciousness of the liberated one is not at all identified with the sensation of the body.

2. He is no more interested in the body. He lives only mechanically in it.

INTRODUCTION TO THE 43rd SŪTRA

TEXT

ननु भूतकञ्चुकित्वमपि अस्य कस्मात् तदेव न निवर्तते ! इत्याह—

TRANSLATION

A doubt arises here. Why does not even his covering of the gross body fall away when he (the *yogī*) is liberated ? In answer to this question, the next *sūtra* says:

SŪTRA—43

नैसर्गिकः प्राणसंबन्धः ॥ ४३ ॥

Naisargikaḥ prāṇasambandhaḥ.

नैसर्गिकः=natural; प्राणसम्बन्धः =the link or association of *prāṇa*—the universal life force, the universal vital principle.

"The link of the universal Life force (with the body) is natural".

COMMENTARY

TEXT

निसर्गात् स्वातन्त्र्यात्मनः स्वभावात् आयातो नैसर्गिकः, प्राणसंबन्धः, संवित् किल भगवती विश्ववैचित्र्यम् अवबिभासयिषुः संकोचावभासपूर्वकं संकुचदशेषविश्वस्फुरत्तात्मकप्राणनारूपग्राहकभूमिकां श्रित्वा ग्राह्यरूपजगदाभासात्मना स्फुरतीति नैसर्गिकः, स्वातन्त्र्यात् प्रथममुद्भासितोऽस्याः प्राणसंबन्धः। तथा च श्रीवाजसनेयायाम्

'या सा शक्तिः परा सूक्ष्मा व्यापिनी निर्मला शिवा।
शक्तिचक्रस्य जननी परानन्दामृतात्मिका॥
महाघोरेश्वरी चण्डा सृष्टिसंहारकारिका।
त्रिवहं त्रिविधं त्रिस्थं बलात्कालं प्रकर्षति॥'

इति संविद एव भगवत्याः प्राणक्रमेण नाडित्रयवाहिसोमसूर्यवह्न्यात्मावस्थिततातीतानागतवर्तमानरूपबाह्यकालोल्लासनविलापनकारित्वमुक्तम्। तदुक्तं स्वच्छन्देऽपि

'प्राणः प्राणमयः प्राणो विसर्गापूरणं प्रति।
नित्यमापूरयत्येष प्राणिनामुरसि स्थितः॥'

इति। प्राणस्य

'हकारस्तु स्मृतः प्राणः स्वप्रवृत्तो हलाकृतिः।'

इत्युक्तनीत्या श्रीस्वच्छन्दभट्टारकरूपप्राणमयत्वात् विसर्गापूरतया सृष्टिसंहारकारित्वमभिहितम् इति युक्तमुक्तम् 'नैसर्गिकः प्राणसंबन्धः' इति । अत एव श्रीभट्टकल्लटेन प्राणाख्यनिमित्तदार्ढ्यम्

'प्राक् संवित् प्राणे परिणता ।'

इति तत्त्वार्थचिन्तामणावुक्तम् ॥ ४३ ॥

TRANSLATION

Naisargika means that which has come from *nisarga* i.e. from nature, in other words from the power of Absolute Free Will of the Lord (*Svātantrya Śakti*). (The link of *prāṇa* with the body is, therefore, unavoidable). The divine consciousness, with a desire to display the variegated panorama of the universe, at first adopts the principle of contraction, assumes the state of limited experients (*jīvas*) who are a form of *prāṇanā*—the universal life force which brings about the manifestation of the entire universe in a limited form and also appears in the form of the world as *grāhya* or object.[1] This link of *prāṇa*, therefore, has been initially brought into manifestation by the Absolute, Free Will of the Lord (*svātantryāt*).

We find the same idea expressed in Vājasaneyā,

"That *Śakti* (Divine Power) who is the highest, subtle, all-pervading, absolutely pure, auspicious, mother of the collective whole of *śaktis*, the highest bliss of the nature of immortality, *mahāghoreśvarī*,[2] *Caṇḍā*[3] (terrible) brings about both manifestation and withdrawal (of the world process), and she forcibly makes manifest and finally withdraws (*prakarṣati*) Time that expresses itself in the form of the three breath-channels[4], (*trivaham*) in three forms[5], (*trividham*) and in three aspects[6], (*triṣṭham*). Thus it is of the divine consciousness that the function of external manifestation and internal withdrawal has been described in the form of the flow of breath in the three channels, the states of moon, sun and fire and the past, future, and present aspects of external time.

The same has been said in *Svacchanda-tantra* also;

"The life-force appears in the individual as *prāṇa* and *apāna* with the function of exhalation and inhalation. Always imparting life, it exists within one's breast. Since it imparts life, therefore, is it known as *prāṇa*." (VII, 25).

In accordance with what *Svacchanda-tantra* says in the following verse:

"*Ha* is said to be *prāṇa* which functions by itself (i.e. is automatic) and is of the form of a plough"[7] (*halākritiḥ*) (IV, 257).

It is of *prāṇa* that the function of manifestation (*sṛṣṭi*) and withdrawal (*saṁhāra*) has been described because of its being of the form of the Highest, Absolutely Free Bhairava and because of its out-going and incoming. Therefore, it has been rightly said that the link of *prāṇa* is natural.

So *Bhaṭṭakallaṭa*, in order to confirm the causality of *prāṇa* has said in *Tattvārtha-cintāmaṇi*—

"Consciousness is, at first, transformed into *prāṇa*."

NOTES

1. For manifestation, the divine consciousness at first transforms itself into *prāṇa*. This *prāṇa* is universal Life-force which brings about both subject (*grāhaka*) and object (*grāhya*).

2. *Mahāghoreśvarī* is here only another name of *Kālasaṅkarṣiṇī Śakti*.

3. *Caṇḍā* is another name of the same *śakti*, She is called *Caṇḍā* (terrible), because she conceals the essential nature of the experient.

4. *Trivaham*—'flow of life-breath in the form of three channels' refers to *iḍā* (the breath channel on the left of the spinal column), *piṅgalā* (the breath channel on the right of the spinal column), *suṣumnā* (the breath channel in the middle of the spinal column).

5. *Trividham* refers to *soma* (moon), *sūrya* (sun), and *agni* (fire) symbolic respectively of *prameya* (object), *pramāṇa* (knowledge) and *pramātā* (subject).

6. *Triṣṭham*—three aspects of time, viz., past, present, future.

7. The letter *ha* is indicative of *visarga śakti* (Creative power). In Śāradā script, the letter *ha* is of the form of a polugh the upper part of which symbolizes exhalation and the lower part symbolizes inhalation. It is constantly and automatically being sounded inwardly in everyone in an *anacka* (vowel-less) and *anāhata* form (i.e. in the form of unstruck sound).

EXPOSITION

It is *saṁvit* or consciousness which is transformed into *prāṇa*. *Prāṇa* in this context does not mean life-breath. It means the universal Life-force which brings about both subject and object. It is the connecting link between consciousness and the various vehicles (*sthūla*, *sūkṣma*, etc) of man. This link is natural. It is this link which maintains the body even when a *yogī* has acquired Self-realization and has constant awareness of the transcendental consciousness. So the question—'Why the body does not fall away when the *yogī* is poised in the transcendental consciousness is meaningless. The body cannot perish so long as the link of *prāṇa* remains. The *yogī* cannot commit suicide.

The universal Life-force assumes mainly two forms in the individual, viz., *prāṇa*-exhalation, and *apāna*-inhalation. *Prāṇa*, the outgoing breath is indicative of *sṛṣṭi*-manifestation of the world process, and *apāna* is indicative of *saṁhāra*—withdrawal of objective manifestation. It is *prāṇa*, the universal life-force that has dual aspect and thus brings about both the manifestation (*sṛṣṭi*) of the objective world and its withdrawal (*saṁhāra*) back to its source.

INTRODUCTION TO THE 44th SŪTRA

TEXT

अतश्च स्थितेऽपि नैसर्गिके प्राणसंबन्धे यस्तदारूढ आन्तरीं कलां विमृशन्नास्ते स लोकोत्तर एव इत्याह—

TRANSLATION

So even while the natural association of *prāṇa* lasts, the *yogī* who is poised in the fourth i.e. the transcendental consciousness being constantly aware of the inward Supreme I-consciousness abides as a transcendental person (lit., beyond the common). This is what the next *sūtra* says.

SŪTRA—44

नासिकान्तर्मध्यसंयमात्, किमत्र, सव्यापसव्यसौषुम्नेषु ॥ ४४ ॥

Nāsikā-antarmadhya-saṁyamāt, kimatra, savyāpasavya-sauṣumneṣu.

नासिका = *prāṇa śakti*; अन्तर्मध्य = centre of the inner consciousness; किमत्र = what is to be said in this matter; सव्य = left; अपसव्य = right; सौषुम्नेषु the *suṣumnā*, the middle *nāḍī*.

"In all the channels left (*iḍā*), right (*piṅgalā*) and *suṣumnā*—the middle one, there is *prāṇa śakti*. By the constant practice of the awareness of Reality that is in the centre of the inner state of *prāṇa śakti*, there abides the awareness of that central Reality viz., the supreme I-consciousness under all circumstances, and in all conditions."

COMMENTARY

TEXT

सर्वनाडीचक्रप्रधानरूपेषु सव्यापसव्यसौषुम्नेषु दक्षिणवाममध्यनाडीपदेषु, या नासिका, नसते कौटिल्येन वहति इति कृत्वा, कुटिलवाहिनी प्राणशक्तिः, तस्याः अन्तरिति आन्तरी संवित्, तस्याः अपि मध्यं सर्वान्तरतमतया प्रधानम् ।

'तस्य देवातिदेवस्य परबोधस्वरूपिणः ।
विमर्शः परमा शक्तिः सर्वज्ञा ज्ञानशालिनी ॥'

इति श्रीकालिकाक्रमोक्तनीत्या यत् विमर्शमयं रूपं तत्संयमात् अन्तर्निभालनप्रकर्षात् ; किमत्र उच्यते, अयं हि सर्वदशासु देदीप्यमानो निर्व्युत्थानः परः समाधिः । तदुक्तं श्रीविज्ञानभैरवे

'ग्राह्यग्राहकसंवित्तिः सामान्या सर्वदेहिनाम् ।
योगिनां तु विशेषोऽयं संबन्धे सावधानता ॥'

इति ॥ ४४ ॥

TRANSLATION

In the main ones of all the *prāṇic* channels, viz., in left (*iḍā*), right (*piṅgalā*), and the middle one viz., *suṣumnā*, there flows the *nāsikā* or *prāṇa śakti*. The word *nāsikā* is derived in the following way—'*nasate*' i.e. that which flows in a zigzag way, that is, *prāṇa-śakti*. *Antar* means the inner aspect of this *prāṇaśakti* i.e. consciousness. *Madhya* means the centre of this inner consciousness i.e. *vimarśa* or I-consciousness. Being the innermost of all, that is the main or central Reality, viz., the Supreme I-consciousness. According to the following verse of *Kālikākrama*, the central I-consciousness is the highest *śakti*.

"Of that God who is greater than all the gods, and who is supreme consciousness itself i.e *prakāśa*, the highest *śakti* is *vimarśa* or I-consciousness, which is omniscient, full of wisdom."

By the *saṁyama*[1] or intensity of repeated inward awareness of that supreme I-consciousness, there is (what is to be said in this matter[2]) in all conditions, radiant, highest *nirvyutthāna-samādhi*[3].

The same idea has been expressed in the following verse in *Vijñāna-bhairava*:

"The consciousness of subject-object relationship is common to all embodied beings. The *Yogīs* have, however, this distinction that they are ever mindful of this relation" (i.e., they are always mindful of the *para-pramātā*, the metaphysical subject without which there can be no such thing as an object". (verse-106).

NOTES

1. *Saṁyama* here is not to be taken in the technical sense of Patañjali's Yoga which means the threefold practice of *dhāraṇā*, *dhyāna* and *samādhi*. Here *saṁyama* means the intensity of repeated inward awareness.

2. *Kimatra* or what is to be said in this matter ? This is an exclamation, an expression of delight.

3. *Nirvyutthāna samādhi* means the ever-present absorption of the mind in the Supreme I-consciousness in the ordinary routine of life even when the *yogī* is not practising formal contemplation.

INTRODUCTION TO THE 45th SŪTRA

TEXT

एवमीदृशस्य योगफलं दर्शयन् प्रकरणमुपसंहरति—

TRANSLATION

The next *sūtra* gives the conclusion of the book by showing the final achievement of the *yoga* of this kind of *yogi*.

SŪTRA—45

भूयः स्यात्प्रतिमीलनम् ॥ ४५ ॥

Bhūyaḥ syāt pratimīlanam.

भूयः=over and over again; स्यात्=there is; प्रतिमीलनम् awareness of the Divine both inwardly and outwardly.

"In the case of this *yogī* there is over and over again the awareness of the Divine both inwardly and outwardly".

COMMENTARY

TEXT

चैतन्यात्मनः स्वरूपात् उदितस्य अस्य विश्वस्य भूयः पुनः, विगलितभेदसंस्कारात्मना बाहुल्येन च प्रतिमीलनम्, चैतन्याभिमुख्येन निमीलनं, पुनरपि चैतन्यात्मस्वस्वरूपोन्मीलनरूपं परयोगाभिनिविष्टस्य योगिनो भवति । तदुक्तं श्रीस्वच्छन्दे

'उन्मनापरतो देवि तत्रात्मानं नियोजयेत् ।
तस्मिन्युक्तस्ततो ह्यात्मा तन्मयश्च प्रजायते ॥'

इति । तथा च

'उद्बोधितो यथा वह्निर्निर्मलोऽतीव भास्वरः ।
न भूयः प्रविशेत्काष्ठे तथात्माध्वन उद्धृतः ॥
मलकर्मकलाद्यैस्तु निर्मलो विगतक्लमः ।
तत्रस्थोऽपि न बध्येत यतोऽतीव सुनिर्मलः ॥'

इति । भूयः स्यादित्यभिदधतोऽयमाशयः, यत् शिवत्वमस्य योगिनो न अपूर्वम्, अपि तु स्वभाव एव, केवलं मायाशक्त्युत्थापितस्वविकल्पदौरात्म्यात् भासमानमपि तत् नायं प्रत्यवम्रष्टुं क्षमः, इत्यस्य उक्तोपायप्रदर्शनक्रमेण तदेव अभिव्यज्यते इति शिवम् ॥ ४५ ॥

'सेयमागमसंवादस्पन्दसंगतिसुन्दरा ।
वृत्तिः शैवरहस्यार्थे शिवसूत्रेषु दर्शिता ॥ १ ॥
शिवरहस्यनिदर्शनसंस्रवन्–
नवनवामृतसाररसोल्बणाम् ।
सुकृतिनो रसयन्तु भवच्छिदे
स्फुटमिमां शिवसूत्रविमर्शिनीम् ॥ २ ॥
इयमरोचकिनां रुचिवर्धिनी
परिणतिं तनुते परमां मतेः ।
रसनमात्रत एव सुधौघवन्–
मृतिजराजननादिभयापहृत् ॥ ३ ॥
देहप्राणसुखादिभिः परिमिताहन्तास्पदैः संवृत–
श्चैतन्यं चिनुते निजं न सुमहन्माहेश्वरं स्वं जनः ।
मध्ये बोधसुधाब्धि विश्वमभितस्तत्फेनपिण्डोपमं
यः पश्येदुपदेशतस्तु कथितः साक्षात्स एकः शिवः ॥ ४ ॥
तरत तरसा संसाराब्धिं विधत्त परे पदे
पदमविचलं नित्यालोकप्रमोदसुनिर्भरे ।
विमृशत शिवप्रोक्तं सूत्रं रहस्यसमुज्ज्वलं
प्रसभविलसत्सद्युक्त्यान्तः समुत्प्लवदायि तत् ॥ ५ ॥

इति श्रीमन्महामाहेश्वराचार्यवर्याभिनवगुप्तपादपद्मोपजीविश्रीक्षेमराज-विरचितायां शिवसूत्रविमर्शिन्यामाणवोपायप्रकाशनं नाम तृतीय उन्मेषः ॥ ३ ॥

समाप्ता चेयं शिवसूत्रविमर्शिनी ॥
कृतिः श्रीक्षेमराजस्य क्षेमायास्तु विमर्शिनाम् ।
शिवस्वात्मैक्यबोधार्था शिवसूत्रविमर्शिनी ॥

TRANSLATION

The *yogī* who is deeply absorbed in the Supreme I-consciousness (*parayogābhiniviṣṭasya*) has a *pratimīlana* of this universe which has arisen from the essential nature of foundational consciousness.

'Pratimīlana'[1] means both inward awareness of the Divine (*nimīlana*), and outward awareness of the Divine (*unmīlana*). He now sees the universe over and over again with an awareness in which the residual traces of difference have completely vanished. (viz. *vigalitabhedasaṁskārātmnā*). The *yogī* has an experience in which he is inwardly absorbed in the Supreme Divine Consciousness (*nimīlana*); again when he turns towards the universe, he experiences it as the same as his own essential Divine Consciousness (*unmīlana*). The same idea has been expressed in the following verse in *Svacchanda-tantra*:

"O Goddess, beyond the *samanā*[2], there is the *unmanā*[3] stage; one should join one's self to it. The self united with that, completely becomes that very *unmanā*," (IV, 332).

Again (in the same Tantra, it has been said),

"Just as kindled fire that has risen pure and radiant from the fuel does not enter it again, even so, the Self that has arisen from the *Ṣaḍadhvā*[4] freed of all *āṇavamala*, (*mala*) *kārma mala* (*karma*) and *māyīya mala* (*kalā*) is past all the fret and fever of life.[5] Even though still remaining in the world, he is not bound by it i.e. is not attracted towards the pleasures of the world because he is now pre-eminently freed of all the *malas* (limitations) and abides perfectly pure." (X, 371-372).

In saying *bhūyaḥ syāt* (is again) the intention of the *sūtrakāra* (composer of the sūtras) is this—that the Divinity (Śivahood) of this *yogī* is not any thing new. It is the very nature of Reality. Only on account of the perversity of one's own thought-constructs brought about by *Māyā-śakti*, the aspirant was not able to recognize it which was there all the while. It is only manifested now by adopting the various means described in this book.

May there be welfare (for all) !

NOTES

1. *Pratimīlana* — *Nimīlana—unmīlana=pratimīlana. Nimīlana* is that *samādhi* in which the *yogī* is completely absorbed inwardly in the supreme I-consciousness. When after coming back to normal consciousness, he turns his attention towards the universe, he experiences the universe also only as an expression of the Divine. This is *unmīlana samādhi.* Having both kinds of experience successively is *pratimīlana.*

2. *Samanā*. Upto *samanā* stage in the upward climb towards the Divine, there is the function of mind, not of the ordinary, normal mind but mind developed to its optimum excellence.

3. *Unmanā* is the stage of consciousness beyond mind. It is entirely divine consciousness. It is a stage where human consciousness has been completely transcended.

4. *Saḍadhvā* (lit. the course of six) includes the entire phenomenal manifestation, three on the subjective side, viz., (i) *varṇa* (2) *mantra* and (3) *pada* and three on the objective side, viz., (a) *kalā* (2) *tattva* and (3) *bhuvana.*

5. The *Ātmā* (spirit) has finished its journey in mundane manifestation. It has crossed the border of human limitation and has become completely divinized. Just as the flame of fire that has risen to the sky does not return to the heap of wood from which it has arisen, even so the soul that has reached the *unmanā* level does not return to the earth. The aspirant that has risen to this height is completely freed of all the three *malas-āṇava, māyīya,* and *kārma.*

Thus is finished the third section describing *āṇavopāya.*

Kṣemarāja's Epilogue.

This commentary on the *Śiva-sūtras* beautified by its harmony with the *Śaiva āgamas,* and by its consistency with the Spandakārikā has been written to expound the secret of *Śaiva yoga.*(1)

May the pious ones enjoy fully well, for cutting out the shackles that bind them to worldly existence, the commentary on the *Śiva Sūtras* named *Vimarśinī* full of everfresh elixir of immortality trickling down from the teaching about the secret doctrine of *Śiva.* (2).

This commentary would stimulate the interest of those who are not interested in the doctrine of *Śiva,* would bring about the most excellent transformation of understanding and remove fear of death, old age, birth etc. like a flood of nectar by mere taste of it. (3)

Environed by the body, *prāṇa,* pleasure etc. due to the limited sense of I-ness, man does not realize the doctrine about one's magnificent divine Self. But he who, owing to this teaching, beholds in the midst of the ocean of (spiritual) awareness the universe as a mass of its foam on all sides is said to be Śiva Himself in sooth. (4)

May you all cross quickly the ocean of transmigratory existence and be established firmly in the highest state full of eternal light and delight. Ponder deeply over the *sūtra* enunciated by *Śiva*, radiant with its mystic truth. Taught by an excellent *guru* (spiritual director), it shines forth vigorously and joyfully enlightens the inner understanding (5).

This is the the third section, viz. *āṇavopāya* of *Śiva-sūtra-vimarśinī* written by Rājānaka Kṣemarāja who is dependent (for his intellectual and spiritual life) on the lotus-feet of (his *guru*) Mahāmāheśvara Rājānaka Abhinavagupta.

This Śiva-sūtra-vimarśinī is finished. This work of Kṣemarāja, viz., Śiva-sūtra-vimarśini is meant for the peace and welfare of those who reflect on life in order that they may understand the identity of their Self with Śiva.

GLOSSARY OF TECHNICAL TERMS

A (अ)

A (अ) : Symbol of Śiva, short form of *anuttara* (the Supreme); the letter pervading all the other letters of the alphabet.

Akala : The experient established in Śiva *tattva* and identified with Śiva.

Akula : *Śiva* or अ (अकारलक्षणं कुलं शरीरमस्य इति आद्यवर्णः ।)

Akrama : Successionless manifestation of the essential nature; Śākta Yoga.

Akhyāti : Primal Ignorance; Mahāmāyā.

Agni (symbolic) : *Pramātā*—knower or subject.

Agniṣomātmikā : The *parāśakti* (highest śakti) that brings about *sṛṣṭi* (manifestation) and *saṁhāra* (withdrawal) of the universe.

Agniṣomamayam : The universe which is of the nature of *pramāṇa* (knowledge) and *prameya* (objects).

Ajñānam : The primal limitation (*mala*); Ajñāna in this system does not mean absence of knowledge, but contracted or limited knowledge. Being inherent in *Puruṣa* on account of which he considers himself as of limited knowledge and limited activity, it is known as *Pauruṣa-Ajñāna*. Being inherent in *Buddhi*, it leads one to form all kinds of *aśuddha vikalpas* (thought-constructs devoid of essential Reality) and is thus known as *Bauddha Ajñāna*.

Aghora : The merciful *Śiva*.

Aghora Śaktis : The *Śaktis* that lead the conditioned experients to the realization of *Śiva*.

Aghoreśa : An aspect of Īśvara below *Śuddha vidyā* giving rise to *aśuddha* tattvas like māyā; Anantanātha.

Adhiṣṭhāna : Substratum, support.

Aṇu : 'Aṇiti śvasiti iti aṇuḥ'—one who breathes i.e. the *jīva*—the empirical individual; the limited, conditioned experient, conditioned by the body, *puryaṣṭaka* and *prāṇa*; the *cittamaya pramātā*, the experient whose predominant nature is the empirical mind; the *Māyā-pramātā*, the experient dominated by Māyā.

Atiśānta padam : The state of *Parama Śiva* beyond the *tattvas*.

Adhvā : Adhvā literally means course or path. *Śuddha Adhvā* is the intrinsic course, the supramundane manifestation. *Aśuddha adhvā* is the course of mundane manifestation.

Anacka : Sounding the consonants without the vowels; esoteric meaning—'concentrating on any mantra back to the source where it is unuttered'.

Anāśrita-śiva : The state of *Śiva* in which there is no objective content yet, in which the universe is negated from Him.

Anantabhaṭṭāraka : The presiding deity of the *Mantra* experients.

Antakoṭi : The last edge or point; it is *dvādaśānta* a measure of twelve fingers.

Antarmukhībhāva : Introversion of consciousness.

Anupāya : Spontaneous realization of Self without any special effort.

Anugraha : Grace.

Anuttara : (1) The Highest; the Supreme; *Parama Śiva*; the Absolute (lit. one than whom nothing is higher). (2) The vowel 'a' (अ).

Anusandhāna : Lit; investigation; tracking a matter to its source. In Yoga, repeated intensive awareness of the Source or essential Reality.

Antarātmā : The conditioned inner soul consisting of *puryaṣṭaka* or subtle body. It is called inner as contrasted with the gross body which is the outer covering of the soul.

Antaḥstha : Lit; standing in between, the letters य, र, ल, व, are known as *antaḥstha* letters. According to Śikṣā (Phonetics) and Vyākaraṇa (Grammar), they are called *antaḥstha*, because they stand between vowels and consonants, they are neither purely vowels, nor purely consonants or they are so called, because they stand between स्पर्श = letters क to म and ऊष्मन् letters (श, ष, स, ह)

According to Kṣemarāja, they are called *antaḥstha* because they are determined by Māyā and her *kañcukas* which operate from within the mind of man.

Abhinavagupta, however, says that since the formation of the *antaḥstha* letters is due to *icchā* and *unmeṣa* śaktis which are inner forces and are identified with the *pramātā* (subject), they are rightly called *antaḥstha*.

Apaśuśakti : One whose bondage has disappeared and who has become a free being (*pati*) like Sadāśiva.

Apāna : The vital *vāyu* that goes in downwards towards the anus; the inhaled air.

Apavarga : Liberation.

Apara : Lower; lowest.

Apavedya suṣupti : Profound sleep in which there is absolutely no awareness of any object whatsoever.

Abuddha : What is known as the awakened state for the common man is from the standpoint of the Yogī *abuddha* or unawakened state i.e. a state of spiritual ignorance.

Amṛta varṇa : the letter 'sa'.

Ambā : The highest Śakti of the Divine.

Amāyīya : Beyond the scope of Māyā. Amāyīya śabda is one which does not depend on convention, in which the word and the object are one.

Alaṁgrāsa : 'Alam' in this context means *atyartham* i.e. to the utmost, and *grāsa* means swallowing, consuming i.e. completely reducing to sameness with Self.

Alaṁgrāsa, therefore, means bringing experienced object completely to sameness with the consciousness of the Self when no impression of *saṁsāra* as separate from consciousness is allowed to remain.

Avadhāna : Constant attentiveness.

Avikalpa (Nirvikalpa) Jñāna : Direct realization of Reality without any mental activity.

Avikalpa (Nirvikalpa) pratyakṣa : Sensuous awareness without any perceptual judgement, unparticularised awareness.

Aviveka : Non-awareness of the Real, *moha* or delusion; ignorance; non-discernment.

Avyakta : Non-manifest.

Aśuddha vidyā : Knowledge of a few particulars; limited knowledge; empirical knowledge.

Asat : Non-being.

Ahaṁkāra : I-making principle, I-feeling.

Ahantā : I-consciousness.

Ā (आ)

Āṇava upāya : The Yoga whereby the individual utilizes his senses, *prāṇa* and *manas* for Self-realization. It consists generally of *uccāra*, *karaṇa*, *dhyāna*, *varṇa*, and *sthāna-kalpanā*. It is also known as *Āṇava yoga*, *Bhedopāya* and *Kriyā-yoga* or *Kriyopāya*.

Āṇava Samāveśa : Identification with the Divine by the above means.

Āṇava mala : Mala or limitation pertaining to *aṇu* or the empirical individual; innate ignorance of the *jīva*; primal limiting condition which reduces universal consciousness to a *jīva*, depriving consciousness of *śakti* and *śakti* of consciousness and thus bringing about a sense of imperfection. This limitation works in two ways—(1) while the sense of doership is present, there is loss of *bodha* or *prakāśa* i.e. considering inconscient things like *śūnya*, *buddhi*, *prāṇa* or body as the Self. (2) While there is *bodha* or *prakāśa*, there is loss of the sense of activity or doership.

Ātmasātkṛ : Reducing to sameness with the Self.

Ātma-viśrānti : Resting in the Self.

Ātma-vyāpti : Realization of the Self without the realization of the all-inclusive *Śiva*-nature.

Ādi koṭi : The first edge or point i.e. the heart from which the measure of breath is determined.

Ānanda : Bliss; the nature of Śakti; the essential nature of Parama Śiva along with *Cit*; the letter 'ā'.

Ānanda-upāya : Realization of Śiva-nature without any yogic discipline. Also known as Ānanda Yoga or Anupāya.

Ābhoga : Expansion; *camatkāra* or spiritual delight.

Āsana : Exoteric meaning—'A particular posture of the body'. Esoteric meaning—'Being established in the Self'.

I (इ)

Ichhā : Will, Representing the letter 'इ' (i).

Ichhā upāya : Śāmbhava-upāya, also known as ichhāyoga.

Ichhā-Śakti : The inseparable innate Will Power of *Parama Śiva* intent on manifestation; that inward state of *Parama*

Śiva in which *jñāna* and *kriyā* are unified; the predominant aspect of Sadāśiva.

Idantā : This—consciousness; objective consciousness.

Indu : *Prameya* or object; *apāna*; *kriyā-śakti.*

I (ई)

Īśāna : Representing the letter 'ī'. The first inner *Śakti* of *Śiva* that acts as the teacher of *Śaiva Śāstra.*

Īśvara-tattva : The fourth tattva, counting from *Śiva.* The consciousness of this *tattva* is 'This am I'. *Jñāna* is predominant in this *tattva.*

Īśvara-bhaṭṭāraka : The presiding deity of the *Mantreśvaras* residing in *Īśvara tattva.*

U (उ)

Uccāra : A particular technique of concentration on Prāṇaśakti under Āṇava upāya. Various aspects of *ānanda* (bliss) are experienced in this concentration.

Ucchalattā : The creative movement of the Divine ānanda in waves bringing about manifestation and withdrawal.

Udāna : The vital *vāyu* that moves upwards. The *Śakti* that moves up in Suṣumnā at spiritual awakening.

Udyama : The sudden spontaneous emergence of the Supreme I-consciousness.

Udyantṛtā : -do-

Udyoga : -do-

Udvamantī : Lit. vomiting; externalizing; manifesting.

Unmeṣa : Lit. Opening of the eye; (1) The externalizing of Ichhā Śakti; the start of the world-process. (2) In Śaiva-yoga—unfolding of the spiritual consciousness which comes about by concentrating on the inner consciousness which is the back-ground of the rise of ideas. (3) Representing the letter 'u'.

Unmanā : The Supramental Śakti of *Parama Śiva* in its primal movement towards manifestation, though inseparable from Him is known as *unmanā* or *unmanī.* Literally it means that which transcends *manas.* This Śakti is *amātra,* measureless and beyond time.

Kṣemarāja in Udyota commentary on Netratantra (Vol. II, p. 285) says about *unmanā mana utkramya gatā anavacchinnaprakāśasphurattā*. It is the *Śakti* that transcends mind and is an uninterrupted Light.

Umā : The Icchā Śakti of the Supreme; U=Śiva; mā=Śakti—श्रो: मा the Śakti of Śiva.

U (ऊ)

Ūnatā : Representing the letter Ū.

Ūṣmā : The letters Śa, ṣa, sa, ha.

E (ए)

Ekāṇavā : *Paśyantī vāk*.

Au (औ)

Aunmukhya : Because of His inherent *ānanda*, the intentness of Śiva towards manifestation; the rising of Icchā Śakti towards creativity.

Ka (क)

Kañcuka : The coverings of Māyā, throwing a pall over pure consciousness (*Śuddha Saṁvid*) and thus converting Śiva into jīva. They are (1) kalā, (2) (aśuddha) Vidyā, (3) Rāga (4) Niyati and (5) Kāla.

Kanda : Mūlādhāra psychic centre.

Karaṇa : (1) The means of *jñāna* and *kriyā—antaḥkaraṇa* and *bahiṣkaraṇa*. (2) One of the *āṇava upāyas* in which the aspirant contemplates over the body and the nervous system as an epitome of the cosmos.

Karaṇeśvarī : *Khecarī*, *gocarī*, *dikcarī* and *bhūcarī cakra*.

Karmendriya : The five powers and organs of action—speaking (*Vāk*), handling (*hasta*), locomotion (*pāda*), excreting (*pāyu*), sexual action (*upastha*).

Kalā : (1) The *Śakti* of consciousness by which all the thirty-six principles are evolved. (2) Part; particle, aspect (3) Limitation in respect of activity (*Kiñcitkartṛtva*). (4) The subtlest aspect of objectivity, viz., *Śāntyatītā*, *śāntā*, *Vidyā*, *Pratiṣṭhā*, and *Nivṛtti*.

Kalācakra : *Mātṛcakra, Śakticakra, Devīcakra*; the group of letters from 'a' to 'kṣa'.

Kalāśarīra : That of which the essential nature is activity; *Kārma mala.*

Ka (का)

Kāraṇa : Cause.

Kārya : Effect.

Kārma mala : *Mala* due to *vāsanās* or impressions left behind on the mind by *Karma* or motivated action.

Kālāgni : Kālāgni-bhuvaneśa—a particular *Rudra* in *Nivṛtti kalā.*

Kāla-adhvā : *Varṇa, mantra* and *pada.*

Kāla pada : The toe of the right foot.

Kāla tattva : Time—past, present, and future determined by the sense of succession.

Kāla śakti : the Śakti or power of the Divine that determines succession.

Ku (कु)

Kuṇḍalī or Kuṇḍalinī : The creative power of Śiva; A distinct śakti that lies folded up in three and a half folds in Mūlādhāra.

Kumbhaka : Retention of *prāṇa.*

Kumārī : One who carries on the play of the world-process or one who brings about an end to the difference-creating Māyā.

Kula : Śakti manifesting herself in 36 *tattvas.*

Kulāmnāya : The Śākta system or doctrine of realizing the Supreme by means of all the letters from अ (a) to क्ष (kṣa).

Kulamārga : The discipline for attaining to the Supreme.

Kū (कू)

Kūṭa-bīja : The letter क्ष (kṣa)

Ke (के)

Kevalī : One whose sole essence of Self consists in being pure consciousness; One who is established in Self.

Kra (क्र)

Krama : Realization of Self by means of *Kriyā Yoga.*

Kriyā Yoga : *Āṇava upāya,* also known as *Kriyopāya.*

Kriyā Śakti : The power of assuming any and every form (*Sarvākārayogitvaṁ Kriyāśaktiḥ*).

Kṣa (क्ष)

Kṣetrajña : The empirical Subject.

Kṣema : Preservation of what is obtained.

Kṣobha : Identification of 'I' with the gross or subtle body.

Kha (ख)

Kha-traya : *Kha*-ākāśa, symbol of consciousness. Kha-traya—The three *ākāśas*, viz; *Śakti*, *vyāpinī*, and *samanā* situated in the head from the Vindu between the eye-brows up to *Brahmarandhra.* Concentrating in the head, one should rise higher by means of the above three *khas.*

Khecarī : Sub-species of *Vāmeśvarī Śakti*, connected with the *pramātā*, the empirical self; Khecarī is one that moves in *Kha* or the vast expanse of consciousness.

Khecarī-cakra : The *cakra* or group of the *śaktis* that move in the expanse of consciousness of the empirical subject.

Khecarī Mudrā : The bliss of the vast expanse of spiritual consciousness, also known as *divya mudrā* or *Śivāvasthā* (the state of Śiva).

Khyāti : Jñāna; knowledge; wisdom;

Ga (ग)

Gaganāṅganā : *Cit-śakti*, consciousness-power.

Garbha : *Akhyāti*, primal ignorance; *Mahāmāyā.*

Guṇa-traya : *Sattva, rajas, tamas.*

Guru-vaktra : Lit. the mouth of the *guru*, *anugraha śakti*; Grace.

Gocarī : Sub-species of *Vāmeśvarī*, connected with the *antaḥkaraṇa* of the experient. '*Go*' means sense; *antaḥkaraṇa* is the seat of the senses; hence *Gocarī* is connected with *antaḥkaraṇa.*

Granthi : Psychic tangle; psychic complex.
Grāhaka : Knower; Subject; Experient.
Grāhya : Known; object of experience.

Gha (घ)

Ghora Śaktis : The *Śaktis* or deities that draw the *jīvas* towards worldly pleasures.
Ghoratarī śaktis : The Śaktis or deities that push the *jīvas* towards a downward path in *saṁsāra.*

Ca (च)

Cakra : The group or Collective whole of *śaktis.*
Cakreśvara : The master or lord of the group of *śaktis.*
Candra : *Prameya* or object of knowledge; the *apāna prāṇa* or *nāḍī* (channel or nerve).
Camatkāra : Bliss of the pure I-consciousness; delight of artistic experience.
Caramakalā : The highest phase of manifestation known as Śāntyatītā or Śāntātītā Kalā.

Ci (चि)

Cit : The Absolute; foundational consciousness; the consciousness that is the unchanging principle of all changes.
Citta : The limitation of the Universal Consciousness manifested in the individual mind, the mind of the empirical individual.
Citi : The consciousness—power of the Absolute that brings about the world-process.
Cidānanda : (1) The nature of ultimate Reality consisting of consciousness and bliss, (2) The sixth stratum of ānanda in *uccāra yoga* of *āṇava upāya.*

Ce (चे)

Cetana : *Parama Śiva,* Self, Conscious individual.
Cetya: Knowable, object of consciousness.

Cai (चै)

Caitanya : The foundational Consciousness which has absolute freedom of knowing and doing, of *jñāna* and *kriyā śakti.*

Cha (छ)

Cheda : Cessation of *prāṇa* and *apāna* by sounding of *anacka* (vowel-less) sounds.

Ja (ज)

Jagat : The world-process.
Jagadānanda : The bliss of the Self or the Divine appearing as the universe, the bliss of the Divine made visible.

Jā (जा)

Jāgrat avasthā : The waking condition.
Jāgrat jñāna : Objective knowledge common to all people in waking condition. *Jāgrat* : Esoteric meaning—'Jñānaṁ Jāgrat'—Enlightenment, undeluded awakening of consciousness at all levels.

Jī (जी)

Jīva : The individual soul; the empirical self whose consciousness is conditioned by the *saṁskāras* of his experience and who is identified with the limitations of his subtle and gross constitution.
Jīvanmukta : The liberated individual who while still living in the physical body is not conditioned by the limitation of his subtle and gross constitution and believes the entire universe to be an expression of *Śiva* or his highest Self.
Jīvanmukti : Experience of liberation while still living in the body.

Jñā (ज्ञा)

Jñāna : Spiritual wisdom; limited knowledge (which is the source of bondage).
Jñāna Yoga : *Śākta upāya.*
Jñāna Śakti : The power of knowledge of the Absolute.

Jya (ज्य)

Jyeṣṭhā : The Śakti of Śiva that inspires the *jīva* for Self-realization or *Śiva*-Consciousness.

Ta (त)

Tattva : Thatness; principle; reality; the very being of a thing;

Tattva-traya : The three tattvas, viz; *Nara, Śakti* and *Śiva* or *Ātmā, Vidyā* and *Śiva.*

Tatpuruṣa : One of the five aspects of Śiva.

Tanmātra : Lit. that only; the primary elements of perception; the general elements of the particulars of sense-perception, viz. *śabda, sparśa, rūpa, rasa, gandha.*

Tamas : One of the constituents of *Prakṛti*—the principle of inertia and delusion.

Tarka śāstra : Logic and dialectics.

Tu (तु)

Turīya or *Turya* : The fourth state of consciousness beyond the states of waking, dreaming and deep sleep and stringing together all the states; the Metaphysical Consciousness distinct from the psychological or empirical self; the *Sākṣī* or witnessing consciousness; the transcendental Self.

Turyātīta : The state of consciousness transcending the *turīya*, the state in which the distinction of the three, viz; waking, dreaming and deep sleep states is annulled; that pure blissful consciousness in which there is no sense of difference, in which the entire universe appears as the Self.

Tri (त्रि)

Trika : The system of philosophy of the triad—*Nara*, *Śakti* and *Śiva* or (1) *para*, the highest, concerned with identity (2) *parāpara*, identity in difference, and (3) *apara*, difference and sense of difference.

Trika (para) : *Prakāśa, Vimarśa* and their *sāmarasya.*

Trika (parāpara) : *Icchā, Jñāna* and *Kriyā.*

Da (द)

Darśana : Seeing; system of philosophy.

Di (दि)

Dik : Space.

Dikcarī : Sub-species of Vāmeśvarī, connected with *bahiṣkaraṇas* or outer senses.

Divya mudrā : *Khecarī mudrā.*

Dī (दी)

Dīkṣā : (1) The gift of spiritual knowledge. (2) The initiation ceremony pertaining to a disciple by which spiritual knowledge is imparted and the residual traces of his evil deeds are purified.

De (दे)

Deśa : Space.

Deśa adhvā : *Kalā*, *tattva*, and *bhuvana*.

Dha (ध)

Dhāraṇā : (1) Meditation (2) The letters य र ल व

Dhruva : (1) *Anuttara* stage (2) The letter अ

Dhyāna Yoga : The highest *dhāraṇā* of *āṇava upāya* in which *pramāṇa* (knowledge), *prameya* (object of knowledge) and *pramātā* (knower) are realized as aspects of *Saṁvid* or foundational consciousness.

Dhvani Yoga : A *dhāraṇā* of *āṇava upāya* consisting of concentration on *anāhata nāda* (unstruck sound) arising within through *prāṇa śakti*. This is also known as *Varṇa Yoga.*

Na (न)

Navavargaka : Letters pertaining to nine classes (1) अ वर्ग (vowels) (2) क वर्ग the letters क, ख, ग, घ, ङ (3) च वर्ग the letters च छ ज झ ञ (4) ट वर्ग, the letters ट ठ ड ढ ण (5) त वर्ग, the letters त थ द ध न (6) प वर्ग, the letters प फ ब भ म (7) य वर्ग the letters य र ल व (8) श वर्ग, the letters श ष स ह and (9) the letter क्ष

Nā (ना)

Nāḍī-saṁhāra : Dissolution of *prāṇa* and *apāna* into *suṣumnā*.

Nāda (1) Metaphysical—The first movement of *Śiva-śakti* towards manifestation. (2) In Yoga—The unstruck sound experienced in *suṣumnā*. (3) When Śakti fills up the whole universe with *Nādānta*, she is designated as *Nāda*. This is also *Sadāśiva tattva* because of the apposition of I and this is in the same principle.

Nāsikā : Prāṇaśakti flowing in a zigzag way in *Prāṇa*, *Apāna* and *Suṣumnā* channels.

Ni (नि)

Nigraha kṛtya : Śiva's act of Self-veiling.

Nijānanda : In *āṇava upāya*, the first stage of *ānanda* arising from concentration on *prāṇa* leading to the resting of the mind on the subject or experient.

Nibhālana : Perception; mental practice.

Nimeṣa : Lit; Closing of the eye-lid, (1) dissolution of the world; (2) the inner activity of *spanda* by which the object is merged into the subject; (3) the dissolution of the Śakticakra in the Self; (4) the involution of Śiva in matter.

Nimīlana Samādhi : The inward meditative condition in which the individual consciousness gets absorbed into the Universal Consciousness.

Niyati : Limitation by cause-effect relation; spatial limitation, limitation of what ought to be done and what ought not to be done.

Nirānanda : The second stage of *ānanda* in *āṇava upāya* resulting from the fixation of *prāṇa-śakti* on *śūnya*.

Nirvāṇa : Dissolution in Śūnya; liberation.

Nirvikalpa : Devoid of all thought-construct or ideation.

Nirvṛti : *Ānanda*.

Nirvyutthāna Samādhi : Samādhi (absorption into the Universal Consciousness) which continues even when one is not engaged in formal meditation.

Pa (प)

Pañcakṛtya : The ceaseless five-fold act of Śiva, viz. manifestation (*sṛṣṭi*), maintenance of manifestation (*sthiti*), withdrawal of manifestation (*saṁhāra*), veiling of Self (*vilaya*); Grace (*anugraha*), or the five-fold act of *ābhāsana, rakti, vimarśana, bījāvasthāpana,* and *vilāpana.*

Pañca mantra : *Īśāna, Tatpuruṣa, Sadyojāta, Vāmadeva, and Aghora.*

Pañca-śakti. The five fundamental *śaktis* (powers) of *Śiva,* viz., *Cit, Ānanda, Icchā, Jñāna,* and *Kriyā.*

Pati : The experient of *Śuddha adhvā*; the liberated individual.

Pati-daśā : The state of liberation.

Para : The Highest; the Absolute.

Para pramātā : The highest experient; Parama Śiva.

Parama Śiva : The Highest Reality, the Absolute.

Parāpara : The intermediate stage, both identical and different; unity in diversity.

Paramārtha : The highest reality; essential truth; the highest goal.

Parānanda : In *āṇava upāya,* the joy of the third stage that ensues by the practice of resting on *prāṇa* and *apāna* in *uccāra yoga.*

Parāmarśa : Seizing mentally; experience; comprehension; remembrance.

Parāvāk : The vibratory movement of the Divine Mind that brings about manifestation; Logos; Cosmic Ideation.

Parāśakti : The Highest Śakti of the Divine; *Citi*; *Parāvāk.*

Pariṇāma : Transformation.

Paśu : The empirical individual bound by *avidyā* or spiritual nescience.

Paśu mātaraḥ : Māheśvarī and other associated *śaktis* active in the various letters, controlling the life of the empirical selves.

Paśyantī : The divine view in undifferentiated form; Vāk śakti, going forth as seeing, ready to create in which there is no difference between *vācya* (object) and *vācaka* (word).

Pāśa : Bondage.

Pidhāna Kṛtya : The act of Self-veiling; same as *vilaya.*

Puṁstattva or Puruṣa tattva: Paśu pramātā; jīva, the empirical Self.

Puryaṣṭaka : Lit., the city of the group of eight i.e. the five *tanmātrās*, *buddhi*, *ahaṁkāra* and *manas*; the *sūkṣma-śarīra* (subtle body).

Pūrṇatva : Perfection.

Pūrṇāhantā : The perfect I-consciousness; non-relational I-consciousness.

Prakāśa : Lit. light; the principle of Self-revelation; consciousness; the principle by which every thing else is known.

Prakṛti or Pradhāna : The source of objectivity from *buddhi* down to earth.

Pramā : Exact knowledge.

Pramāṇa : Knowledge; means of knowledge.

Pramātā : Knower; subject; experient.

Prameya : Known; object of knowledge; object.

Prath : To expand; unfold; appear; shine.

Prathā : The mode of appearance.

Pratibhā : (1) Ever creative activity of consciousness; (2) The spontaneous Supreme I-consciousness; (3) Parā Śakti.

Pratimīlana : Both *nimīlana* and *unmīlana* i.e. turning of the consciousness both within i.e. into *Śiva* and outside i.e. the *Śakti* of *Śiva*, experience of divinity both within and outside.

Pratyabhijñā : Recognition.

Pratyāhāra : (1) Comprehension of several letters into one syllable effected by combining the first letter of a *sūtra* with its final indicatory letter. (2) In yoga, withdrawal of the senses from their objects.

Pratyavamarśa : Self-recognition.

Prabuddha : One greatly awakened to the higher spiritual consciousness.

Pralaya : Dissolution of manifestation.

Pralayākala : or Pralayakevalī : One resting in Māyātattva, not cognizant of anything; cognizant of *śūnya* or void only.

Prasara : Expansion; manifestation of *Śiva* in the form of the universe through His *śakti*.

Prāṇa : Generic name for the vital power; vital energy; life energy; specifically it is the vital *vāyu* in expiration.

Prāṇa-pramātā : The subject considering *prāṇa* to be the Self.

Prāṇa-bīja : The letter 'ha'.

Prāṇāyāma : Breath control.

Prāsāda : The *mantra Sauḥ*.

Prithivi : The earth *tattva*.

Pauruṣa ajñāna : The innate ignorance of Puruṣa regarding his real Self.

Pauruṣa jñāna : Knowledge of one's Śiva nature after the ignorance of one's real Self has been eliminated.

Ba (ब)

Bandha (1) Bondage; (2) Limited knowledge (3) Knowledge founded on primal ignorance (4) Yogic practice in which certain organs of the body are contracted and locked.

Bala : *Cid-bala*, power of Universal Consciousness or true Self.

Bindu or Vindu : (1) A point, a metaphysical point. (2) Undivided Light of Consciousness. (3) The compact mass of *śakti* gathered into an undifferentiated point ready to create (4) Paraḥ pramātā, the Highest Self or Consciousness. (5) Anusvāra or nasal sound (in अहं) indicated by a dot on the letter ह, suggesting the fact that *Śiva* in spite of the manifestation of the universe is undivided. (6) A specific *teja* or light appearing in the centre of the eye-brows by the intensity of meditation.

Bahirmukhatā : Externalization, extroversion.

Brahma : (In Śāṅkara Vedānta) Pure foundational Consciousness without activity; unlimited knowledge devoid of activity. (In Śaiva Philosophy) Pure foundational consciousness full of *svātantrya śakti* i.e. unimpeded power to know and do any and every thing; *parama Śiva*.

Brahmanāḍī : *Suṣumnā* or the central prāṇic channel or nerve.

Brahmanirvāṇa : Resting in pure *jñāna tattva* devoid of activity; the state of *Vijñānākala*.

Brahmarandhra : The *Sahasrāra Cakra*.

Brahmavāda : Śāṅkara Vedānta.

Brahmānanda : The fourth stage of ānanda (joy) in *āṇavopāya* experienced by resting of consciousness on *Samāna prāṇa* resulting from the unified combination of multifarious objects.

Bīja : (1) *Viśva Kāraṇaṁ sphurattātmā parāśaktiḥ* i.e., the active light of the highest Śakti which is the root cause of the universe. (2) vowel. (3) The mystical letter forming the essential part of the *mantra* of a deity. (4) The first syllable of a mantra.

Buddha : One awakened to the light of consciousness.

Buddhi : The ascertaining intelligence; the intuitive aspect of consciousness by which the essential Self awakens to truth.

Buddhīndriya : The five powers of sense-perception, viz., smelling, tasting, seeing, feeling by touch, hearing, also known as *jñānendriya*.

Baindavī kalā : *Baindavī*—pertaining to *Bindu* or the knower, *Kalā*—will power. *Baindavī kalā* is that freedom of *Parama Śiva* by which the knower always remains as the knower and is never reduced to the known, *svātantrya śakti*.

Bauddha ajñāna : The ignorance inherent in Buddhi by which one considers his subtle or gross body as the Self on account of *aśuddha vikalpas*.

Bauddha jñāna : Considering oneself as Śiva by means of *śuddha vikalpas*.

Bha (भ)

Bhakti (aparā) : Devotion; intense feeling and will for being united with Śiva.

Bhakti (parā) The constant feeling of being united with Śiva and the supreme bliss of. that consciousness.

Bhāva : Existence both internal and external; object.

Bhāvanā : The practice of contemplating or viewing mentally oneself and everything else as *Śiva*; *jñāna yoga*; *Śākta-upāya*; creative contemplation; apprehension of an inner, emergent divine consciousness.

Bhāva-śarīra : Consideration of sound, etc. as one's Self.

Bhuvana : Becoming; place of existence; abode.

Bhuvana adhvā : The third spatial existence, namely world. There are 108 *bhuvanas*.

Bhūta : Gross physical element.

Bhūtakaivalya : Withdrawal of the mind from the elements.

Bhūta-jaya : Control over the elements.

Bhūta-pṛthaktva : Detachment of the essential Self from the elements.

Bhūta-śarīra : Consideration of the gross physical body as the Self.

Bhūcarī : Sub-species of Vāmeśvari, connected with the bhāvas or existent objects.

Bhūmikā : Role.

Bhairava (apara) : Siddhas who have unity-consciousness and consider the whole world as identical with Self.

Bhairava (para) : *Parama Śiva*; the Highest Reality. This is an anacrostic word, *bha*, indicating *bharaṇa*, maintenance of the world, *ra*, *ravaṇa* or withdrawal of the world, and va, *vamana* or projection of the world.

Bhairava Āgama : Sixty-four *Śaiva Āgamas* that teach non-dualism.

Bhairava (Teachers) : Liberated *Śivas* who are established in unity-consciousness and teach the sixty-four non-dualistic *śāstras*.

Bhairava mudrā or Bhairavī mudrā : This is a kind of psycho-physical condition brought about by the following practice 'Attention should be turned inwards; the gaze should be turned outwards, without the twinkling of the eyes'.

Bhairava Samāpatti : Identity with *Parama Śiva*.

Bhoga : Experience, some times used in the narrow sense of 'enjoyment'.

Bhoktā : Experient.

Ma (म)

Maṭhikā : The four traditions of *Śaiva* religion.

Madhya : (1) The central Consciousness; the pure I-consciousness. (2) The Suṣumnā or central *prāṇic nāḍī*.

Madhyadhāma : The central *nāḍi* in the *prāṇamayakośa*, also known as *brahmanāḍī* or *Suṣumnā*.

Madhyamā : *Śabda* in its subtle form as existing in the *antaḥ-karaṇa* prior to its gross manifestation.

Madhyamaka : Buddhist philosophy that teaches that Reality lies in the middle and not in any of the tetralemma;

Madhyaśakti : Saṁvit-śakti, the central Consciousness-power.

Manas : That aspect of mind which co-operates with the senses in building perceptions, and which builds up images and concepts, intention and thought-construct.

Mantra : (1) Sacred word or formula to be chanted (2) In Śāktopāya that sacred word or formula by which the nature of the Supreme is reflected on as identical with the Self. It is called *mantra*, because it induces *manana* or reflection on the Supreme and because it provides *trāṇa* or protection from the whirlgig of transmigratory life. In Śāktopāya, the *citta* itself assumes the form of *mantra*. (3) The experient who has realized the *Śuddha Vidyātattva*.

Mantra-maheśvara : The experient who has realized *Sadāśiva tattva*.

Mantra-vīrya : The perfect and full I-consciousness; Śiva-Consciousness, the experience of *parā-vāk*.

Mantreśvara : The experient who has realized *Īśvara tattva*.

Manthāna Bhairava : Bhairava that churns i.e. dissolves all objects into Self-consciousness; Svacchanda Bhairava.

Marīci : Sakti.

Mala : Dross; limitation; ignorance that hampers the free expression of the spirit.

Maheśvara : The highest lord; *parama Śiva*.

Mahānanda : In *āṇavopāya*, the fifth stage of *ānanda* resulting from the resting of consciousness on *udāna agni* that devours all the *pramāṇas* and *prameyas*.

Mahārtha : The greatest end; the highest value; the pure I-consciousness; the Kaula discipline.

Mahāmantra : The great *mantra* of pure consciousness, of Supreme I-consciousness.

Mahāmāyā (aparā) : The state below *Śuddha Vidyā* and above *Māyā* in which resides the vijñānākala. In this state there is only prakāśa without vimarśa;

Mahāmāyā (parā) : The lower stratum of *Śuddha vidyā* in which reside the *vidyeśvaras* who, though considering themselves as of the nature of pure consciousness take the world to be different from the Self.

Mahāhrada : The highest, purest I-consciousness. It is called *mahāhrada* or the great lake because of its limpidity and depth.

Mātṛkā : (1) The little unknown mother, the letter and word-power which is the basis of all knowledge (2) The *parāvāk śakti* that generates the world.

Mātṛkā-cakra : The group of *Śaktis* pertaining to *Mātṛkā.*

Mādhyamika : The follower of the Buddhist Madhyamaka philosophy.

Māyā tattva : The principle that throws a veil over pure consciousness and is the material cause of physical manifestation, the source of the five *kañcukas.*

Māyā (In Śāṁkara Vedānta) : The beginningless cause that brings about the illusion of the world.

Māyā-śakti : The *śakti* of Śiva that displays difference in identity and gives rise to *māyā tattva*; the finitising power of the Infinite.

Māyā pramātā : The empirical self, governed by Māyā.

Māyīya mala : The limitation due to Māyā which gives to the soul its gross and subtle body, and brings about a sense of difference.

Mālinī : *Śakti* of letters which holds the entire universe within itself and in which the letters are arranged in an irregular way from 'na' to 'pha'.

Māheśvarya : The power of Maheshvara, the supreme lord;

Māheśvaryādayaḥ : Māhesvarī and other deities presiding over the groups of letters.

Mukta-śiva : The classes of experients who have acquired Śiva-Consciousness *Mantra*, *Mantreśvara*, *Mantramaheśvara*, and experients known as *Śiva*, *Rudra* and *Bhairava.*

Mukti : Liberation from bondage; acquisition of Śiva-consciousness : *Jīvan-mukti*-Liberation while living i.e. acquisition of Śiva-consciousness while the physical, biological and psychic life are still going on. *Videha-mukti*-establishment in Śiva-consciousness after the mortal body has been dissolved.

Mudrā : (1) *Mud* (joy), *ra* (to give); it is called *mudrā,* because it gives the bliss of spiritual consciousness or because it seals up (*mudraṇāt*) the universe into the being of *turīya-*

consciousness (2) Yogic control of certain organs as help in concentration.

Mudrā-krama or Krama-mudrā : The condition in which the mind by the force of *samāveśa* swings alternately between the internal (Self or Śiva) and the external (the world which now appears as the form of Śiva).

Mudrā-vīrya : The power by which there is emergence of the Supreme I-consciousness; *mantra-vīrya*; *khecarī state*.

Mūrti : Most manifest *Kriyā-śakti.*

Meya (prameya) : Object.

Moha : Delusion by which one regards the body as the self; Māyā.

Mokṣa : Same as mukti.

Ya (य)

Yoga : (1) Acquisition of what is not yet acquired. (2) Communion, Communion of the individual soul with the Supreme; discipline leading to this communion (3) (In Patañjali) Samādhi, cessation of mental fluctuations (*yuji samādhau*).

Yoginyaḥ : The *śaktis-Khecarī, Gocarī, Dikcarī, Bhūcarī* etc.

Yoni : (1) womb, source. (2) The nine classes of consonants; in the context of letters, *śakti* is *yoni*, and *Śiva* is *bīja.* (3) The four *śaktis*, viz., *Ambā, Jyeṣṭhā, Raudrī, Vāmā* (4) *Māyā-śakti.*

Yonivarga : *Māyā* and its progeny; *māyīya mala.*

Ra (र)

Rajas : The principle of motion, activity and disharmony—a constituent of Prakṛti.

Ravi : *Pramāṇa* (knowledge); *prāṇa.*

Raśmi : *Śakti.*

Rāga : One of the *kañcukas* of Māyā on account of which there is limitation by desire; passionate desire.

Rudra (kālāgni) : Rudra residing in the lowest plane of Nivṛtti kalā;

Rudrāḥ : The deities that are responsible for manifestation, maintenance of manifestation, and withdrawal of manifestation of the world-process; the souls that have evolved to the status of *pati* or selves that have realized Śiva-consciousness.

Rudra pramātā : *Mukta Śiva.*

Rudrāḥ (teachers) : Exponents of 18 Śaivāgamas who are *mukta Śiva.*

Rekhinī : The *śakti* that forms a straight line in the formation of the letter.

Rodhinī. The *śakti* that obstructs the passage to *mokṣa.*

Raudrī : The *śakti* that induces the pleasure-seeking souls to be confined to their pleasures.

La (ल)

Laya : Interiorization of consciousness; dissolution.

Loka : Plane of existence.

Va (व)

Varga : Classes of letters like *kavarga, cavarga,* etc.

Varṇa : (1) Letter (2) Object of concentration known as *dhvani* in āṇavopāya; *anāhata nāda* (unstruck sound experienced in suṣumnā).

Vācaka : Word; indicator; *mantra, varṇa* and *pada.*

Vācya : Object, indicated; *kalā, tattva, bhuvana.*

Vāmā or Vāmeśvarī : The divine Śakti that emits (from *vam* to emit) or projects the universe out of the Absolute and produces the reverse (*vāmā*) consciousness of difference (whereas there is non-difference in the divine).

Vāsanā : Residual traces of actions and impressions retained in the mind; habit energy.

Vāha : Flow; channel; the prāṇa flowing in the *iḍā nāḍī* on the left and *apāna* flowing in the *piṅgalā nāḍī* on the right of *suṣumnā* are together known as *vāha.*

Vikalpa : Difference of perception; distinction; option; an idea as differentfrom another idea; ideation; fancy; imagination, thought-construct.

Vikalpa-Kṣaya : The dissolution of all *vikalpas.*

Vikalpanam : The differentiation-making activity of the mind;

Vikalpa-(*śuddha*) : The fixed idea that I am Śiva.

Vikāsa : Unfoldment; development.

Vigraha : Individual form or shape; body.

Vigrahī : The embodied.

Vijñānākala : The experient below *Ś*uddha Vidyā but above Māyā who has pure awareness but no agency. He is free of *kārma* and *māyīya mala* but not free of *āṇava mala.*

Vitarka : The thought that I am Śiva, the Self of the universe (I, 17).

Vidyā : (1) *Śuddha vidyā tattva*; (2) *Unmanā śakti*, *Sahaja vidyā* (3) Limited knowledge, a *kañcuka* of Māyā.

Vidyāśarīra : Śabdarāśi—the group of letters and words (sūtra 3, Section II).

Vināyakāḥ : Beings who create obstacles in spiritual progress by offering temptations.

Vimarśa : Self-consciousness or awareness of *Parama Śiva* full of *jñāna* and *kriyā* which brings about the world-process.

Vivarta: (In Śāṅkara Vedānta) Appearance of the Real as something different.

Viśva: The universe; the all.

Viśvamaya, Viśvātmaka: Immanent.

Viśvottīrṇa : Transcendent.

Visarga : Emanation; creation.

Visargabhūmi : Two dots simultaneously, representing Śakti's external manifestation of the universe and the internal assimilation of the same into *Śiva.*

Vīreśa : The lord or master of the senses that are intent on removing all sense of difference inasmuch as the lord of the senses has now experienced the delight of the transcendental consciousness. The senses are called *vīra,* because they are now *śaktis.*

Vedaka : Experient.

Vedya : Object.

Vaikharī : *Śakti* as gross physical word.

Vyāna : The pervasive *prāṇa.*

Vyāpakatva : All-pervasiveness.

Vyāmohitatā : Delusion.

Vyutthāna : Lit., rising, coming to normal consciousness after *samādhi* or meditative absorption.

Śa (श)

Śakti : (1) The power of *Śiva* to manifest, to maintain the manifestation and to withdraw it. (2) The *spanda* or creative pulsation of Śiva or foundational consciousness.

Śakti-Cakra : The group of the twelve *mahākālīs*; the goddesses responsible for creation, etc; the group of Śaktis of the senses; group of *mantras*; the group of *Khecarī*, etc., the group of the goddess *Sṛṣṭi*, etc. (सृष्ट्यादि शक्तिचक्र).

Śakti tattva : The *vimarśa* aspect, or the foundational I-consciousness of *Śiva*; the intentness of Śiva's I-consciousness to manifest in the form of the universe; the second of the 36 tattvas.

Śakti-pañcaka : The five foundational *śaktis* of *Śiva*, viz., *cit*, *ānanda*, *icchā*, *jñāna*, and *kriyā*.

Śakti-pāta : Descent of Śakti; Divine grace by which the empirical individual turns to and realizes his essential divine nature.

Śaktimān Maheśvara; Śiva.

Śabda : sound; word.

Śabda-brahma : Ultimate Reality in the form of thought-vibration in which state thought and word are identical.

Śabda-rāśi : The group of letters from *a* to *kṣa*.

Śākta-upāya : The ever-recurring contemplation of the pure thought-construct of oneself being essentially Śiva or the Supreme I-consciousness.

Śākta-japa : The constant remembrance of the Supreme I-consciousness.

Śākta-samāveśa : Identification with Supreme Consciousness by means of *Śākta-upāya*.

Śākta-Yoga : Same as *Śākta-upāya*, *jñāna-yoga*.

Śāmbhava upāya : Sudden emergence of Śiva-Consciousness without any thought-construct (*vikalpa*) by a mere hint that one's essential Self is Śiva; also known as *Śāmbhava Yoga* or *Icchopāya* or *Icchā-Yoga*.

Śāmbhava-pramātā : One established in Śiva-Consciousness, also known as *Śiva-pramātā*.

Śāmbhava-samāveśa : Identification with *Śiva* without any

thought-construct born out of profound insight or *śāmbhava upāya.*

Śiva : The good; the name of the Divine in general; the foundational *prakāśa* or divine light.

Śiva (*parama*): The Absolute; the transcendent divine principle.

Śiva Tattva : The first of the 36 *tattvas*; the primal divine light, the source of all manifestation.

Śuddha Adhvā : The course of extra-mundane manifestation from *Śiva* upto *Śuddha Vidyā.*

Śuddha tattva : *Parama Śiva.*

Śuddha Vikalpa : The thought of one's self being essentially *Śiva.*

Śuddha Vidyā : The fifth tattva, counting from Śiva. In this *tattva,* the consciousness of both I and This is equally prominent. Though the germinal universe is seen differently, yet identity runs through it as a thread. There is identity in diversity at this stage. *Kriyā* is predominent in this *tattva.* The consciousness of this state is 'I am I and also this.'

Śūnya (Bauddha) : A state in which there is no distinct consciousness of knower, knowledge and known; an indefinable state of Reality.

Śūnya (Śaiva) : A state in which no object is experienced.

Śūnya-pramātā : The experient who is identified with objectless consciousness; *pralayākala.*

Śaiva āgama : The ten dualistic *śāstras*, eighteen *śāstras* which teach identity in difference, and sixty-four non-dualistic *śāstras* expounded by *Śiva.*

Śaiva yoga or Sādhanā : *Āṇava upāya, Śākta upāya* and *Śāmbhava upāya.*

Ṣa (ष)

Ṣaḍadhvā : The six forms of manifestation—three on the subjective side viz., *mantra, varṇa* and *pada* and three on the objective side, viz., *Kalā, tattva* and *bhuvana.*

Ṣaṇḍha-bīja : The four letters ऋ ॠ ऌ ॡ—which are unable to give rise to any other letter.

Ṣaṣṭha-vaktra : Lit., the sixth organ or *meḍhra-kāṇḍa*, near the root of the rectum.

Sa (स)

Saṅkoca : Contraction, limitation.

Sandhāna : Lit., joining; union, union of the individual consciousness with the universal Consciousness through fixed, intensive awareness or one-pointedness.

Saṁghaṭṭa : Meeting; mental union; concentration.

Saṁvāhya : One who is carried from one form of existence to another : *karmātmā, paśu.*

Sambodha : *Samyak bodha*, full or perfect knowledge of the essential nature of Reality as a mass of consciousness and bliss which is the essential nature of Self.

Saṁvit : Supreme consciousness in which there is complete fusion of *prakāśa* and *vimarśa, jñāna-śakti*; *svātantrya-śakti*; the supreme I-consciousness.

Saṁvit-devatā : From the macrocosmic point of view *Saṁvit-devatās* are *khecarī, gocarī, dikcarī* and *bhūcarī*. From the microcosmic point of view, the internal and external senses are said to be *saṁvit*-devatā.

Saṁsāra or saṁsṛti : Transmigratory existence, the world process.

Saṁhāra kṛtya : The withdrawal or reabsorption of the Universe into *Śiva.*

Saṁhāra : Assimilation to the Highest Consciousness.

Saṁsārin : Transmigratory being.

Sakala : All limited experients.

Sat : Existence which is consciousness.

Sattva : (1) The principle of being; light and harmony, a constituent of Prakṛti (2) The inner essential Self. (III, 12).

Satya pramātā : *Para Śiva.*

Sadvidyā : *Śuddha Vidyā.*

Sadāśiva (*Sādākhya tattva*) : The third *tattva*, counting from Śiva. At this stage, the I-experience is more prominent than this experience—This *tattva* is also known as Sādākhya inasmuch as *sat* or being is posited at this stage. Ichhā or Will is predominant in this *tattva.*

Samanā : When the *unmanā śakti* begins to display herself in the form of the universe beginning with *śūnya* and ending with earth, then descending from the highest state of Pramātā (knowing Self), she is known as Samanā inasmuch as she has started the mentation of all that is thinkable (*aśeṣa-mananamātrarūpatvāt samanā*—Udyota, p. 286)

Samaraṣa : One having the same feeling or consciousness.

Samādhi : Collectedness of mind in which there is cessation of the fluctuations of the mind.

Samādhi-sukha : The bliss that is experienced in being established in pramātṛ-pada i.e. in the state of the essential Self or subject.

Samāna : The vital *vāyu* that helps in the assimilation of food etc., and brings about equilibrium between *prāṇa* and *apāna.*

Samācāra : *Sam-samyak*; *ā-īṣat*; *cāra-prasaraṇa*—external expansion of the properly evolved *prāṇa* (III, 22).

Samāpatti : Sometimes a synonym of *samādhi*; consummation; attainment of psychic at-onement.

Samāveśa : Being possessed by the Divine, absorption of the individual consciousness in the Divine.

Sarvakartṛtva : Omnipotence.

Sārvajñatva : Omniscience.

Savikalpa jñāna : Knowledge which is acquired through the judgement of Buddhi.

Sahaja : Innate essenital nature.

Sahaja-vidyā : Knowledge of the innate essential nature; *unmanā*; pure divine consciousness in which mental consciousness ceases, pervasion into Śiva-consciousness (*Śiva-vyāpti*).

Sāmarasya : Unison of Śiva and Śakti; identity of Consciousness; identical state in which all differentiation has disappeared.

Sāyujya : The state in which the aspirant realizes identity with the Divine in the midst of difference.

Sārūpya : The state in which the aspirant realizes complete identity with the Divine.

Sālokya : The state in which the aspirant lives on the same plane with his chosen deity.

Sākṣāt upāya : Śāmbhava upāya.

Sākṣātkāra : Direct intuitive experience of the essential Self.

Sugata : The Buddha.

Suprabuddha : One who has awakened to the transcendental state of consciousness and in whom that consciousness is constantly present.

Suṣupti : Sound, dreamless sleep.

Suṣupti (savedya) : Sound sleep in which there remains a slight trace of the sense of pleasure, lightness etc.

Suṣupti (apavedya) : Very deep sleep in which there is complete absence of all objective consciousness.

Suṣuptatā or sauṣuptam : Delusive condition caused by primal ignorance.

Sūkṣma Śarīra : The inner subtle body, *puryaṣṭaka.*

Sūrya (symbolic) : *Prāṇa, pramāṇa* (knowledge), *Jñāna-śakti.*

Sūrya nāḍī : The *Iḍā nāḍī* carrying prāṇa.

Sṛṣṭi-bīja : *Mantra-bīja,* the Supreme I-consciousness which brings about manifestation.

Soma (symbolic) : *Prameya* or object, *apāna.*

Soma nāḍī : The *Piṅgalā nāḍī* carrying *apāna.*

Saugata : Follower of Buddha, a Buddhist.

Sauṣupta Sṛṣṭi : The sṛṣṭi in which *pralayākalas remain.*

Sthāna-Kalpanā : A mode of *āṇava upāya* concerned with concentration of external things.

Sthiti Kṛtya : Maintenance of manifestation.

Sthūla bhūtāni : Gross elements—ether, air, fire, water and earth.

Sthūla Śarīra : Gross physical body.

Spanda : Apparent motion in the motionless Śiva which brings about the manifestation, maintenance and withdrawal of the universe; Svātantrya Śakti, creative pulsation.

Sphurattā : Gleam; a throb-like gleam of the absolute Freedom of the Divine bringing about the world-process; spanda; the light of the spirit.

Svatantra : The Absolute, of unimpeded Will.

Svacchanda : The absolutely Free Being, *Śiva*; *Bhairava.*

Svapna : Dream; dreaming condition; *vikalpas* or fancies limited to particular individuals;

Svapna sṛṣṭi : The plane of existence in which the *bhuvana,* body and objects are subtle like dream.

Svarūpa : Essential nature.

Svarūpāpatti : Attaining one's essential nature or true Self.

Svalakṣaṇa : An object limited in its particular space and time.
Svasaṁvedana : An intuitive apprehension of oneself without the aid of internal and external sense.
Svācchandya : Absolute Freedom of the Supreme.
Svātantrya : Absolute Freedom of Will; *Vimarśa Śakti.*
Svātma-sātkṛ : To assimilate to oneself; to integrate to oneself.
Svecchā : Śiva's or Śakti's own Will, synonymous with *svātantrya.*

Ha (ह्)

Ha : Symbol of Śakti or divine power.
Haṭhapāka : Persistent process of assimilating experience to the central consciousness of the experient.
Hṛdaya : Lit., heart; the central consciousness; Light of Central Consciousness which is the substratum of all manifestation; *citprakāśa.*
Hetu : Cause.
Hetumat : Effect.
Hrada : Lit., Lake; the Supreme Spiritual awareness; It is called a lake, because it is clear, uncovered by anything, deep, and infinite.
Haṁsa— the *jīva,* the soul
Haṁsajapa : The consciousness of *nāda-kalā*

SUBJECT-INDEX

ABSOLUTE : Ātmā — Caitanya — Parama Śiva 6-12, its proof 13; Ātmā as the individual self 126-128; ātmā as an actor 152-154; antara-ātmā as the stage 155; senses as the spectator 156-157.

BONDAGE : Māyīya mala, Kārma mala, āṇava mala 16-20; 128-130; 132-133.

LIBERATION :

(1) ŚĀMBHAVA UPĀYA 29-31; Śakticakra-sandhā as help 32-34. Effect to Śāmbhava Yoga — the joyous experience of the turīya or the fourth state of consciousness 36-40, 48; the development of Icchā Śakti 53-55; All phenomena like the Yogī's body are the form of his consciousness, 59-60: disappearance of the binding power of the limited self 61-63; delight of samādhi 66-68: the power of creating any kind of body 69-71, acquisition of powers of separating and uniting the elements 71-74; acquisition of śuddha vidyā or unmanā avasthā 75-77 experience of the supreme I-consciousness, the generative source of all mantras 78-80.

(2) ŚĀKTOPĀYA, śakti as *mantra*, *citta* becoming *mantra* 82-84; perfect I-consciousness inherent in words is the secret of *mantra* 88-93; emergence of Śiva-Consciousness from I-consciousness 99-101; *Guru*, the help in acquiring this consciousness 102-104; enlightenment regarding mātṛkā from the *Guru* 104-110; Effects of this enlightenment 119-122.

(3) ĀṆAVOPĀYA dissolution of the *tattva*s in the body 134; *uccāra karaṇa*, *dhyāna*, *varṇa*, *sthāna-kalpanā*, the chief aspects of *āṇava yoga* 135-138; aids for *dhyāna* and powers gained from these aids 139-142; effects of the conquest of *moha* 147-150 powers arising from the realization of *āṇava yoga* 157-170, caution regarding the maintenance of *śuddha vidyā* 174-178; condition of the *yogī* who has attained transcendental consciousness 185-205 207-208; vitalization of the body, the senses and external things with the

Index to Important Sanskrit Words

An Alphabetical Index to the Sūtras

——ooo——